Proteomics of the Nervous System

Edited by
Hans Gerd Nothwang and
Steven E. Pfeiffer

Related Titles

Müller, H. W. (ed.)

Neural Degeneration and Repair

Expression Profiling, Proteomics, and Systems Biology

2007
ISBN: 978-3-527-31707-3

Westermeier, R., Naven, T., Höpker, H.-R.

Proteomics in Practice

A Guide to Successful Experimental Design

2007
ISBN: 978-3-527-31941-1

Van Eyk, J. E., Dunn, M. J. (eds.)

Clinical Proteomics

From Diagnosis to Therapy

2007
ISBN: 978-3-527-31637-3

Hamacher, M., Marcus, K., Stühler, K., van Hall, A., Warscheid, B., Meyer, H. E. (eds.)

Proteomics in Drug Research

2006
ISBN: 978-3-527-31226-9

Thiel, G. (ed.)

Transcription Factors in the Nervous System

Development, Brain Function, and Diseases

2006
ISBN: 978-3-527-31285-6

Proteomics of the Nervous System

Edited by
Hans Gerd Nothwang and
Steven E. Pfeiffer

WILEY-
BLACKWELL

WILEY-VCH Verlag GmbH & Co. KGaA

The Editors

Prof. Hans Gerd Nothwang
TU Kaiserslautern
Abteilung Tierphysiologie
Gottlieb-Daimler-Str. 47
67653 Kaiserslautern
Germany

Prof. Steven E. Pfeiffer
Department of Neuroscience
University of Connecticut
Medical School
263, Farmington Avenue
Farmington, CT 06030-3205
USA

Library of Congress Card No.: applied for
British Library Cataloguing-in-Publication Data
A catalogue record for this book is available
from the British Library.

**Bibliographic information published by
the Deutsche Nationalbibliothek**
Die Deutsche Nationalbibliothek lists this
publication in the Deutsche National-
bibliografie; detailed bibliographic data are
available on the Internet at
<http://dnb.d-nb.de>.

Composition   Laserwords Private Ltd.,
Chennai, India

Printing   Betz-Druck GmbH, Darmstadt

Bookbinding   Litges & Dopf GmbH,
Heppenheim

Cover Design   Adam Design, Weinheim

Printed in the Federal Republic of Germany
Printed on acid-free paper

ISBN: 978-3-527-31716-5

Contents

Proteomics of the Nervous System. Edited by H.G. Nothwang and S.E. Pfeiffer
Copyright © 2008 WILEY-VCH Verlag GmbH & Co. KGaA, Weinheim
ISBN: 978-3-527-31716-5

2   Common Methods in Proteomics   19
*Henning Urlaub, Mads Grønborg, Florian Richter, Timothy
D. Veenstra, Thorsten Müller, Florian Tribl, Helmut E. Meyer and
Katrin Marcus*

**3   Proteomic Technologies for the Analysis of Protein
            Complexes   35**
Ming Zhou and Timothy D. Veenstra

Preface

Proteomic technologies have substantially expanded the toolbox for molecular neurobiologists over the last decade. Although still evolving in many methodological aspects, proteomics already provide exciting insight into molecular mechanisms underlying the development and function of the nervous system. Equally important, it has also shed light on the pathogenesis of some of the most devastating human conditions such as neurodegenerative disorders. Therefore we felt that this is the appropriate time to present the current stage of proteomics of the nervous system.

Of course, there are no specific "neuroproteomics" techniques and one might therefore wonder what warrants the focus of this book. First, although the basic lay-out of proteomic approaches is similar for different cell types, organs, or organisms, there are subtle but important differences such as sample complexity and sample preparation. Taking them into account in the experimental design will make the difference between success and failure. Second, the sheer numbers of the publications on proteomics in the nervous system merit *per se* a compilation of the magnificent work in this field; this book provides a flavor of what is currently being done. We believe that this focus on proteomics reflects the important current and future roles of this approach in molecular analysis of the nervous system.

The book is divided into three parts. The first chapters introduce the basic technologies used in proteomic approaches and the rapidly expanding vocabulary in this field. The latter point should not be underestimated. Because of limited space in many scientific journals, proteomic methods are only briefly described with "cryptic" abbreviations. This makes it often difficult for the reader to follow the experimental design, which, however, is necessary to judge the quality of the information provided. The second part provides examples of various proteomics techniques applied to decipher the molecular secrets of the nervous system. In the third part, the focus is on biomedical questions, although, in practice, there is not always a clear-cut distinction between basic and biomedical research. In the latter two parts, a short introduction to the scientific enquiry being pursued by the respective authors is combined with the detailed protocols being followed. This should enable experienced scientists to apply the technique of interest directly, whereas novices can better estimate the time and effort required to implement the respective protocol into lab routines.

We hope that this book will serve as a source of inspiration and will assist to make proteomics a popular and valuable tool in neuroscience.

Farmington, Oldenburg   *Hans Gerd Nothwang*
July 2008   *Steven E. Pfeiffer*

Abbreviations

ENO1	alpha-enolase
AD	Alzheimer's disease
APS	ammonium persulfate
APP	amyloid precursor protein
ALS	amyotropic lateral sclerosis
ankB	ankyrinB
ApoE	apolipoprotein E
AICD	APP intracellular domain
BACs	bacterial artificial chromosomes
BAC	16-benzyldimethyl-*n*-hexadecyl-ammonium chloride
16-BAC	Benzyldimethyl-*n*-hexadecylammonium chloride
BN	blue native
BDNF	brain-derived neurotrophic factor
JNKs	c-Jun N-terminal kinases
CBP	calcium-binding protein
CBP	calmodulin-binding peptide
CE	capillary electrophoresis
cICAT	carbon isotope-coded affinity tags
CA2	carbonic anhydrase II
CAMs	cell adhesion molecules
CNS	central nervous system
CSF	cerebrospinal fluid
CTAB	cetyltrimethylammoniumbromide
CCK	cholecystokinin
ChAT	choline acetyl transferase
CCV	clathrin-coated vesicles
CRMP-2	collapsin response mediator protein 2
CID	collision induced dissociation
CN	colorless-native
ConA	concanavalin A
CBB	Coomassie Brilliant Blue

Proteomics of the Nervous System. Edited by H.G. Nothwang and S.E. Pfeiffer
Copyright © 2008 WILEY-VCH Verlag GmbH & Co. KGaA, Weinheim
ISBN: 978-3-527-31716-5

CCD	countercurrent distribution
CMC	critical monomer concentration
COX-2	cyclooxygenase-2
DDA	data-dependent acquisition
DRMs	detergent-resistant membranes
DIGE	difference in-gel electrophoresis
DRP-2	dihydropyrimidinase related protein-2
DNPH	2,4-dinitrophenylhydrazine
Dlx1	distal-less homeobox 1
DTT	dithiothreitol
ESI	electrospray ionization
ED	embryonic day
ER	endoplasmic reticulum
FDR	false discovery rate
fALS	familial amyotrophic lateral sclerosis
FACS	fluorescence-activated cell sorting
FDA	Food and Drug Administration
GENSAT	Gene Expression Nervous System Atlas
GFAP	glial fibrillary acidic protein
G6PI	glucose-6-phosphate isomerase
GADs	Glutamate decarboxylases
GST	glutathione S-transferase
GAPDH	glyceraldehyde 3-phosphate dehydrogenase
GRAVY	grand average of hydrophobicity
GFP	green fluorescing protein
His_6	hexahistidine
HPLC	High-performance liquid chromatography
hrCN	high-resolution clear native
HBPP	Human Brain Proteome Project
HUPO	Human Proteome Organization
HD	Huntington's disease
HIC	hydrophobic interaction chromatography or
HNE	4-hydroxy-2-*trans*-nonenal
IMAC	immobilized metal-ion affinity chromatography
IAC	Immunoaffinity chromatography
iNOS	inducible nitric oxide synthase
ID	inner diameter
IF	intermediate filament
IEX	ion-exchange chromatography

iTRAQ	isobaric tags for relative and absolute quantification
IEF	isoelectric focusing
pI	isoelectric point
ICAT	isotope-coded affinity tags
KCC	K^+/Cl^- cotransporters
LDV	large-dense core vesicles
LCM	Laser capture microdissection
LSCM	laser scanning confocal microscopy
LC	liquid chromatography
LC-MS	liquid chromatography coupled to mass spectrometry
LC-MS/MS	Liquid chromatography coupled to tandem mass spectrometry
LC-MS	liquid chromatography–mass spectrometry
LAMP	lysosomal-associated membrane protein
MRI	magnetic resonance imaging
MBP	maltose binding protein
MS	mass spectrometry
m/z	mass-to-charge ratio
MALDI-TOF	Matrix assisted laser desorption ionization-time of flight
MALDI	matrix-assisted laser desorption/ionization
MALDI-TOF/TOF	matrix-assisted laser desorption/ionization coupled to tandem time-of-flight mass spectrometry
MPC	Medizinisches Proteom-Center
µRP-HPLC	micro-reversed-phase liquid chromatography
MCI	Mild cognitive impairment
MELC	multi-epitope-ligand cartography
MARS	multiaffinity removal system
MuD-PIT	multidimensional protein identification technology
MAD	multiple-wavelength anomalous diffraction
TEMED	N, N, N, N'-tetramethyl-ethylenediamine
nanoLC-MS/MS	nano liquid chromatography coupled with tandem MS
nanoLC	nano-liquid chromatography
NGFN	National Genome Research Network
NS	nervous system
ENO2	neuron-specific enolase
nNOS	neuronal NOS
NPY	neuropeptide Y
Ni-NTA	nickel-nitrilotriacetic acid
3-NT	3-nitrotyrosine
NF-κB	nuclear factor-kappa B

NMR	nuclear magnetic resonance
NOE	nuclear Overhauser effect
1D- or 2D-PAGE	one- and two-dimensional polyacrylamide gel electrophoresis
1D-PAGE	one-dimensional gel electrophoresis
1D-SDS-PAGE	one-dimensional sodium dodecyl sulfate polyacrylamide-based gel electrophoresis
OD	outer diameter
ppm	part per million
PNGase F	peptide-N-glycosidase F
PBMCs	peripheral blood mononuclear cells
PMSF	phenylmethyl sulfonylfluoride
PGK1	phosphoglycerate kinase 1
PGAM	phosphoglycerate mutase
PGM1	phosphoglycerate mutase 1
PM	plasma membrane
PMCA	Plasma membrane-bound Ca^{2+} ATPases
PEG	poly(ethylene glycol)
PAGE	polyacrylamide gel electrophoresis
PDMS	polydimethylsiloxane
PCR	polymerase chain reaction
PET	positive emission tomography
PSD	postsynaptic density
PTMs	posttranslational modifications
PGE_2	prostaglandin E2
PSA	prostate-specific antigen
PDB	Protein Data Bank
q	quadrupole
QUICK	quantitative immunoprecipitation combined with knockdown
RNS	reactive nitrogen species
ROS	reactive oxygen species
RT-PCR	reverse transcriptase polymerase chain reaction
RPC	reversed-phase chromatography
SERCA	sarcoplasmic/endoplasmic Ca^{2+} ATPases
SPECT	single photon emission computer tomography
SAD	single-wavelength anomalous diffraction
SEC	size-exclusion chromatography
SDS	sodium dodecyl sulfate

SDS-PAGE	sodium dodecyl sulfate polyacrylamide-based gel electrophoresis
SST	Somatostatin
SILAC	stable isotope labeling with amino acids in cell culture
SCX	strong cation exchange
SCN	suprachiasmatic nuclus
SLS	Swiss Light Source
SV	synaptic vesicle
MS/MS	tandem mass spectrometry
TOF	time-of-flight
TROS	transverse relaxed optimized spectroscopy
TCA	trichloroacetic acid
TFA	trifluoroacetic acid
TPI	triosephosphate isomerase
2D-DIGE	two-dimensional fluorescence difference in-gel electrophoresis
2D-IEF	two-dimensional isoelectric focusing
2D-LC-MS	two-dimensional liquid chromatography-based mass spectrometry
2D-PAGE	two-dimensional polyacrylamide gel electrophoresis
UCH-L1	Ubiquitin C-terminal hydrolase L1
UPS	ubiquitin proteasome system
vATPs	vacuolar proton pumps
VIP	vasoactive intestinal peptides
VAMP	vesicle-associated membrane protein or
VGLUT	vesicular glutamate transporter
VDAC-1	voltage-dependent anion channel protein 1
WGA	wheat germ agglutinin
ZnT	zinc transporters

List of Contributors

Richard R. Burgess
University of Wisconsin
School of Medicine and
Public Health, Oncology
1400 University Ave
Madison, WI 53706
USA

D. Allan Butterfield
University of Kentucky
Department of Chemistry and
Sanders-Brown Center on Aging
Center of Membrane Sciences
Lexington, KY 40506
USA

Lutz Andreas Eichacker
Ludwig-Maximilians-Universität
Department Biologie I
München
Germany

Mads Grønborg
Max-Planck Institute
for Biophysical Chemistry
Department of Neurobiology and
Department of Bioanalytical
Mass Spectrometry
Am Faßberg 11
37077 Göttingen
Germany

Michael Hamacher
Ruhr-Universität Bochum
Medizinisches Proteom-Center
Universitätsstr. 150
44780 Bochum
Germany

Udo Heinemann
Max Delbrück Center for
Molecular Medicine
Robert-Rössele-Str. 10
13125 Berlin
Germany

Matthew Holt
Max-Planck Institute for
Biophysical Chemistry
Department of Neurobiology
Am Faßberg 11
37077 Göttingen
Germany

Haleem J. Issaq
Laboratory of Proteomics and
Analytical Technologies
SAIC-Frederick, Inc.
National Cancer Institute at Frederick
Frederick, MD 21702-1201
USA

Proteomics of the Nervous System. Edited by H.G. Nothwang and S.E. Pfeiffer
Copyright © 2008 WILEY-VCH Verlag GmbH & Co. KGaA, Weinheim
ISBN: 978-3-527-31716-5

Reinhard Jahn
Max-Planck Institute for
Biophysical Chemistry
Department of Neurobiology
Am Faßberg 11
37077 Göttingen
Germany

K.W. Li
Vrije Universiteit
Center for Neurogenomics and
Cognitive Research
Faculty of Earth and Life Sciences
De Boelelaan 1085
1081 HV Amsterdam
The Netherlands

Katrin Marcus
Ruhr-Universität Bochum
Medizinisches Proteom-Center
Universitätsstr. 150
44780 Bochum
Germany

Helmut E. Meyer
Ruhr-Universität Bochum
Medizinisches Proteom-Center
Universitätsstr. 150
44780 Bochum
Germany

Gary M. Muschik
Laboratory of Proteomics and
Analytical Technologies
SAIC-Frederick, Inc.
National Cancer Institute at Frederick
Frederick, MD 21702-1201
USA

Thorsten Müller
Ruhr-Universität Bochum
Medizinisches Proteom-Center
Universitätsstr. 150
44780 Bochum
Germany

Thomas A. Neubert
New York University
Skirball Institute of
Biomolecular Medicine and
Department of
Pharmacology
School of Medicine
New York, NY 10016
USA

Shelley F. Newman
University of Kentucky
Department of Chemistry and
Sanders-Brown Center on Aging
Center of Membrane Sciences
Lexington, KY 40506
USA

Hans Gerd Nothwang
University of Kaiserslautern
Tierphysiologie
Gottlieb-Daimler-Str. 47
67653 Kaiserslautern
Germany

Yasuhiro Ogawa
University of Connecticut
Department of Neuroscience
Health Center
263 Farmington Avenue
Farmington, CT 06032
USA

Matthew N. Rasband
University of Connecticut
Department of Neuroscience
Health Center
263 Farmington Avenue
Farmington, CT 06032
USA

Veronika Reisinger
Ludwig-Maximilians-Universität
Department Biologie I
Großhaderner Str. 4
82152 Martinsried
Germany

Florian Richter
Max-Planck Institute for
Biophysical Chemistry
Department of Bioanalytical
Mass Spectrometry
Am Faßberg 11
37077 Göttingen
Germany

Dietmar Riedel
Max-Planck Institute for
Biophysical Chemistry
Department of Neurobiology
Am Faßberg 11
37077 Göttingen
Germany

A.B. Smit
Vrije Universiteit
Center for Neurogenomics and
Cognitive Research
Faculty of Earth and Life Sciences
De Boelelaan 1085
1081 HV Amsterdam
The Netherlands

Daniel S. Spellman
New York University
Skirball Institute of Biomolecular
Medicine and Department of
Pharmacology
School of Medicine
New York, NY 10016
USA

Rukhsana Sultana
University of Kentucky
Department of Chemistry and
Sanders-Brown Center on Aging
Center of Membrane Sciences
Lexington, KY 40506
USA

Shigeo Takamori
Tokyo Medical and Dental University
21st century COE Program
Department of Neurology and
Neurological Science
Graduate School of Medicine
Tokyo 113-8519
Japan

Florian Tribl
Ruhr-Universität Bochum
Medizinisches Proteom-Center
Universitätsstr. 150
44780 Bochum
Germany

Andrew P. Turnbull
Cancer Research Technology
Birckbeck College
University of London
Malet Street
London WC1E 7HX
UK

Henning Urlaub
Max-Planck Institute for
Biophysical Chemistry
Department of Bioanalytical
Mass Spectrometry
Am Faßberg 11
37077 Göttingen
Germany

André van Hall
Ruhr-Universität Bochum
Medizinisches Proteom-Center
Universitätsstr. 150
44780 Bochum
Germany

Timothy D. Veenstra
Laboratory of Proteomics and
Analytical Technologies
SAIC-Frederick, Inc.
Advanced Technology Program
NCI-Frederick
Frederick, MD 21702
USA

Kojiro Yano
Cambridge University
Department of Physiology
Development and Neuroscience
Downing Street
Cambridge CB2 3EG
UK

Ming Zhou
Laboratory of Proteomics and
Analytical Technologies
SAIC-Frederick, Inc.
Advanced Technology Program
NCI-Frederick
Frederick, MD 21702
USA

Color Plates

Hydrogen bonds

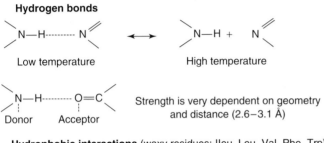

Low temperature   High temperature

Donor   Acceptor   Strength is very dependent on geometry
and distance (2.6–3.1 Å)

Hydrophobic interactions (waxy residues: Ileu, Leu, Val, Phe, Trp)

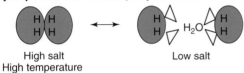

High salt   Low salt
High temperature

Ionic interactions (charged residues: Asp- Glu- S- Lys+ Arg+ His+)

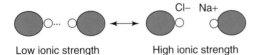

Low ionic strength   High ionic strength

Figure 1.2 Hydrogen bonds, hydrophobic interactions, ionic interactions. (This figure also appears on page 3.)

Proteomics of the Nervous System. Edited by H.G. Nothwang and S.E. Pfeiffer
Copyright © 2008 WILEY-VCH Verlag GmbH & Co. KGaA, Weinheim
ISBN: 978-3-527-31716-5

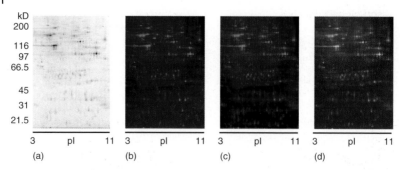

Figure 2.2 Various staining methods for two-dimensional gels. (a) 150 μg of whole human brain extracts were analyzed on a 2D gel using isoelectric focusing for the first dimension (pH 3–11; non-linear) and size-directed protein separation for the second dimension (21.5–200 kDa). Subsequently gel was silver-stained. (b, c) Samples and separation technique were identical to (a). However, mouse brain extracts were stained before separation with either Cy5 (green, e.g. transgenic mouse sample) or Cy3 (red, e.g. control mouse sample). Subsequently, the gel was scanned twice at corresponding wavelengths for the Cy5 and Cy3 channel. Comparison of spot intensities of labeled proteins (Cy3 to Cy5; overlay, d) reveal levels of different protein expression. (This figure also appears on page 21.)

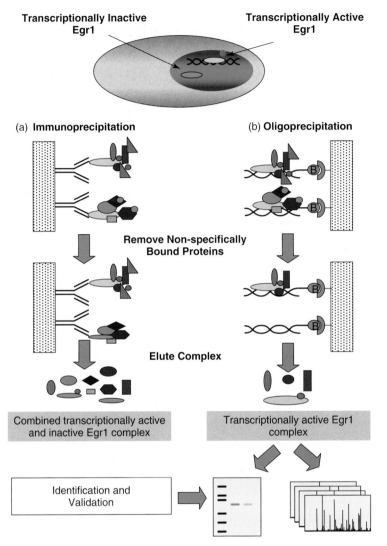

Transcriptionally Inactive Egr1

Transcriptionally Active Egr1

(a) **Immunoprecipitation**

(b) **Oligoprecipitation**

Remove Non-specifically Bound Proteins

Elute Complex

Combined transcriptionally active and inactive Egr1 complex

Transcriptionally active Egr1 complex

Identification and Validation

Figure 3.1 Comparison of oligoprecipitation of an active transcription factor protein to an immunoprecipitation of the same target protein. In this schematic using early growth response protein 1 (Egr1) as an example, the oligoprecipitation approach targets the transcriptionally active, phosphorylated version of Egr1. The immunoprecipitation method results in the isolation of protein complexes built around both the active and inactive forms of Egr1. (This figure also appears on page 39.)

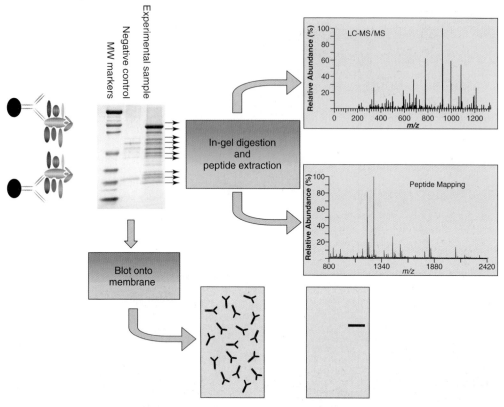

Figure 3.2 Discovery and hypothesis-driven methods of identifying interacting partners of target proteins. In a discovery-driven approach, a target protein and its binding partners are extracted from cells using a technique such as immunoprecipitation. The extracted proteins are separated by gel electrophoresis and stained bands are excised and processed for analysis by peptide mapping or liquid chromatography coupled on-line with tandem mass spectrometry (LC-MS/MS). In a hypothesis-driven approach, the proteins from the gel are blotted onto a membrane, which is interrogated with an antibody specific for a protein that is believed to interact with the target protein. (This figure also appears on page 41.)

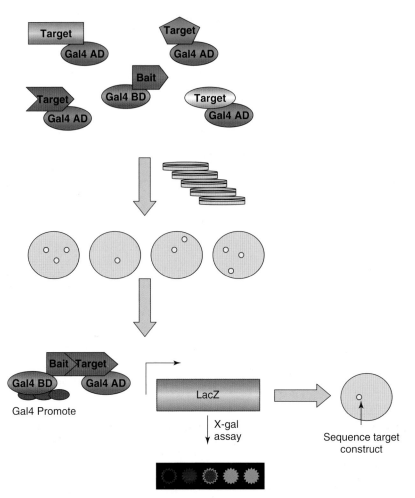

Figure 3.3 Schematic of the yeast two-hybrid method. In the yeast-two hybrid method, a plasmid containing a bait pro-tein fused to the DNA-binding domain of a transcription factor (Gal4 in this example) is constructed. This construct is trans-formed into yeast cells containing a library of plasmids containing target proteins fused to the activation domain of the same transcription factor. The transformed cell population is cultured on a series of plates containing the appropriate growth medium. The interaction of the bait with a target protein brings the two domains of the transcription factor together, resulting in the expression of a reporter gene (i.e. LacZ). Colonies that have an activated reporter gene are selected and the plasmid inserts sequenced to identify the target protein that interacted with the bait protein. (This figure also appears on page 44.)

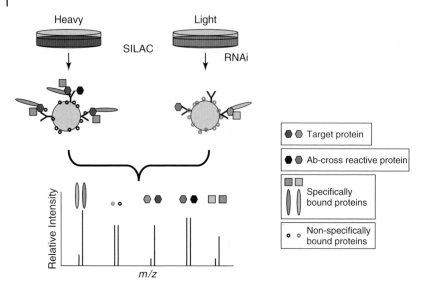

Figure 3.4 Principles of quantitative immunoprecipitation combined with knockdown (QUICK). Proteins are differentially labeled with stable isotopes by culturing cells in medium containing light or heavy amino acids (SILAC). The expression of the target protein is knocked down in one of the cultures using RNA interference (RNAi). After extraction of the target protein complex by immunoprecipitation, the samples are combined and analyzed by liquid chromatography coupled directly on-line with tandem mass spectrometry (LC-MS/MS). Proteins that non-specifically bind to components of the immunoprecipitation apparatus (i.e. beads, antibody) will be represented in the mass spectrum by peaks of equal intensity. Proteins that specifically interact with the target protein, as well as the target protein itself, will produce peaks of lesser relative intensity from the cells in which RNAi was used to knock down the expression of the target protein. (This figure also appears on page 45.)

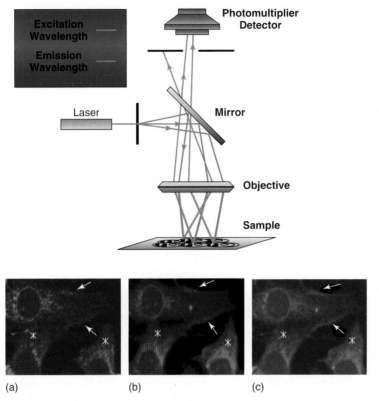

(a) (b) (c)

Figure 3.5 Principles of laser scanning confocal microscopy (LSCM). Top: In LSCM, the sample of interest is irradiated using a laser with a wavelength of light that causes excitation within a fluorophore that is associated with a protein of interest. The emission wavelength of the excited compound is then recorded. Bottom: To determine whether or not proteins co-localize, proteins are tagged with fluorophores that have different excitation and emission wavelengths. Overlaying of the two images results in a color combination that suggests the two proteins of interest occupy the same space within the cell. (This figure also appears on page 48.)

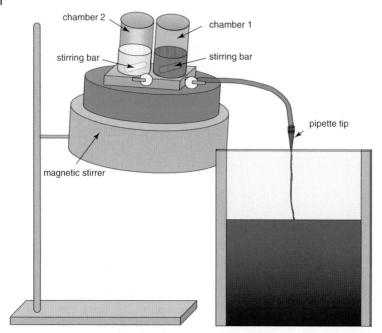

chamber 2

chamber 1

stirring bar

stirring bar

pipette tip

magnetic stirrer

Figure 4.1 Schematic setup for casting of gradient gels from the top. The gradient mixer is placed in such a way that chamber 1 is positioned at the center of a magnetic stirrer which shows a moderate decline towards the casting stand. This will ensure the directed flow of the gel solutions. Chamber 1 is filled with the heavy acrylamide solution, chamber 2 with the light acrylamide solution. Both chambers contain a stirring bar. The gradient mixer is connected to the glass plate sandwich by a cut pipette tip. To start gradient formation, all ports are closed and the magnetic stirrer is switched on. The port between the chambers is opened and after liquid connection between both chambers, the port connecting the chamber 1 to the glass plate sandwich is opened. (This figure also appears on page 59.)

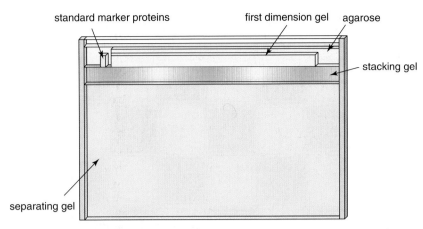

Figure 4.2 Transfer of the first dimension BN-PAGE strip to the second dimension SDS-PAGE. After solubilization, a strip of the first dimension gel is transferred onto a second dimension stacking gel. The strip is positioned centrally on top of the second dimension. A piece of Whatman filter paper soaked with SDS-PAGE standard marker proteins is positioned next to the first dimension strip onto the stacking gel. The gel strip and the SDS size marker are fixed with agarose. (This figure also appears on page 67.)

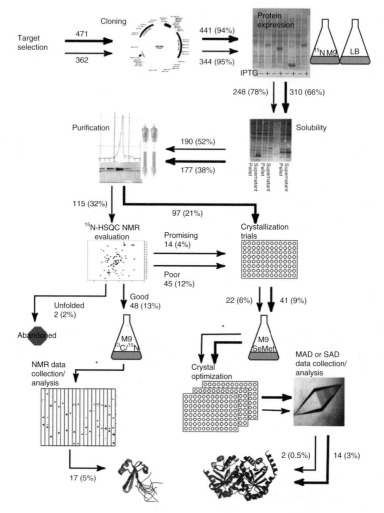

Figure 5.1 Schematic flow diagram of the strategies employed in structural genomics initiatives, using *Methanobacterium thermoautotrophicum* as an example. The number of protein targets after each step and the percentage relative to the number of starting targets are indicated in brackets. Thin arrows and italicized numbers are for smaller molecular weight proteins, and wide arrows and bold numbers are for larger molecular weight proteins. (Diagram taken from Yee *et al.*, 2003.) (This figure also appears on page 72.)

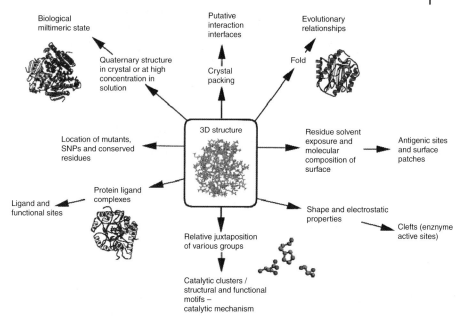

Figure 5.2 Summary of the information deriving from the three-dimensional structure of a protein relating to its biological function. (Taken from Thornton *et al.*, 2000.) (This figure also appears on page 73.)

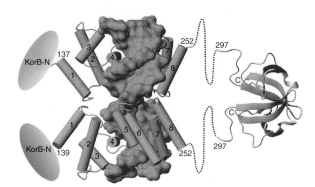

Figure 5.3 Natively disordered regions in the bacterial trancriptional regulator and partitioning protein KorB. The KorB DNA-binding domains (KorB-O, center) are connected by flexible linkers to N-terminal domains of unknown structure and function (KorB-N, left), and the KorB dimerization domains (KorB-C, right). (Picture taken from Khare *et al.*, 2004.) (This figure also appears on page 75.)

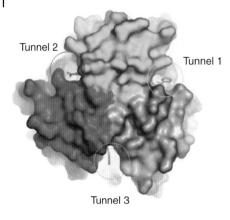

Tunnel 2

Tunnel 1

Tunnel 3

Figure 5.4 Crystal structure of the trimeric human protein, hp14.5. Benzoate molecules picked up from the crystallization buffer bind in the inter-subunit tunnels and mark putative hydrolytic active sites (Manjasetty *et al.*, 2004). (Picture with permission from Dr B.A. Manjasetty.) (This figure also appears on page 75.)

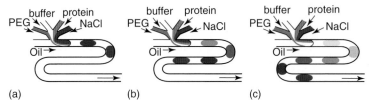

(a)   (b)   (c)

Figure 5.5 Droplet-based microfluidic system for protein crystallization. (a–c) A schematic illustration: As the flow rate of the NaCl stream is decreased and the flow rate of the buffer stream is increased, the volume of NaCl solution injected into each droplet decreases, and the concentration of NaCl in each droplet decreases. The shade of the droplets represents NaCl concentration. Each successive droplet represents a trial that tests a different ratio of stock solutions. (Taken from Zheng *et al.*, 2003.) (This figures also appears on page 80.)

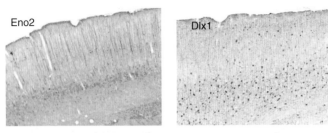

Figure 6.2 GENSAT images of neuron-specific enolase (ENO2)- and distal-less homeobox 1 (Dlx1)-expressing cells in cerebral cortex. (This figure also appears on page 103.)

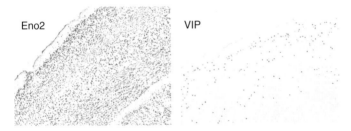

Figure 6.3 Images of neuron-specific enolase (ENO2)- and (VIP)-expressing cells in cerebral cortex from Allen's Brain Atlas. (This figure also appears on page 104.)

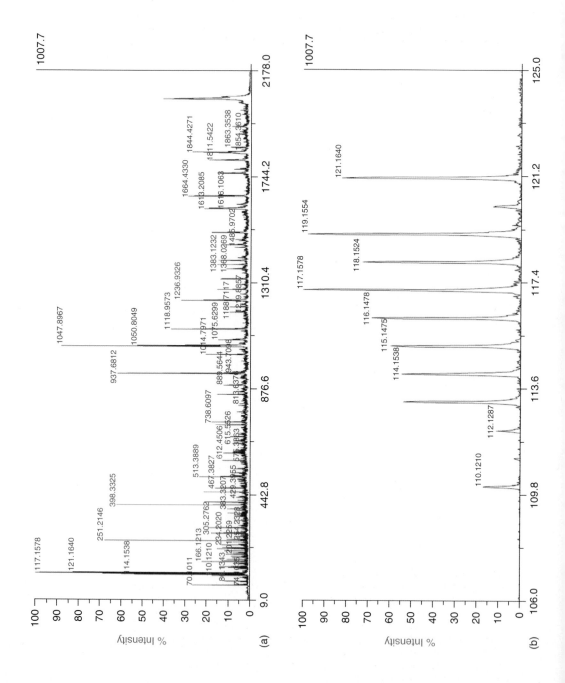

◀ **Figure 9.1** Representative example of an 8-plex iTRAQ reagents-based quantitative analysis of a sample with control and experimental treated groups. Upper panel shows an MS/MS spectrum of iTRAQ reagent-labeled peptide with good ion series for peptide sequencing. Lower panel focuses on the mass range encompassing the reporter ions used for quantitation. The reporter ions of 113.1–116.1 represent four independent biological replicates of the control group; the reporter ions of 117.1–119.1 and 121.1 the experimental treated group. Comparison of the reporter ions reveals upregulation of this protein in the treated group. The x-axis is mass-to-charge ratio; y-axis is in arbitrary units with the most intense peak set to 100%. (This figure also appears on page 170.)

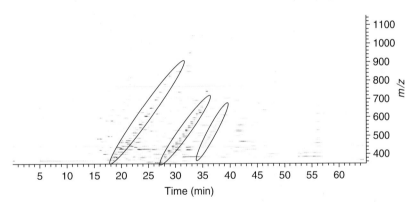

Figure 10.1 Electrospray ionization mass spectrometric analysis of a peptide extract from an invertebrate nerve. Peptides were extracted from the nerve by homogenization in a 1.5-mL reaction tube with acidic solvent. After centrifugation, the supernatant was injected into a nano-C18 column and eluted with an increasing gradient of acetonitrile. The eluents were electrosprayed on-line into a LTQ-Orbitrap mass spectrometer. There were many endogenous peptides scattered across the whole elution time and *m/z* value. Three well-defined clusters of singly charged polymers were also prominently present (enclosed in elliptical circles), and they may interfere with the analysis of the peptides. The x-axis is elution time from the column; y-axis is mass-to-charge ratio. (This figure also appears on page 186.)

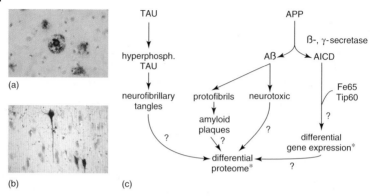

(a)

(b)   (c)

Figure 12.1   Neuropathological hallmarks and putative pathophysiological pathways in Alzheimer's disease. Reliable diagnosis of Alzheimer's disease is based upon immunohistochemical detection of extracellular amyloid plaques (a) as well as intracellular neurofibrillar tangles (b). Plaques consist of β-amyloid, which is cleaved off from the amyloid precursor protein by β- and γ-secretases (c). The intracellular domain of APP (AICD; another APP cleavage product) is believed to enter the nucleus and to alter gene expression pattern (in concert with the proteins Fe65 and Tip60). Neurofibrillary tangles mainly consist of hyperphosphorylated tau protein. (This figure also appears on page 211.)

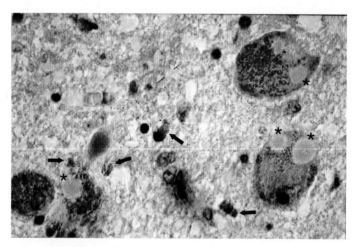

Figure 12.2   Neuromelanin and Parkinson's disease. Neurodegeneration of the substantia nigra pars compacta in Parkinson's disease is accompanied by massive loss of the pigmented neurons. During this process, the pigment neuromelanin is liberated from the neurons and phagocytosed by glial cells (arrows). Some pigmented neurons exhibit pathophysiological α-synuclein-containing protein aggregates, so-called Lewy bodies (asterisks). This figure was kindly provided by Prof. Dr. W. Paulus, Münster, Germany, and was published by the German Neuroscience Society. (This figure also appears on page 216.)

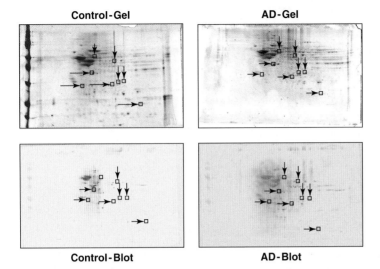

Figure 14.2 Images of Sypro Ruby-stained 2D gels (a and c) and blots probed for protein carbonyls (b and d) from control and Alzheimer's disease subjects, respectively. The arrows within the boxed areas indicate a number of oxidized proteins, both in a qualitative and quantitative manner. (This figure also appears on page 259.)

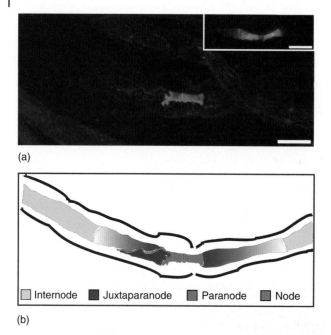

(a)

(b)

Internode Juxtaparanode Paranode Node

Figure 15.1 Myelinated axons are divided into polarized membrane domains including nodes, paranodes, juxtaparanodes, and internodes. (a) Nodes of Ranvier in the peripheral nervous system are characterized by a high density of Nav channels (red) flanked by paranodal junctions consisting of the cell adhesion molecules Caspr (green), contactin, and NF-155. Inset: CNS node of Ranvier immunostained using antibodies against juxtaparanodal Kv1 channels (red), paranodal Caspr (green), and nodal Nav channels (blue). (b) Cartoon illustrating the different domains of a myelinated axon. The black outline delineates the outer aspect of the myelin sheath. Scale bars = 10 μm. (This figure also appears on page 272.)

1
Protein Purification

Richard R. Burgess

1.1
Introduction

The magnitude of the challenge of protein purification becomes clearer when one considers the mixture of macromolecules present in a cell extract. In addition to the protein of interest, several thousand other proteins with different properties are present in the extract, along with nucleic acids (DNA and RNA), polysaccharides, lipids, and small molecules. The proteins present in the bacterium *Escherichia coli* may be dramatically visualized after resolution by two-dimensional gel electrophoresis as shown in Figure 1.1. A given protein may be present at more than 10% or at less than 0.001% of the total protein in the cell. Enzymes are found in different states and locations: soluble, insoluble, membrane-bound, DNA-bound, in organelles, cytoplasmic, periplasmic, and nuclear. The challenge, therefore, is to separate the protein of interest from all of the other components in the cell, especially the unwanted contaminating proteins, with reasonable efficiency, speed, yield, and purity, while retaining the biological activity and chemical integrity of the polypeptide.

Sections 1.1–1.6 provide background on classical protein fractionation and purification; that is, the isolation of a protein from its natural source. Sections 1.7 and 1.8 give a brief introduction to overproduction and purification of recombinant proteins cloned and overexpressed in a bacterial host expression system.

1.2
Types of Molecular Interactions and Variables that Affect Them

With regard to protein structure and stability and the interaction between an individual protein and other proteins, DNA, or materials used in protein purification, one must understand the molecular forces involved and how the strength of these forces varies as one varies conditions such as temperature, pH, and ionic strength of a solution. The atomic interactions that seem to be

Proteomics of the Nervous System. Edited by H.G. Nothwang and S.E. Pfeiffer
Copyright © 2008 WILEY-VCH Verlag GmbH & Co. KGaA, Weinheim
ISBN: 978-3-527-31716-5

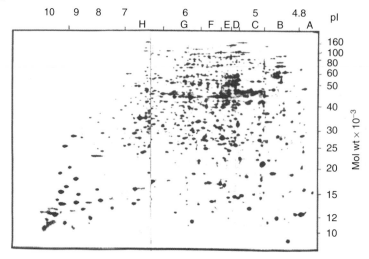

Figure 1.1 *E. coli* proteins resolved on a two-dimensional gel. The approximate isoelectric point and molecular weight scales are indicated. *E. coli* K12 strain W3110 was labeled with $^{35}SO_4$ during growth in glucose minimal medium at 37°C. A composite autoradiogram was made from non-equilibrium (left side) and pH 5–7 (right side) isoelectric focusing gels. (Adapted, with permission, from Neidhardt and Phillips (1985).)

the most important with regard to protein interactions are hydrogen bonds, hydrophobic interactions, and ionic interactions. These are described briefly below (Also see Creighton, 1993).

1.2.1
Hydrogen Bonds

Hydrogen bonds (Figure 1.2) occur when a proton is shared between a proton donor (NH and OH) and a proton acceptor (OC and N). Optimal hydrogen bonds have a linear geometry and a distance between the donor and acceptor atoms between 2.6 and 3.1 Å. Hydrogen bonds are stronger at low temperature and are weakened as the temperature is raised.

1.2.2
Hydrophobic Interactions

Non-polar residues (isoleucine, leucine, valine, phenylalanine, and tryptophan) cannot make favorable hydrogen bonds with water. In order to avoid water, they tend to come together in a so-called hydrophobic interaction (see Figure 1.2), usually resulting in their being buried in the interior of a protein. Hydrophobic interactions are strengthened at high salt levels and high temperature.

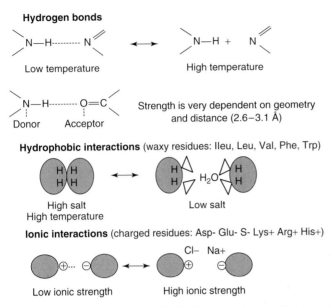

Figure 1.2 Hydrogen bonds, hydrophobic interactions, ionic interactions. (Please find a color version of this figure in the color plates.)

1.2.3
Ionic Interactions

Ionic interactions (see Figure 1.2) occur between charged molecules, with like charges repelling and opposite charges attracting. The force of the electrostatic interaction is given by an approximation of Coulomb's law, $E = Z_A Z_B e^2 / Dr_{AB}$, where r_{AB} is the distance between two charges, A and B, Z_A, and Z_B are their respective number of unit charges, e is one unit of electronic charge, and D is the dielectric constant of the solvent. The strength of ionic interactions is therefore inversely proportional to the distance between the charges and the dielectric constant of the solvent, which varies from 2 in non-polar solvents like hexane to 80 in highly polar solvents such as water. Ionic interactions are weakened as the ionic strength of the solvent increases and the charge is shielded by counterions. Ionic interactions are affected by the pH of the solution, since pH determines the number of charged residues.

1.2.4
Variables that Affect Molecular Forces

Conditions can be varied to affect the relative strength of the above molecular forces. Temperature, ionic strength, ion type, dielectric constant, and pH, for example, can all be varied. In a few cases, researchers have also varied pressure.

1.3
Protein Properties that can be Used as Handles for Purification

A single protein can be purified from a mixture of thousands of proteins because proteins vary tremendously in a number of their physical and chemical properties. These properties are the result of proteins having different numbers and sequences of amino acids. The amino acid residues attached to the polypeptide backbone may be positively or negatively charged, neutral and polar, or neutral and hydrophobic. In addition, the polypeptide is folded in a very definite secondary structure (α-helices, β-sheets, and various turns) and tertiary structure to create a unique size, shape, and distribution of residues on the surface of the protein. By exploiting the differences in properties between the protein of interest and other proteins in the mixture, a rational series of fractionation steps can be designed. These properties include: size, shape, charge, isoelectric point, charge distribution, hydrophobicity, solubility, density, ligand binding, metal binding, reversible association, posttranslational modifications and specific sequences or structures

1.3.1
Size

Proteins may vary in size from peptides of a few amino acids (with molecular weights of a few hundred) to very large proteins containing over 10 000 amino acids (with molecular weights of over 1 000 000). Most proteins have molecular weights in the range 10 000–150 000 (see Figure 1.1). Proteins that are part of multi-subunit complexes may reach much larger sizes. Proteins are often fractionated on the basis of size (really on the basis of effective radius or Stokes' radius) by passing down a gel-filtration column (or size-exclusion column, SEC). The column is filled with porous beads with characteristic pore sizes. The largest proteins cannot penetrate into the bead and are excluded and elute first in what is called the void or excluded volume. Very small proteins and salts easily pass in and out of the beads and see the entire volume of the column (the column volume). Other intermediate-sized proteins elute between the void and the column volume based on how much time they spend outside and inside the beads.

1.3.2
Shape

Protein shapes range from approximately spherical (globular) to quite asymmetric. The shape of a protein influences its movement through a solution during centrifugation, through small pores in membranes, into beads during gel filtration, or through gels during electrophoresis. For example, consider two monomeric proteins of the same mass where one is spherical and the other is cigar shaped. During centrifugation through a glycerol gradient, the spherical protein will have a smaller Stokes' radius and, thus, will encounter less friction as it sediments through the solution. It will sediment faster, and thus, appear to be larger than the cigar-shaped protein. On the other hand, during size-exclusion chromatography, the same spherical protein with its smaller Stokes' radius will more readily diffuse into the pores of a gel-filtration bead and will elute later, thus appearing smaller than the cigar-shaped protein.

1.3.3
Charge

The net charge of a protein is determined by the sum of the positively and negatively charged amino acid residues. If a protein has a preponderance of aspartic and glutamic acid residues, it has a net negative charge at pH 7 and is termed an acidic protein. If it has a preponderance of lysine and arginine residues, it is considered to be a basic protein. The equilibrium between charged and uncharged groups and hence the charge of a protein is determined by the pH of the solution. The charge of the ionizable groups found on unmodified proteins as a function of pH is shown in Table 1.1. In general, a positively charged resin (an anion-exchange column) is used to bind a negatively charged protein and a negatively charged resin (a cation-exchange column) to bind a positively charged protein. The protein is bound to the column at low salt (e.g. 0.1 M NaCl) and eluted with an increasing salt gradient. At some stage, the ionic attraction of the protein to the column resin will become weak enough to cause the protein to dissociate from the column and elute.

Table 1.1 The charge of the ionizable groups found on unmodified proteins as a function of pH.

Ionizable group	pK$_a$[a]	pH 2										pH 7										pH 12
C-terminal (COOH)	4.0	0	0	0	0	0	–	–	–	–	–	–	–	–	–	–	–	–	–	–	–	–
Aspartate (COOH)	4.5	0	0	0	0	0	0	–	–	–	–	–	–	–	–	–	–	–	–	–	–	–
Glutamate (COOH)	4.6	0	0	0	0	0	0	–	–	–	–	–	–	–	–	–	–	–	–	–	–	–
Histidine (imidazole)	6.2	+	+	+	+	+	+	+	+	+	0	0	0	0	0	0	0	0	0	0	0	0
N-terminal (amino)	7.3	+	+	+	+	+	+	+	+	+	+	+	0	0	0	0	0	0	0	0	0	0
Cysteine (SH)	9.3	0	0	0	0	0	0	0	0	0	0	0	0	0	0	0	–	–	–	–	–	–
Tyrosine (phenol)	10.1	0	0	0	0	0	0	0	0	0	0	0	0	0	0	0	0	0	–	–	–	–
Lysine (amino)	10.4	+	+	+	+	+	+	+	+	+	+	+	+	+	+	+	+	+	0	0	0	0
Arginine (guanido)	12.0	+	+	+	+	+	+	+	+	+	+	+	+	+	+	+	+	+	+	+	+	0

[a] pK$_a$ is the pH at which the ionizable group is half ionized. The precise pK$_a$ value for a given ionizable group can be influenced by the immediate local environment.

1.3.4
Isoelectric Point

The isoelectric point is the pH at which the charge on a protein is zero and is determined by the number and titration curves of the positively and negatively charged amino acid residues on the protein. Protein pI values generally range from 4 to 10 (Figure 1.1). An example of a theoretical titration curve and pI determination of *E. coli* RNA polymerase transcription factor, sigma32 (σ^{32}), is shown in Figure 1.3.

1.3.5
Charge Distribution

The charged amino acid residues may be distributed uniformly on the surface of the protein or they may be clustered such that one region is highly positive while another region is highly negative. Such non-random charge distribution can be used to discriminate among proteins. An example is the *E. coli* σ^{32} protein (Figure 1.3). At pH 7.9, σ^{32} has a negative charge of −46 and a positive charge of +40, giving a net charge of −6. It is able to bind reasonably tightly

Isoelectric of: Ecorpoh. Pep Ck: 9825 1 to 285 December 2, 1991 15:34

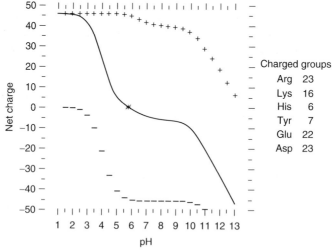

Figure 1.3 Titration curve and isoelectric point (pI) of *E. coli* σ^{32}. This graph shows theoretical plots of the number of positively charged and negatively charged groups and the net charge as a function of pH for the *E. coli* RNA polymerase transcription factor σ^{32}, based on its amino acid sequence. The pI is indicated by the asterisk and is 5.78. The charged groups are Arg (23), Lys (16), His (6), Tyr (7), Glu (22), and Asp (23). This plot was generated using the Genetics Computer Group Sequence Analysis Software package.

to both anion- and cation-exchange columns, apparently because its charged residues are not evenly distributed on the surface. This property can be used to purify this protein because most proteins will not bind to both types of ion-exchange columns under a single solvent condition.

1.3.6
Hydrophobicity

Most hydrophobic amino acid residues are buried on the inside of a protein, but some are found on the surface. The number and spatial distribution of hydrophobic amino acid residues present on the surface of the protein determine the ability of the protein to bind to hydrophobic column materials (as in hydrophobic interaction chromatography or HIC) and, therefore, can be exploited in fractionation. In general, a protein mixture is loaded onto an HIC column at high salt (e.g. 1 M ammonium sulfate), where hydrophobic interactions are strongest, and then eluted with a decreasing salt gradient to successively elute more and more tightly bound proteins.

1.3.7
Solubility

Proteins vary dramatically in their solubility in different solvents, all the way from being essentially insoluble ($<10\ \mu g\ mL^{-1}$) to being very soluble ($>300\ mg\ mL^{-1}$). Key variables that affect the solubility of a protein include pH, ionic strength, the nature of the ions, temperature, and the polarity of the solvent. Proteins are generally less soluble at their isoelectric point where there is less charge repulsion. Proteins are commonly fractionated by adding higher and higher concentrations of the mild salt ammonium sulfate. In general, the solubility of a given protein will decrease about 10-fold as the ammonium sulfate increases about 6% in saturation. (It takes about 760 g of ammonium sulfate added to a liter of water to give a 100% saturated solution, which is about 4.1 M, at 20 °C.) Since ammonium sulfate is mild and stabilizing to proteins, relatively inexpensive and pure, and highly soluble, it is the most common material used to fractionate proteins on the basis of solubility.

1.3.8
Density

The density of most proteins is between 1.3 and $1.4\ g\ cm^{-3}$ and this is not generally a useful property for fractionating proteins. However, proteins containing large amounts of phosphate (e.g. phosvitin, density $= 1.8\ g\ cm^{-3}$) or lipid moieties (e.g. β-lipoprotein, density $= 1.03\ g\ cm^{-3}$) are substantially different in density compared with the average protein and may be separated from the bulk of proteins using density methods.

1.3.9
Ligand Binding

Many enzymes bind substrates, effector molecules, cofactors, or DNA sequences quite tightly. This binding affinity can be used to bind an enzyme to a column to which the appropriate ligand or DNA sequence has been immobilized. For example, the transcription factor AP-1 is purified by binding to a specific DNA affinity column.

1.3.10
Metal Binding

Many enzymes bind certain chelated metal ions (e.g. Cu^{2+}, Zn^{2+}, Ca^{2+}, Co^{2+}, and Ni^{2+}) quite tightly, usually through interactions with cysteine or histidine residues. This binding can be used to bind an enzyme to a column to which the appropriate chelated metal ion has been immobilized. See Section 1.3.15 on the use of a metal-chelate column for purification of protein tagged by the addition of 6–10 terminal histidines.

1.3.11
Reversible Association

Under certain solution conditions, some enzymes aggregate to form dimers, tetramers, and so on. For example, the ability of *E. coli* RNA polymerase to be a dimer under one condition (0.05 M NaCl) and a monomer under another condition (0.3 M NaCl) can be used if two fractionations based on size are carried out sequentially under those two different conditions (Burgess, 1969).

1.3.12
Posttranslational Modifications

After protein synthesis, many proteins are modified by the addition of carbohydrates, acyl groups, phosphate groups, or a variety of other moieties. In many cases, these modifications provide handles that can be used in fractionation. For example, proteins containing carbohydrates on their surface can often be bound to columns containing plant lectins, which are molecules capable of binding tightly to certain carbohydrate moieties on glycoproteins. Phosphoproteins will in some cases bind to a chelated Fe^{2+} column.

1.3.13
Specific Sequence or Structure

The precise geometric presentation of amino acid residues on the surface of a protein can be used as the basis of a separation procedure. For example, an antibody that recognizes only a particular site (epitope) on a protein can usually be obtained. An immunoaffinity column can be prepared by attaching a monospecific antibody (which binds only to the protein of interest) to a resin. Immunoaffinity chromatography (IAC) can result in highly selective separation and provides a very effective purification step (Burgess and Thompson, 2002). A protein of interest can also be immobilized and used to specifically bind another protein out of a complex protein extract. This process is called protein affinity chromatography.

1.3.14
Unusual Properties

In addition to the types of properties mentioned above, certain proteins have unusual properties that can be exploited during their purification—an example is unusual thermostability. Most proteins unfold and coagulate or precipitate when heated to 95 °C. A protein that remains soluble and active after such heat treatment can be separated easily from the bulk of the other cellular proteins. Another such property is unusual resistance to proteases. These two properties often go hand in hand. An interesting example of a purification involving these properties is that of *E. coli* alkaline phosphatase. The cellular extract is heated and the insoluble coagulated proteins are removed by centrifugation. The supernatant that contains the phosphatase is then treated with a protease, which digests the remaining contaminating proteins, leaving an essentially pure preparation of alkaline phosphatase.

1.3.15
Genetically Engineered Purification Handles

With the advent of genetic engineering, it has become relatively easy to clone the cDNA encoding a given protein. It is then possible to construct an over-producing strain of *E. coli* that can be induced to produce large amounts of a desired gene product. Recently, it has become common to alter the cDNA in such a way as to add a few extra amino acids on the N-terminus or the C-terminus of the protein being expressed. This added "tag" can be used as an effective purification handle. One of the most popular tags is addition of 6–10 histidines onto the N-terminus of a protein (Hochuli *et al.*, 1988; Ford *et al.*, 1991; Porath, 1992). The protein is then purified by its ability to bind tightly to a column containing chelated Ni^{2+} or Co^{2+} in which it can be washed and then eluted with free imidazole or by lowering the pH to 5.9, where histidine becomes fully protonated and no longer binds to chelated metal.

1.3.16
What Can Be Learnt from the Amino Acid Sequence of a Protein that is Useful in Purification?

These days it is common to purify a protein in which the gene has been sequenced. Thus, one can easily deduce the amino acid sequence of the corresponding protein. Can this knowledge help in designing a purification scheme? The answer is that it can be somewhat, but not very, helpful. It is easy to determine the precise molecular weight of the polypeptide chain, but not to predict whether it forms dimers or tetramer or is part of a multi-subunit complex. Its charge versus pH and its isoelectric point can be determined as shown in Figure 1.3, which gives some idea as to which type of ion-exchange column to use, but again this will only be useful if it is not associated with other proteins. It is possible to calculate its extinction coefficient on the basis of its tryptophan and tyrosine content, which is very useful when it is pure (Gill and von Hippel, 1989). It is possible to determine if it has membrane-spanning regions or it has potential modification sites. One may be able to deduce that it is a member of a larger family of proteins by sequence alignment or by the presence of conserved sequence motifs that suggest cofactor affinity. However, its shape is not known, since the three-dimensional structure from sequence cannot yet be reliably predicted. Its multi-subunit features cannot be predicted, nor can its ammonium sulfate precipitation properties or its surface features such as hydrophobic patches, charge distribution, or antigenic sites. Therefore, it must be concluded that protein purification is still an empirical science.

1.4
Types of Separation Methods

There are a large number of separation processes that can be utilized to fractionate proteins on the basis of the properties listed above. These are summarized in Table 1.2. The sequential use of several of these separation processes will allow the progressive purification of almost any protein. If the processes are chosen carefully, and if proper attention is paid to separation conditions, and to maintaining the stability of the protein, the purification will result in reasonable efficiency, speed, yield, and purity, while retaining the biological activity and chemical integrity of the polypeptide (See Burgess, 1987; Coligan *et al.*, 1997; Deutscher, 1990).

An example of a hypothetical protein fractionation scheme is shown in Figure 1.4. This scheme relies on three of the most common fractionation methods, ammonium sulfate precipitation, ion-exchange chromatography, and gel-filtration or size-exclusion chromatography. The purification summary in Table 1.3 is a typical way of summarizing the yield and specific activity of each of the major steps in a purification scheme.

1.5
Protein Inactivation and How to Prevent It

A protein purification scheme will generally not be considered successful if the result is a protein that is pure, but inactive. Therefore, one of the key considerations in working with a protein is to prevent it from becoming inactivated. Table 1.4 summarizes some of the main reasons why a protein might become

Table 1.2 Separation processes that can be utilized to fractionate proteins.

Separation process	Basis of separation
Precipitation	
Ammonium sulfate	Solubility
Acetone	Solubility
Polyethyleneimine	Charge, size
Isoelectric	Solubility, pI
Phase partitioning (e.g. with polyethylene glycol)	Solubility
Chromatography	
Ion exchange (IEX)	Charge, charge distribution
Hydrophobic interaction (HIC)	Hydrophobicity
Reverse-phase HPLC	Hydrophobicity, size
Affinity	Ligand-binding site
DNA affinity	DNA-binding site
Lectin affinity	Carbohydrate content and type
Immobilized metal affinity (IMAC)	Metal binding
Immunoaffinity (IAC)	Specific antigenic site
Chromatofocusing	pI
Gel filtration/size exclusion (SEC)	Size, shape
Electrophoresis	
Gel electrophoresis (PAGE)	Charge, size, shape
Isoelectric focusing (IEF)	pI
Centrifugation	Size, shape, density
Ultrafiltration	Size, shape

inactivated and what can be done to prevent this inactivation. In general, working quickly and at low temperature (in a cold room or ice bucket) will help to avoid proteolytic degradation. Avoiding foaming or undue exposure to oxygen and adding a reducing agent should prevent oxidation. A buffer is used to maintain pH and a chelating agent like EDTA to protect against heavy-metal ions. Addition of 5% glycerol seems to stabilize most proteins and reduce adsorption to the walls of the container. A low salt concentration (e.g. 100 mM) helps increase solubility and prevent ionic adsorption to surfaces. Table 1.5 gives a good all-purpose buffer that in most cases will keep a protein active and happy.

1.6
Protein Purification Strategy

How a purification scheme is designed will, in large part, determine how successful it will be in achieving the goal of a protein purification: getting a high yield of highly pure and active protein in the minimal number of steps. Achieving a high final yield requires a high recovery at each step. Four steps at 80% step yield will be $(0.8)^4 = 0.41 = 41\%$ final yield, while four steps at 60% step yield will give a 13% final yield. Final purity will be guided by the intended

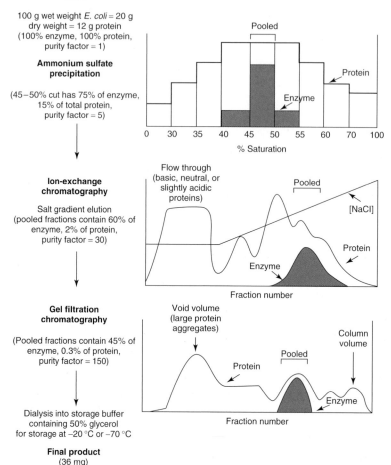

Start

100 g wet weight *E. coli* = 20 g
dry weight = 12 g protein
(100% enzyme, 100% protein,
purity factor = 1)

**Ammonium sulfate
precipitation**

(45–50% cut has 75% of enzyme,
15% of total protein,
purity factor = 5)

**Ion-exchange
chromatography**

Salt gradient elution
(pooled fractions contain 60% of
enzyme, 2% of protein,
purity factor = 30)

**Gel filtration
chromatography**

(Pooled fractions contain 45% of
enzyme, 0.3% of protein,
purity factor = 150)

Dialysis into storage buffer
containing 50% glycerol
for storage at –20 °C or –70 °C

Final product
(36 mg)

Figure 1.4 A hypothetical purification scheme.

use of the protein, but it should be free of major contaminants and any traces
of enzymes that interfere with the intended use. High activity will depend on
maintaining the stability of the protein as discussed in Section 1.5. By choosing
high-resolution fractionation steps, a given fold purification can be achieved
in fewer steps. For example, if the target protein is 0.01% of the total protein
in the extract, it will require a 10^4-fold purification. This can be achieved in
four steps, each giving a 10-fold purification, or three steps with a 22-fold
purification, or two steps capable of 100-fold purification. The fewer the steps,
the faster the preparation, the lower the protein losses, and the lower the cost
of the purification procedure. Some of the key considerations in designing a
purification procedure are (i) to have a convenient assay to follow purification;
(ii) choose a starting material rich in protein; (iii) take precautions to minimize
damage, inactivation or loss; (iv) use the minimal number of steps; (v) remove

Table 1.3 Summary of hypothetical purification in Figure 1.4.

Fraction	Total protein (mg)	Total activity (%)	Specific activity	Step yield (%)	Overall yield (%)
Extract	12 000	100	= 1	75	= 100
Ammonium sulfate precipitation (45–50%)	1800	75	5	80	75
IEC (pooled peak)	240	60	30	75	60
Gel filtration (peak)	36	45	150-fold purification		45 final yield
Pure standard			150		

IEC, ion exchange chromatography.

Table 1.4 Protein inactivation and ways of preventing it.

Reasons for inactivation	How to prevent it
Oxidation, foaming	Add DTT or TCEP, store under argon
Protease degradation	Add protease inhibitors, cooler, purer
Adsorption to container	Use polypropylene tubes, BSA carrier, glycerol, non-ionic detergent, protein more concentrated
Aggregation and precipitation	Store less concentrated, add salt, pH away from pI
Heavy metals	Add EDTA, cleaner tube, reagents
Temperature inactivation	Store cooler, add ligand or glycerol to stabilize
Bacterial growth	Use Tris, EDTA, azide, avoid PO_4, OAc^-
Enzymatic reaction (phosphatase)	Cooler, purer, add specific inhibitor
Dissociation of subunits/cofactors	Store more concentrated
pH changed	Avoid CO_2 in room, Tris changes pH with temperature
Inactive/misfolded conformation	Incubate at 37 °C to anneal the structure

the bulk of material quickly; (vi) avoid unnecessary duplication, dialysis, and delay; (vii) generally use fractionation steps in the order: precipitation, ion exchange, affinity, sizing; and (viii) use high-resolution steps where possible.

1.7
Overproducing Recombinant Proteins

The advent of genetic engineering has given us the ability to routinely clone genes and overproduce their gene products. This has changed the way we

Table 1.5 A good all-purpose buffer for keeping proteins happy.

TGED + 0.1 M NaCl	
Buffer	50 mM Tris-HCl, pH 7.9 at 20 °C
Stabilizer	5% glycerol
Chelator	0.1 mM EDTA
Reducing agent	0.1 mM DTT (dithiothreitol)
Salt	0.1 M NaCl

Storage buffer—similar to above but has 50% glycerol. Will not freeze at −20 °C. Best stored at −70 °C.

think about protein purification. For most protein purifications, it is no longer necessary to start with large amounts of naturally occurring material. Instead, the gene of interest can be cloned, inserted into a suitable expression vector and the vector transformed into a suitable expression host (e.g. *E. coli*). The cells can then be grown, transcription of the gene of interest induced, the cells harvested, the cells broken open and the overproduced recombinant protein purified. By using an expression vector where the target gene has a strong, inducible promoter, it is possible to express the target to levels as high as 20–40% of the total cellular protein.

The most commonly used bacterial expression system was developed by Bill Studier and colleagues at Brookhaven National Laboratory (Studier *et al.*, 1990). The host strain BL21(DE3) is a derivative of *E. coli* B that is deficient in several proteases to help prevent proteolysis of the recombinant protein and that has an inducible copy of the T7 phage RNA polymerase integrated as a phage lambda lysogen in the bacterial chromosome. The T7 RNA polymerase is kept repressed by the lactose operon repressor due to the placement of a lac operator near the promoter. The gene of interest is inserted into a multicopy expression vector under the control of a T7 RNA polymerase promoter, also with a lac operator to keep it off. The vector also contains an extra copy of the lac repressor gene to enhance repression. The repressor and the presence of an additional plasmid (pLysS, that encodes a T7 lysozyme to inhibit low levels of T7 RNA polymerase activity) help keep uninduced transcription of the target gene low. When the cells have been grown to the desired cell density, the lac operon inducer, IPTG, is added to about 1 mM, causing the repressor to dissociate from the lac operators and allowing expression of the T7 RNA polymerase. The T7 RNA polymerase in turn actively transcribes the many copies of the plasmid-encoded recombinant gene and the resulting mRNA is efficiently translated into the protein of interest. The result can be the production of very large amounts of the recombinant protein, to as much as 20–40% of the total cell protein within about 4 h after induction. This means that it is possible to purify as much as 30–50 mg of recombinant protein from 1 g of wet weight bacterial cell paste.

Several refinements have been introduced in the last few years to improve the chances that overproduction will be successful, especially if it is a mammalian,

Table 1.6 Problems of poor recombinant protein expression and their solutions.

Problem	Solution
1. Target gene contains rare *E. coli* codons	Supplement host *E. coli* with rare tRNAs (Novy *et al.*, 2001)
2. Target mRNA is degraded	Use *E. coli* strain deficient in RNase E (Lopez *et al.*, 1999)
3. Target protein is toxic to host cells	Use tighter repression, lower copy plasmid
4. Target protein is a membrane protein	Use a strain that has extra internal membranes (Miroux and Walker, 1996)
5. Target protein needs to form disulfide bonds	Use strain that is deficient in several key reductases, Gor, TrxB (Bessette *et al.*, 1999)
6. Product normally forms stable heterodimers	Simultaneous coexpression of two different proteins in one *E. coli* strain (Held *et al.*, 2003)

plant, or archaeal protein that is being overproduced. One problem is that human proteins often use codons that are rarely used in *E. coli*. These codons correspond to *E. coli* tRNAs that are very low in abundance in the cell. When overexpression of a gene containing many of these rare codons is attempted, the result is that very little, if any, of the protein is produced. This problem was originally solved by changing the DNA sequence of the recombinant gene so that it did not contain rare codons, but it contained the preferred *E. coli* codons. A much easier and more elegant solution has now been developed and is marketed by several biotechnology research products companies. This involves creation of an improved host bacterial strain that has had 3–5 of its rare tRNAs augmented. Many poorly expressed proteins can now be expressed at very high levels. Table 1.6 lists this and several other problems that have been encountered in protein overexpression in *E. coli* along with how these problems have been solved or alleviated. There are a wide variety of elegantly engineered expression vectors and bacterial expression hosts available from many different biotechnology research products companies worldwide. In addition to many *E. coli*-based expression hosts, there are also expression hosts such as: *Bacillus subtilis*, *Pichia pastoris*, *Aspergillus* spp., baculovirus/insect cells, mammalian cells, plants, and animals.

1.8
Refolding Proteins Solubilized from Inclusion Bodies

One of the most common problems in overexpressing a recombinant protein in *E. coli* is the fact that while large amounts of the protein are produced, most of it is not soluble, but is found as an insoluble inclusion body.

Apparently, the newly synthesized protein, when partially folded into its native structure, exposes some hydrophobic regions and is quite sticky and prone to interaction with other partially folded proteins, leading to aggregation and inclusion body formation. There are two main approaches to dealing with inclusion bodies: (i) try to increase the proportion of the overproduced protein that is soluble (Schein, 1989); and (ii) purify the inclusion body, solubilize it by dissolving it in a protein denaturant, and then refold it into its native structure (Marschak *et al.*, 1996).

1.8.1
Increasing Production of Soluble Protein

To purify the soluble material, it is necessary to increase as much as possible the proportion of the overproduced protein that is soluble. The most common approach is to induce the overproduction in cells growing at 20–25 °C. Apparently, the slower growth rate and lower temperatures results in more refolded protein and less aggregation and inclusion body formation. People have tried coexpressing cloned chaperone proteins to facilitate proper folding, but this is not common as it is only effective in some cases. An elegant recent approach has been to grow the cells at 37 °C, shift the temperature briefly to 42 °C to induce the heat shock response, and then shift the cells to 20 °C for induction. Often if two proteins that normally form stable heterodimers are individually overexpressed they are insoluble, but if coexpressed in the same cell they form soluble, native heterodimers. Finally, many proteins remain soluble when overexpressed as genetic fusions with known proteins that readily fold to form stable native structures (protein fusion partners like NusA, GST, TrxA, and maltose binding protein, MBP).

1.8.2
Refolding Inclusion Bodies

If a protein solubilized from inclusion bodies is to be refolded, it is common to first wash the inclusion bodies with a non-ionic detergent like Triton X-100 to solubilize membranes and break any unbroken cells. The washed inclusion body is then almost pure, and is ready to be solubilized. The real challenge is not the purification, but the refolding. The key to refolding without reaggregation and precipitation is to refold under low protein concentration. Under these conditions, the concentration of sticky, partially refolded material is lower, decreasing the opportunity for interaction and aggregation. However, for larger preparations, the large volumes become a major problem. Usually, refolding conditions can be found that give efficient refolding yields at reasonable protein concentrations.

1.8.3
A General Procedure for Refolding Proteins from Inclusion Bodies

A general method that the author has found to be quite effective for many proteins is given below.

1. Grow cells and induce overexpression of target protein.
2. Harvest cells, weigh cell pellet, store frozen at $-80\,°C$.
3. Break cells by sonication (pLysS cells are easy to break because of the presence of some T7 lysozyme). Otherwise adding lysozyme helps.
4. Centrifuge cell lysate, wash the inclusion body pellet with 1% Triton X-100 to solubilize membranes and membrane proteins, then wash with buffer to remove Triton X-100.
5. Solubilize inclusion bodies with a denaturant such as 6 M guanidium hydrochloride or 0.3% Sarkosyl to about 1 mg protein mL^{-1}. Difficult-to-refold proteins may need to be diluted to 0.1 mg mL^{-1} in denaturant; 8 M urea can also be used, but there is a risk of carbamylation of the protein.
6. Centrifuge out any undissolved material and slowly drip dilute the solubilized protein into 15–60 volumes of suitable refolding buffer. Additives or various buffer variables are often used to improve folding efficiency of a particular protein. These include 0.5 M arginine, 25% glycerol, varying the pH, temperature, presence of divalent ions, and presence of redox buffers.
7. Pass dilute refolded protein over a suitable high-resolution ion-exchange column, wash the column, and then elute with an increasing salt gradient. This step accomplishes several important things: (i) it concentrates the dilute protein; (ii) it removes the denaturant; (iii) it removes impurities that do not bind to the column or bind weaker or stronger than the target protein; and finally (iv) it often separates refolded monomer from soluble multimers that tend to bind tighter and elute later in the gradient.
8. The resulting protein is usually fully active, homogeneous, and capable of forming crystals suitable for three-dimensional structure determination.

References

Bessette, P.H., Aslund, F., Beckwith, J. and Georgiou, G. (1999) Efficient folding of proteins with multiple disulfide bonds in the E. coli cytoplasm. *Proceedings of the National Academy of Sciences of the United States of America*, **96**, 13703–13708.

Burgess, R.R. (1969) A new method for the large-scale purification of E. coli DNA-dependent RNA polymerase. *Journal of Biological Chemistry*, **244**, 6160–6167.

Burgess, R.R. (1987) Protein Purification, in *Protein Engineering* (eds D. Oxender and C.F. Fox), A.R. Liss, New York, pp. 71–82.

Burgess, R.R. and Thompson, N.E. (2002) Advances in gentle immunoaffinity chromatography. *Current Opinions in Biotechnology*, **13**, 304–308.

Coligan, J.E., Dunn, B.M., Ploegh, H.L., Speicher, D.W. and Wingfield, P. (1997) *Current Protocols in Protein Science*, John Wiley & Sons, Inc., New York.

Creighton, T.E. (1993) *Proteins: Structures and Molecular Properties*, 2nd edn., W.H. Freeman, San Francisco, CA.

Deutscher, M.P. (1990) *Guide to Protein Purification, Methods in Enzymology*, vol. 182, Academic Press, New York.

Ford, C.F., Suominen, I. and Glatz, C.E. (1991) Fusion tails for the recovery and purification of recombinant proteins. *Protein Expression and Purification*, **2**, 95–107.

Gill, S. and von Hippel, P. (1989) Calculation of protein extinction coefficients from amino acid sequence data. *Biochemistry*, **182**, 319–326.

Held, D., Yaeger, K. and Novy, R. (2003) Co-expression vectors. *Innovations*, **18**, 4–6.

Hochuli, E., Bannworth, W., Dobeli, R., Gentz, R. and Studber, D. (1988) Genetic approach to facilitate purification of recombinant proteins with a novel metal chelate adsorbent. *Biotechnology*, **6**, 1321–1325.

Lopez, P.J., Marchand, I., Joyce, S.A. and Dreyfus, M. (1999) RNase E, the C-terminal half of which organizes the *E. coli* degradosome, participates in mRNA degradation but not rRNA processing in vivo. *Molecular Microbiology*, **33**, 188–199.

Marschak, D., Kadonaga, J., Burgess, R., Knuth, M., Brennan, W. and Lin, S.-H. (1996) *Strategies for Protein Purification and Characterization: A Laboratory Manual*, Cold Spring Harbor Press, Cold Spring Harbor.

Miroux, B. and Walker, J. (1996) Over-production of proteins in *E. coli*: mutant hosts that allow synthesis of some membrane proteins and globular proteins at high levels. *Journal of Molecular Biology*, **260**, 289–298.

Neidhardt, F.C. and Phillips, T.A. (1985) The protein catalog of E. coli, in *Two-Dimensional Gel Electrophoresis of Proteins* (eds J.E. Celis and R. Bravo), Academic Press, New York, pp. 417–444.

Novy, R., Drott, D., Yaeger, K. and Mierendorf, R. (2001) Overcoming codon bias of E. coli for enhanced protein expression. *Innovations*, **12**, 1–3.

Porath, J. (1992) Immobilized metal ion affinity chromatography. *Protein Expression and Purification*, **3**, 206–281.

Schein, C.H. (1989) Production of soluble recombinant proteins in bacteria. *Biotechnology*, **7**, 1141–1149.

Scopes, R. (1994) *Protein Purification: Principles and Practice*, 3rd edn., Springer-Verlag, New York.

Simpson, R.J. (ed.) (2004) *Purifying Proteins for Proteomics: A Laboratory Manual*, Cold Spring Harbor Press, Cold Spring Harbor.

Studier, W., Rosenberg, A., Dunn, J. and Dubendorff, J. (1990) Use of T7 RNA polymerase to direct expression of cloned genes. *Methods in Enzymology*, **185**, 60–89.

2
Common Methods in Proteomics

Henning Urlaub, Mads Grønborg, Florian Richter, Timothy D. Veenstra,
Thorsten Müller, Florian Tribl, Helmut E. Meyer and Katrin Marcus

2.1
Introduction

A typical proteomics workflow comprises protein separation using polyacrylamide-based gel electrophoresis (PAGE) or liquid chromatography, digestion of proteins, and finally identification by mass spectrometry and a database search (Figure 2.1). This workflow is widely accepted in neuroproteomics as well as in the other divergent fields of proteomic research. In this chapter, we outline the principles of the underlying techniques and comment on the most important aspects.

2.2
Protein Separation by Polyacrylamide Gel Electrophoresis

Despite rapid progress in gel-free separation methods for proteins and peptides, gel-based separation techniques continue to prevail in proteomics. Their major advantages are ease, availability in most laboratories, low costs of set-up and performance, and the robustness of one- and two-dimensional polyacrylamide gel electrophoresis (1D- or 2D-PAGE).

2.2.1
Two-dimensional Polyacrylamide Gel Electrophoresis

The combination of isoelectric focusing (IEF) and sodium dodecyl sulfate (SDS)-PAGE is currently the most common technique in proteomic analysis, with a resolution of up to 10 000 protein spots per gel (Klose, 1999). IEF separates proteins according to their isoelectric point. Most often, IEF is performed with immobilized pH gradients (Gorg *et al.*, 2000). Alternatively, carrier ampholytes are often used to establish the pH gradient during the

Proteomics of the Nervous System. Edited by H.G. Nothwang and S.E. Pfeiffer
Copyright © 2008 WILEY-VCH Verlag GmbH & Co. KGaA, Weinheim
ISBN: 978-3-527-31716-5

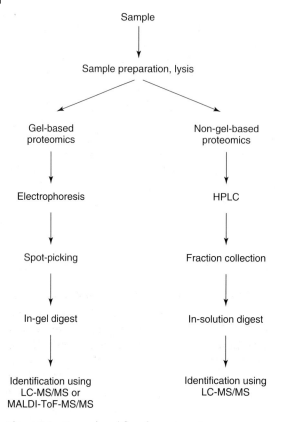

Figure 2.1 General workflow for proteomics.

IEF process (Klose, 1975; Klose and Kobalz, 1995). In the second dimension, the focused proteins are separated by SDS-PAGE according to their apparent molecular weight.

A drawback of 2D-PAGE is the fact that it is less suitable for the separation of integral membrane proteins. Only membrane proteins with a low grand average of hydrophobicity (GRAVY) score and a few transmembrane domains will be detected (Fischer *et al.*, 2006). Hydrophobic and membrane proteins exhibit incomplete solubility in the buffers used for 2D-PAGE. Moreover, such proteins can precipitate, thus inhibiting their transfer from the first to the second dimension. Alternative strategies for gel-based analysis of membrane proteins are (i) protein separation by 1D-PAGE combined with nano liquid chromatography coupled with tandem MS (nanoLC-MS/MS) or with off-line matrix-assisted laser-desorption ionization (MALDI) tandem MS (MALDI-MS/MS), and (ii) protein analysis by two-dimensional 16-BAC/SDS-PAGE gel electrophoresis (see Chapter 8). 16-BAC/SDS-PAGE separates the proteins in the first dimension using an acidic buffer system and the cationic detergent benzyldimethyl-*n*-hexadecylammonium chloride (16-BAC) and in the second dimension by SDS-PAGE (Macfarlane, 1989; Hartinger *et al.*, 1996). This technique has previously been demonstrated to work very well for the fractionation of integral membrane proteins (Dreger *et al.*, 2001; Diao *et al.*, 2003; Guillemin *et al.*, 2005; Takamori *et al.*, 2006).

After separation by electrophoresis, the proteins must be visualized in the gel by using organic stains (e.g. Coomassie R 250 and Coomassie G 250), silver, reverse stains (e.g. zinc imidazole and copper chloride) or fluorescence dyes (e.g. Sypro Ruby, Sypro Orange) (Rabilloud and Charmont, 1999). An example of a silver-stained 2D-PAGE image is shown in Figure 2.2a (Dzandu *et al.*, 1988; Shaw *et al.*, 2003). Note that protocols using silver in combination with glutaraldehyde for fixing the proteins within the gel are not compatible with MS, so that alternative silver-staining protocols have to be used (Shevchenko *et al.*, 1996; Yan *et al.*, 2000).

In addition, several staining techniques are available for the analysis of posttranslational modifications when using 1D- or 2D-PAGE. The oxidative modification of proteins catalyzed by metal ions introduces carbonyl groups at lysine, arginine, proline, or threonine residues (Stadtman, 1993). These carbonyl groups can be used to detect oxidized proteins by subsequent modification with 2,4-dinitrophenylhydrazine (DNPH) (Levine *et al.*, 1994; Boyd-Kimball *et al.*, 2005) followed by gel-electrophoretic separation. After transfer of the proteins from the gel to a membrane by standard blotting procedures, the DNPH-modified proteins are detected with an anti-DNPH antibody (see Chapter 14). Phosphorylated proteins can be detected either by immunoblot analysis using anti-tyrosine, anti-serine, or anti-threonine

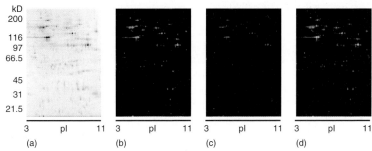

Figure 2.2 Various staining methods for two-dimensional gels. (a) 150 μg of whole human brain extracts were analyzed on a 2D gel using isoelectric focusing for the first dimension (pH 3–11; non-linear) and size-directed protein separation for the second dimension (21.5–200 kDa). Subsequently, the gel was silver-stained. (b, c) Samples and separation technique were identical to (a). However, mouse brain extracts were stained before separation with either Cy5 (green, e.g. transgenic mouse sample) or Cy3 (red, e.g. control mouse sample). Subsequently, the gel was scanned twice at corresponding wavelengths for the Cy5 and Cy3 channel. Comparison of spot intensities of labeled proteins (Cy3 to Cy5; overlay, d) reveal levels of different protein expression. (Please find a color version of this figure in the color plates.)

antibodies or by the Pro-Q Diamond staining method (Invitrogen) which visualizes phosphoserine-, phosphothreonine-, and phosphotyrosine-containing proteins (Steinberg *et al.*, 2003). After separation, the phosphorylated proteins are stained specifically with a fluorescent dye and detected in a fluorescence scanner. The staining of phosphorylated proteins is fully compatible with MALDI and electrospray ionization (ESI)-MS, as the Pro-Q Diamond fluorescent dye does not bind covalently to the phosphorylated residues (Schulenberg *et al.*, 2003). Comparable to the Pro-Q Diamond stain for phosphoproteins, the Pro-Q Emerald glycoprotein stain reacts with periodate-oxidized carbohydrate groups, creating a fluorescent signal on glycoproteins. By using this stain, it is possible to detect as little as 4 ng of glycoprotein per band, depending upon the nature and the degree of glycosylation. The Pro-Q Emerald stain binds only to carbohydrate groups at glycosylation sites. After trypsin digestion, the non-glycosylated peptides, which are not stained, can be identified directly by standard MS techniques. Details of mass-spectrometric identification of posttranslationally modified peptides are given in Chapter 11.

2.2.2
2-D Fluorescence Difference in-Gel Electrophoresis

The two-dimensional fluorescence difference in-gel electrophoresis (2D-DIGE) (GE Healthcare) technique is often used for differential proteome analysis. Proteins from two different samples and a standard sample are initially each labeled with spectrally distinct fluorescent dyes with matching mass and charge (CyDyes: one sample with Cy2, another with Cy3, and the standard with Cy5). The samples are then pooled and separated by 2D-PAGE (Unlu *et al.*, 1997). The dye-labeled proteins are viewed on the gel by scanning it at the (different) fluorescence wavelengths of each dye (Figure 2.2b–d). Image-analysis software generates a stackable gel image for each dye and volume ratios for each spot that are used to calculate relative concentration levels. The key benefit of the DIGE technology is the introduction of an internal standard (preferably a mixture of all samples used in the differential study) labeled with the third CyDye. The internal standard is used to match the protein pattern across the gels, minimizing quantification errors caused by inter-gel variation. Drawbacks of the technique are that DIGE can be laborious and time-consuming, and that the co-migration or partial co-migration of proteins can compromise the results of quantification.

2.2.3
In-Gel Digestion

After the resolution of proteins by gel electrophoresis, the protein spots/lanes of interest have to be excised from the gel. Trypsin is normally the preferred endoproteinase for the in-gel digestion of proteins for several reasons: (i) It cleaves specifically on the C-terminal side of arginine and lysine. Thus, the peptide (precursor) generated automatically carries a positively charged amino acid (Arg or Lys) at its C-terminus and its ionization is thus favored under acidic conditions. (ii) Most of the tryptic peptides generated have a mass-to-charge ratio (m/z) in a range suitable for MS analysis ($m/z = 350$–1400). (iii) It is active in the presence of a variety of denaturing agents, including urea, guanidinium hydro-chloride, and SDS. (iv) It is relatively inexpensive. Moreover, non-modified trypsin (sequencing grade) produces well-characterized autoproteolytic fragments, which can serve both as internal standards—giving excellent reproducibility of retention times in the liquid chromatography system—and as calibration standards for increased mass accuracy in the subsequent database search.

Since membrane proteins contain stretches of highly hydrophobic transmembrane domains that lack an adequate number of arginine and lysine residues, the sequence coverage of membrane proteins can be relatively poor when only trypsin is used as a proteinase. To circumvent this problem, different endoproteinases and solvents can be used in combination with both in-gel and in-solution digestion procedures; this can help to increase the number of detectable peptides in the MS analysis (Wu and Yates, 2003; Fischer *et al.*, 2006).

2.3
Liquid Chromatography-Based Separation Techniques

Many limitations of the 2D-PAGE system can be overcome by using non-gel-based LC (Wang and Hanash, 2003). Hydrophobic and membrane proteins and highly acidic and basic proteins in particular can be analyzed by LC techniques (Dixon *et al.*, 2006). The versatility of this technique is increased greatly by the wide variety of stationary and mobile phases and chromatography types that it offers, for example, size-exclusion chromatography (SEC), affinity chromatography, ion-exchange chromatography (IEX), and reversed-phase chromatography (RPC) (Wang and Hanash, 2003). State-of-the-art LC techniques use peptides rather than proteins for analysis because of their improved separation properties and their higher solubility (Issaq *et al.*, 2002). In the multidimensional protein identification technology (MuDPIT), for instance, protein samples are digested with proteases and loaded onto a biphasic microcapillary column packed with strong cation-exchange and reversed-phase material. Sequentially, eluted peptides are detected and identified on a tandem mass spectrometer (Washburn *et al.*, 2001). Unfortunately, most of the LC approaches at present available fail to perform sufficiently well in separating complex biological mixtures (Issaq, 2001). For this reason, pre-fractionation of proteins is gaining prominence in LC-based proteome analysis.

2.3.1
Automated NanoLC-MS/MS Analysis

2.3.1.1 Chromatography System(s)

Automated nanoLC-MS/MS is currently the method of choice for protein analysis. The chromatography set-up can be coupled either on-line to an ESI-MS (Section 2.4.1) or off-line to a MALDI-MS target-spotter (Section 2.4.2). A frequently used automated nanoLC-MS/MS set-up (off-line and on-line) consists of a one-dimensional RPC system that utilizes an autosampler with a capillary loading pump working at a flow rate of $1-2500 \, \mu L \, min^{-1}$ (for initial desalting of the samples on a pre-column), a nano-pump system working in the flow range of $0.05-1 \, \mu L \, min^{-1}$ (for separation of the sample on the analytical column) and a 6-port or 10-port nano-valve for connecting the pre- and analytical columns. Typical pre- and analytical columns have an inner diameter of 75–300 and 50–120 µm, respectively. Note that desalting of the sample (after in-gel digestion) is essential before it is subjected to MS analysis. The above set-up is required when relatively large volumes of non-desalted samples are applied. No loading pump and pre-columns are required when the samples are desalted before chromatography (Rappsilber *et al.*, 2003).

The workflow for the procedures described above, including a desalting step with a pre-column, contains the following steps: (i) loading the sample onto the pre-column at high flow rates ($\geq 10 \, \mu L \, min^{-1}$) for trapping and desalting of the sample, (ii) elution of the sample by backflush (switching of the 6- or 10-port valve) from the pre-column onto the analytical column and subsequent separation of the captured peptides by an acetonitrile gradient using the nanopump system. The duration of the gradient can vary from 15 min to several hours, depending on the columns, the flow rates, and the complexity of the sample. As a rule of thumb, on an "ordinary" column of 75 µm inner diameter and 10 cm length a good starting point for further optimization is a 60-min gradient.

Pre- and analytical columns of diverse sizes can be purchased from various manufacturers or, alternatively, they can be packed in the laboratory with a variety of materials. Since the performance of the chromatography is very dependent upon the column material, for best results it is recommended that several trial runs, employing different reverse-phase materials, be conducted. A protocol for preparing and packing reverse-phase columns for nanoLC-MS/MS is provided in Chapter 8.

2.3.1.2 On-Line Coupled ESI Mass Spectrometry

On-line coupling of nanoLC to an ESI mass spectrometer is a fast and powerful way to obtain peptide sequence information. The chromatography system greatly reduces the complexity of the sample, and the direct coupling to the source ensures that the peptides eluted are immediately ionized and analyzed in the instrument.

Most state-of-the-art mass spectrometers use data-dependent acquisition (DDA) to analyze the peptide mixture that is eluted from the LC system. The DDA cycle (duty cycle) consists of two main steps: First, an MS scan over a certain mass range (typically 350–1500 m/z) is performed to detect singly, doubly, triply, and quadruply charged peptides, and second, only doubly, triply, and quadruply charged peptide precursors are selected for MS/MS analysis (fragmentation). Importantly, after the initial MS scan, several peptide precursors can be selected for subsequent MS/MS analysis, which allows the most intense precursor signals in the MS spectrum to be sequenced. Note that while the instrument is occupied with MS/MS experiments no MS scans can be performed; therefore, during this time, peptides that are eluted from the column into the instrument cannot be detected and sequenced. Consequently, instruments with a short duty cycle can sequence more peptides in a given time than instruments with a long duty cycle.

Despite the separation power of modern LC techniques, in complex samples a multitude of peptides are still eluted every second from the column, and even modern mass spectrometers cannot register all of these in the time available. Therefore, a successful analysis is also dependent upon an initial separation of the complex protein/peptide mixture; this is achieved by two-dimensional liquid chromatography-based mass spectrometry (2D-LC-MS) of complex peptide mixtures, for example, strong cation exchanger in the first dimension, reversed-phase high-performance liquid chromatography (HPLC) in the second dimension, or separation of proteins by SDS-gel electrophoresis and subsequent LC-MS/MS of extracted peptides derived from the in-gel hydrolyzed proteins. A further important factor is the acquisition speed (duty cycle) of the mass spectrometer. In general, ion-trap instruments have a faster duty cycle as compared with qQ-ToF instruments and they are therefore frequently used for the analysis of very complex mixtures. On the other hand, the quality of the MS/MS spectra derived from qQ-ToF instruments is considerably better, so that the number of MS/MS spectra that can be used to assign a peptide sequence correctly is higher (Elias *et al.*, 2005; Domon *et al.*, 2006).

2.3.1.3 Off-Line-Coupled MALDI-ToF MS/MS

State-of-the-art MALDI mass spectrometers provide the opportunity to select ions for MS/MS experiments. Thanks to this capability, MALDI-MS/MS can also be combined with the separation of complex peptide mixtures by LC. For this purpose, an LC set-up can be coupled to a fractionator that spots very small volumes (fractions) eluting from the analytical column (in the nl range) onto a MALDI sample plate (named the target). The fractions are either mixed with the MALDI matrix solution during the spotting or, alternatively, the matrix can be pre-spotted onto the target and the fractions are then spotted on top of the matrix.

One potential drawback of off-line coupled MALDI-MS compared with on-line ESI-MS analysis is a longer analysis time. In addition to the chromatographic separation time, the subsequent MS- and MS/MS-analysis time must be added to the total analysis time. However, several advantages also exist for off-line LC-MALDI-MS/MS including (i) it can be fully automated, that is, complex peptide mixtures can be spotted onto the target and the targets can be stored over a longer period and then analyzed automatically one after the other and (ii) the sample can be re-investigated as in most cases the spotted fraction is not completely used up. This has an important consequence: fractions derived from very complex mixtures can be analyzed once and the identified proteins can then be put onto an "exclusion list;" the samples can then be re-investigated, whereby only those peptides (precursors) are sequenced that do not belong to the set of proteins already identified (i.e. those on the exclusion list).

Importantly, off-line MALDI-MS/MS analysis provides a strong complementary approach in the analysis of membrane proteins. In particular, large hydrophobic peptides derived from transmembrane regions of proteins are not readily ionized by ESI and thus give poor signals in ESI-MS. MALDI-MS has the advantage that it can cover a larger mass range, that is, it is better suited for larger peptides. Furthermore, peptides that are derived from cleavage of membrane proteins with endoproteinases other than trypsin yield more reliable sequence information in MALDI-MS/MS. This is due to the fact that ESI-MS/MS requires doubly and triply charged peptides for sequence analysis, and this is especially favored by digestion of proteins with trypsin. Singly charged peptides give almost no sequence information in ESI-MS/MS, and the number of singly charged peptides becomes higher when endoproteinases such as Glu-C, chymotrypsin, Asp-N and so on, are used (as the generated peptides do not contain a basic amino acid at their C-terminus).

2.4
Mass Spectrometry and Data Analysis

Mass spectrometers represent one of the most important tools in proteomics and have largely displaced Edman sequencing, which was used for the identification of proteins before the development of MS for this application. Advantages of MS are the short analysis time, high sensitivity, and feasible automation. For sensitive detection of proteins and peptides, different types of high-sensitivity mass spectrometers (e.g. time-of-flight (ToF), triple quadrupole and ion-trap MS) are currently used with various ionization types (e.g. MALDI or ESI) (Karas and Hillenkamp, 1988; Fenn *et al.*, 1989). Within the mass spectrometer, the peptides are ionized and separated, and the mass-to-charge ratio (m/z) is determined. By using protein databases and automated search algorithms, the proteins are identified (Steen and Mann, 2004; Shadforth *et al.*, 2005).

2.4.1
Electrospray Ionization

ESI is a continuous ionization method whereby multiply charged biomolecules (e.g. $[M + 2H]^{2+}$ to $[M + n\,H]^{n+}$) are produced in solution from a capillary electrode placed at high voltage with respect to a grounded counter electrode (Fenn *et al.*, 1989). A so-called "electrospray" is generated. The "sprayed" ions are first desolvated while they are guided into the interface of the mass spectrometer, where they are subsequently separated according to their *m/z* value and analyzed. Because of their size, most peptides become doubly, triply, or quadruply charged.

2.4.2
Matrix-Assisted Laser Desorption Ionization

In contrast to ESI, matrix-assisted laser desorption ionization time-of-flight (MALDI-ToF) is a pulsed ionization technique (Karas and Hillenkamp, 1988). Analyte molecules (peptides and proteins) are first embedded in a light-absorbing matrix (e.g. 2,5-dihydroxybenzoic acid or α-cyano-cinnamic acid) and are subsequently desorbed by a laser pulse, whereby mainly singly charged (i.e. $[M + H]^+$) peptides/proteins are generated by charge transfer (i.e. H^+) from the matrix molecules to the analyte molecules. An electric field is applied, which accelerates the charged molecules through a high-vacuum tube towards the detector. The time the analyte molecules need to reach the detector is directly proportional to their molecular weight.

2.4.3
Database Searches and Data Validation

Once the raw data for MS analysis have been recorded, a "peak list" is generated. A peak list contains information about (i) the masses of the precursors selected for MS/MS analysis, (ii) the masses of the fragment ions from the precursors selected for MS/MS analysis, and (iii) the intensity of the fragment ions for each MS/MS spectrum. Identification of the peptide/protein is performed by using a search engine to search the peak list against a database of proteins "digested *in silico*." The latter term refers to a two-step computer prediction: first the proteome is scanned and all possible proteolytic products (oligopeptides) are noted, and then the fragmentation pattern of each oligopeptide is predicted. The database search is therefore only possible when the genome and the protein sequences of a particular organism are available in the database. When organisms are investigated whose genomes have not yet been sequenced, a sequence analysis *de novo* must be performed: this entails manual annotation and interpretation of the MS/MS spectra in order to obtain enough information about the peptides' sequences.

Several search engines are available, for example, Mascot, SEQUEST, and XTandem. However, Mascot and SEQUEST currently are the most widely used search engines in the proteomic community. Even though Mascot and SEQUEST apply similar search algorithms to assign peptides in a sequence database to the measured MS/MS spectra, they use fundamentally different principles in their mathematical operations. Mascot uses a probability-based system to access the likelihood that a fragmented peptide will give rise to an observed spectrum (Elias *et al.*, 2005), whereas SEQUEST uses empirical and correlation measurements to score the alignments between observed and predicted spectra (Yates *et al.*, 1995). The use of either Mascot or SEQUEST as a search algorithm has recently been demonstrated to play a role in the total number of peptides identified from a large-scale proteomics dataset, depending on the type of instrument used for the analysis (i.e. ion-trap versus qQ-ToF hybrid instrument) (Elias *et al.*, 2005). While the scoring functions for the two search algorithms showed similar results for MS/MS data obtained from an ion-trap instrument (>85% overlap) Mascot was significantly better in interpreting MS/MS data from a hybrid instrument (QSTAR) (Elias *et al.*, 2005). To some extent, the total number of proteins identified can be increased when the MS/MS spectra are searched by both Mascot and SEQUEST. However, the sequence coverage of peptides, and the total number of proteins identified, can be increased significantly if (i) the samples are analyzed by using different instruments and (ii) they are analyzed several times (20–30% more proteins identified) (Elias *et al.*, 2005). In Table 2.1 the suggested default search settings for an ion-trap and a hybrid-type instrument are presented. They should, of course, be modified for specialized searches.

As described above, there are several points that one should take into consideration when planning an experiment in respect both of instrument type (e.g. ion-trap versus qQ-ToF hybrid instrument) and of search algorithm (e.g. Mascot versus SEQUEST). However, even though these factors are essential for maximizing the output in terms of proteomics results, a final validation of the search results is a critical step in the proteomic analysis. A stringent validation ensures that the final list of proteins identified contains

Table 2.1 Suggested database search settings for an ion-trap and a hybrid-type (qQ-ToF) instrument.

Instrument type	Peptide tolerance	MS/MS tolerance	Missed cleavages	Fixed modifications	Variable modifications
Hybrid (Q-ToF)	0.2 Da	0.2 Da	2	Carbamido-methylation on cysteines	Oxidation of methionine
Ion trap (triple quad)	0.8 Da	1.2 Da	2	Carbamido-methylation on cysteines	Oxidation of methionine

a minimum of (or no) false positives. Manual interpretation of the MS/MS data of the proteins positively identified by the search algorithm is regarded as the "gold standard" of validation. However, recent validation approaches have also included searches in both a normal protein database and a "reversed" or "randomized" protein database in which the sequences have been reversed or randomized (Elias *et al.*, 2005; Takamori *et al.*, 2006). Since one does not expect to get any real matches from the "decoy" database, the number of matches that are found is an excellent estimate of the number of false positives that are present in the results from the real database. By comparing then the number of proteins positively identified from the two searches (normal versus "reversed" or "randomized") the "false discovery rate" (FDR) can be calculated (Peng *et al.*, 2003), which describes the number of false positives in the dataset. The FDR is usually below 1% in larger proteomics datasets. Instructions how to create a "decoy" database can be found for example, under http://www.matrixscience.com/search_form_select.html.

2.5
Protein Quantification Methods

The power of proteomics has been greatly enhanced by the development of relative and absolute quantitative proteomic methods. This has been demonstrated by using traditional quantitative approaches such as two-dimensional electrophoresis and the related DIGE technique (Hu *et al.*, 2005; Wilson *et al.*, 2005). More recently, gel-free quantitative methods including chemical, enzymatic, and metabolic labeling of specific protein populations with different isotopes and subsequent quantification by MS have gained popularity, as they show increased sensitivity compared with gel-based methods. They include carbon isotope-coded affinity tags (cICAT) (Gygi *et al.*, 1999), isobaric tags for relative and absolute quantification (iTRAQ) (Ross *et al.*, 2004), enzymatic labeling with protein hydrolysis in the presence of heavy (i.e. ^{18}O-containing) water (^{18}O/^{16}O proteolytic labeling) (Yao *et al.*, 2001; Staes *et al.*, 2004) and stable isotope labeling with amino acids in cell culture (SILAC) (Ong *et al.*, 2002). Basically, in all chemical labeling approaches proteins derived from different samples are hydrolyzed, and the corresponding peptide pool is chemically labeled with reagents that differs in mass due to the incorporation of different heavy stable isotopes like ^{13}C, ^{15}N, or ^{2}D. After mixing, the thus differently labeled samples are analyzed by MS. Importantly, the intensity in the MS of the same but differently labeled peptides derived from the various sample can be directly compared and reflects the relative quantities of the particular peptide and therefore of the particular protein in different samples. Chemical labeling is mostly used on the peptide level, that is, labeling takes place after the proteins are digested with specific endoproteinases. cICAT has been originally reported for labeling on the protein level and in principal all reagents also should work on the protein level. The advantage of the chemically labeling strategy is the fact that it can be used for MS-based quantification approaches in tissues (e.g. brain). SILAC, although a highly efficient labeling approach as labeled ^{13}C- and ^{15}N-labeled amino acids (e.g. ^{13}C-lysine, ^{13}C-arginine) are incorporated into proteins nearly to 100% during growth of cell-in-cell cultures, is restricted to the investigation of cells growing in culture (e.g. HeLa cells).

More recently, label-free quantification by MS has also shown great promise; this uses techniques such as spectral counting (Old *et al.*, 2005) and ion-current measurement (Wiener *et al.*, 2004).

Recent analyses have revealed that combining these approaches increases the number of proteins identified as showing different expression levels. In a comparative study of DIGE, cICAT, and iTRAQ, the iTRAQ method was more sensitive than cICAT, which in turn was more sensitive than DIGE (Wu *et al.*, 2006). In addition, the three techniques identified different proteins *per se*, suggesting the complementary nature of these methods. Another study used the cICAT and ^{16}O/^{18}O labeling methods together to maximize the number of proteins identified and quantified from biological samples (Blonder *et al.*, 2006).

2.5.1
Carbon Isotope-Coded Affinity Tags

The cICAT method (Gygi *et al.*, 1999; Wu *et al.*, 2006) involves labeling of proteins from two different biological samples with heavy (^{13}C) and light (^{12}C) reagents, followed by enzymatic digestion, affinity isolation, sample pooling, HPLC separation, and finally detection and quantification of the labeled pairs by tandem MS. The cICAT reagents label the cysteine residues in proteins and will not detect proteins that do not contain cysteine. Information on any posttranslational modification is lost, because many posttranslationally modified peptides are not retained during the affinity-chromatography step. The traditional cICAT method uses strong ion-exchange and avidin affinity steps for sample clean-up. Recently, alternative cICAT clean-up procedures were evaluated in which an Oasis MXC mixed-mode extraction cartridge, a strong cation-exchange ZipTip, and a self-packed monomeric avidin column were used for the first step (Yu *et al.*, 2004).

2.5.2
Isobaric Tags for Relative and Absolute Quantification

The iTRAQ method (Ross *et al.*, 2004; Wu *et al.*, 2006) involves protein reduction and alkylation, enzymatic digestion, labeling up to four different samples with heavy and light isotope labeled reagents, sample pooling, HPLC separation, and finally detection and quantification by tandem MS. The iTRAQ reagent is an amine-specific reagent that labels peptide N-termini and lysine side-chains with multiplex (4-plex) isobaric mass tags, that is, tags with identical masses. Fragmentation of the tag attached to the peptides generates a low molecular mass reporter ion, which is unique to the tag used to label each of the samples. Measurement of the intensity of these reporter ions enables relative quantification of the peptides in each sample (see Chapter 9 and also e.g. Ross *et al.*, 2004). Multiplexing can save time during the quantification of samples taken at several time points, and information on posttranslational modification is not lost using the iTRAQ method. The confidence in protein identification and detection using iTRAQ versus cICAT is increased because of the greater abundance of lysine than of cysteine residues in proteins. However, as it is not restricted to cysteine-containing proteins, the iTRAQ method does not reduce the sample complexity (in contrast to cICAT), and this places greater demands upon the separation step before tandem MS.

2.5.3
Labeling with Heavy Water

The $^{16}O/^{18}O$ method involves protein isolation, tryptic digestion, trypsin-catalyzed $^{16}O/^{18}O$ labeling, sample pooling, HPLC separation, and MS/MS detection and quantification. When trypsin, Glu-C, or Lys-C protease is used for protein digestion in the presence of $H_2^{18}O$, up to two ^{18}O atoms are incorporated into the resulting peptide-terminal carboxyl group. The ^{18}O-labeled carboxyl group does not back-exchange in the presence of unlabeled water under normal conditions of sample handling, HPLC separation, and MS/MS analysis. The resulting peptide pairs (e.g. normal versus disease states) observed in the mass spectrometer will have a mass difference of 4 atomic mass units.

2.6
Summary

In conclusion, proteomics is a highly dynamic field with many promising technical improvements currently being implemented. This will provide researchers on the one hand with an unprecedented battery of possibilities to identify and characterize proteins. On the other hand, these many possibilities require a careful consideration before getting started to adopt the approach best suited to address a given problem. Furthermore, each of the many different techniques will require an intense know-how, causing the field of proteomics to split into specialized sections and groups. In this respect, the emergent field of neuroproteomics does not require a particular set of "neuroproteomic techniques" but uses—like other proteome studies—the range of "state-of-the-art" protein identification technologies to its full extent.

References

Blonder, J., Yu, L.R., Radeva, G., Chan, K.C., Lucas, D.A., Waybright, T.J., Issaq, H.J., Sharom, F.J. and Veenstra, T.D. (2006) Combined chemical and enzymatic stable isotope labeling for quantitative profiling of detergent-insoluble membrane proteins isolated using Triton X-100 and Brij-96. *Journal of Proteome Research*, **5**, 349–360.

Boyd-Kimball, D., Castegna, A., Sultana, R., Poon, H.F., Petroze, R., Lynn, B.C., Klein, J.B. and Butterfield, D.A. (2005) Proteomic identification of proteins oxidized by Abeta(1–42) in synaptosomes: implications for Alzheimer's disease. *Brain Research*, **1044**, 206–215.

Diao, A., Rahman, D., Pappin, D.J.C., Lucocq, J. and Lowe, M. (2003) The coiled-coil membrane protein golgin-84 is a novel rab effector required for Golgi ribbon formation. *Journal of Cell Biology*, **160**, 201–212.

Dixon, S.P., Pitfield, I.D. and Perrett, D. (2006) Comprehensive multi-dimensional liquid chromatographic separation in biomedical and pharmaceutical analysis: a review. *Biomedical Chromatography: BMC*, **20**, 508–529.

Domon, B. and Aebersold, R. (2006) Mass spectrometry and protein analysis. *Science*, **312**, 212–217.

Dreger, M., Bengtsson, L., Schoneberg, T., Otto, H. and Hucho, F. (2001) Nuclear envelope proteomics: Novel integral membrane proteins of the inner nuclear membrane. *Proceedings of the National Academy of Sciences of the United States of America*, **98**, 11943–11948.

Dzandu, J.K., Johnson, J.F. and Wise, G.E. (1988) Sodium dodecyl sulfate-gel electrophoresis: staining of polypeptides using heavy metal salts. *Analytical Biochemistry*, **174**, 157–167.

Elias, J.E., Haas, W., Faherty, B.K. and Gygi, S.P. (2005) Comparative evaluation of mass spectrometry platforms used in large-scale proteomics investigations. *Nature Methods*, **2**, 667–675.

Fenn, J.B., Mann, M., Meng, C.K., Wong, S.F. and Whitehouse, C.M. (1989) Electrospray ionization for mass spectrometry or large biomolecules. *Science*, **243**, 64–71.

Fischer, F., Wolters, D., Rogner, M. and Poetsch, A. (2006) Toward the complete membrane proteome: high coverage of integral membrane proteins through transmembrane peptide detection. *Molecular & Cellular Proteomics: MCP*, **5**, 444–453.

Gorg, A., Obermaier, C., Boguth, G., Harder, A., Scheibe, B., Wildgruber, R. and Weiss, W. (2000) The current state of two-dimensional electrophoresis with immobilized pH gradients. *Electrophoresis*, **21**, 1037–1053.

Guillemin, I., Becker, M., Ociepka, K., Friauf, E. and Nothwang, H.G. (2005) A subcellular prefractionation protocol for minute amounts of mammalian cell cultures and tissue. *Proteomics*, **5**, 35–45.

Gygi, S.P., Rist, B., Gerber, S.A., Turecek, F., Gelb, M.H. and Aebersold, R. (1999) Quantitative analysis of complex protein mixtures using isotope-coded affinity tags. *Nature Biotechnology*, **17**, 994–999.

Hartinger, J., Stenius, K., Hogemann, D. and Jahn, R. (1996) 16-BAC/SDS-PAGE: a two-dimensional gel electrophoresis system suitable for the separation of integral membrane proteins. *Analytical Biochemistry*, **240**, 126–133.

Hu, Y., Malone, J.P., Fagan, A.M., Townsend, R.R. and Holtzman, D.M. (2005) Comparative proteomic analysis of intra- and interindividual variation in human cerebrospinal fluid. *Molecular & Cellular Proteomics: MCP*, **4**, 2000–2009.

Issaq, H.J. (2001) The role of separation science in proteomics research. *Electrophoresis*, **22**, 3629–3638.

Issaq, H.J., Conrads, T.P., Janini, G.M. and Veenstra, T.D. (2002) Methods for fractionation, separation and profiling of proteins and peptides. *Electrophoresis*, **23**, 3048–3061.

Karas, M. and Hillenkamp, F. (1988) Laser desorption ionization of proteins with molecular masses exceeding 10 000 daltons. *Analytical Chemistry*, **60**, 2299–2301.

Klose, J. (1975) Protein mapping by combined isoelectric focusing and electrophoresis of mous tissue: a novel approach to testing for induced proint mutations in mammals. *Humangenetik*, **26**, 231–243.

Klose, J. (1999) Large-gel 2-D electrophoresis. *Methods in Molecular Biology*, **112**, 147–172.

Klose, J. and Kobalz, U. (1995) Two-dimensional electrophoresis of proteins: an updated protocol and implications for a functional analysis of the genome. *Electrophoresis*, **16**, 1034–1059.

Levine, R.L., Williams, J.A., Stadtman, E.R. and Shacter, E. (1994) Carbonyl assays for determination of oxidatively modified proteins. *Methods in Enzymology*, **233**, 346–357.

Macfarlane, D.E. (1989) Two dimensional benzyldimethyl-n-hexadecylammonium chloride-sodium dodecyl sulfate preparative polyacrylamide gel electrophoresis: a high capacity high resolution technique for the purification of proteins from complex mixtures. *Analytical Biochemistry*, **176**, 457–463.

Old, W.M., Meyer-Arendt, K., Aveline-Wolf, L., Pierce, K.G., Mendoza, A., Sevinsky, J.R., Resing, K.A. and Ahn, N.G. (2005) Comparison of label-free methods for quantifying human proteins by shotgun proteomics. *Molecular & Cellular Proteomics: MCP*, **4**, 1487–1502.

Ong, S.E., Blagoev, B., Kratchmarova, I., Kristensen, D.B., Steen, H., Pandey, A. and Mann, M. (2002) Stable isotope labeling by amino acids in cell culture, SILAC, as a simple and accurate approach to expression proteomics. *Molecular & Cellular Proteomics: MCP*, **1**, 376–386.

Peng, J., Elias, J.E., Thoreen, C.C., Licklider, L.J. and Gygi, S.P. (2003) Evaluation of multidimensional chromatography coupled with tandem mass spectrometry (LC/LC-MS/MS) for large-scale protein analysis: the yeast proteome. *Journal of Proteome Research*, **2**, 43–50.

Rabilloud, T. and Charmont, S. (1999) Detection of proteins on two-dimensional electrophoresis gels, in *Proteome Research: Two-dimensional Gel Electrophoresis and Identification Methods* (ed. T. Rabilloud), Springer-Verlag, Heidelberg, pp. 107–126.

Rappsilber, J., Ishihama, Y. and Mann, M. (2003) Stop and go extraction tips for matrix-assisted laser desorption/ionization, nanoelectrospray, and LC/MS sample pretreatment in proteomics. *Analytical Chemistry*, **75**, 663–670.

Ross, P.L., Huang, Y.N., Marchese, J.N., Williamson, B., Parker, K., Hattan, S., Khainovski, N., Pillai, S., Dey, S., Daniels, S., Purkayastha, S., Juhasz, P., Martin, S., Bartlet-Jones, M., He, F., Jacobson, A. and Pappin, D.J. (2004) Multiplexed protein quantitation in Saccharomyces cerevisiae using amine-reactive isobaric tagging reagents. *Molecular & Cellular Proteomics: MCP*, **3**, 1154–1169.

Schulenberg, B., Aggeler, R., Beechem, J.M., Capaldi, R.A. and Patton, W.F. (2003) Analysis of steady-state protein phosphorylation in mitochondria using a novel fluorescent phosphosensor dye. *Journal of Biological Chemistry*, **278**, 27251–27255.

Shadforth, I., Crowther, D. and Bessant, C. (2005) Protein and peptide identification algorithms using MS for use in high-throughput, automated pipelines. *Proteomics*, **5**, 4082–4095.

Shaw, J., Rowlinson, R., Nickson, J., Stone, T., Sweet, A., Williams, K. and Tonge, R. (2003) Evaluation of saturation labelling two-dimensional difference gel electrophoresis fluorescent dyes. *Proteomics*, **3**, 1181–1195.

Shevchenko, A., Wilm, M., Vorm, O. and Mann, M. (1996) Mass spectrometric sequencing of proteins from silver stained polyacrylamide gels. *Analytical Chemistry*, **68**, 850–858.

Stadtman, E.R. (1993) Oxidation of free amino acids and amino acid residues in proteins by radiolysis and by metal-catalyzed reactions. *Annual Review of Biochemistry*, **62**, 797–821.

Staes, A., Demol, H., Van Damme, J., Martens, L., Vandekerckhove, J. and Gevaert, K. (2004) Global differential non-gel proteomics by quantitative and stable labeling of tryptic peptides with oxygen-18. *Journal of Proteome Research,* **3**, 786–791.

Steen, H. and Mann, M. (2004) The ABC's (and XYZ's) of peptide sequencing. *Nature Reviews. Molecular Cell Biology,* **5**, 699–711.

Steinberg, T.H., Agnew, B.J., Gee, K.R., Leung, W.Y., Goodman, T., Schulenberg, B., Hendrickson, J., Beechem, J.M., Haugland, R.P. and Patton, W.F. (2003) Global quantitative phosphoprotein analysis using multiplexed proteomics technology. *Proteomics,* **3**, 1128–1144.

Takamori, S., Holt, M., Stenius, K., Lemke, E.A., Gronborg, M., Riedel, D., Urlaub, H., Schenck, S., Brugger, B., Ringler, P., Muller, S.A., Rammner, B., Grater, F., Hub, J.S., De Groot, B.L., Mieskes, G., Moriyama, Y., Klingauf, J., Grubmuller, H., Heuser, J., Wieland, F. and Jahn, R. (2006) Molecular anatomy of a trafficking organelle. *Cell,* **127**, 831–846.

Unlu, M., Morgan, M.E. and Minden, J.S. (1997) Difference gel electrophoresis: a single gel method for detecting changes in protein extracts. *Electrophoresis,* **18**, 2071–2077.

Wang, H. and Hanash, S. (2003) Multi-dimensional liquid phase based separations in proteomics. *Journal of Chromatography. B, Analytical Technologies in the Biomedical and Life Sciences,* **787**, 11–18.

Washburn, M.P., Wolters, D. and Yates, J.R. (2001) Large-scale analysis of the yeast proteome by multidimensional protein identification technology. *Nature Biotechnology,* **19**, 242–247.

Wiener, M.C., Sachs, J.R., Deyanova, E.G. and Yates, N.A. (2004) Differential mass spectrometry: a label-free LC-MS method for finding significant differences in complex peptide and protein mixtures. *Analytical Chemistry,* **76**, 6085–6096.

Wilson, K.E., Marouga, R., Prime, J.E., Pashby, D.P., Orange, P.R., Crosier, S., Keith, A.B., Lathe, R., Mullins, J., Estibeiro, P., Bergling, H., Hawkins, E. and Morris, C.M. (2005) Comparative proteomic analysis using samples obtained with laser microdissection and saturation dye labelling. *Proteomics,* **5**, 3851–3858.

Wu, C.C. and Yates, J.R., III (2003) The application of mass spectrometry to membrane proteomics. *Nature Biotechnology,* **21**, 262–267.

Wu, W.W., Wang, G., Baek, S.J. and Shen, R.F. (2006) Comparative study of three proteomic quantitative methods, DIGE, cICAT, and iTRAQ, using 2D gel- or LC-MALDI TOF/TOF. *Journal of Proteome Research,* **5**, 651–658.

Yan, J.X., Wait, R., Berkelman, T., Harry, R.A., Westbrook, J.A., Wheeler, C.H. and Dunn, M.J. (2000) A modified silver staining protocol for visualization of proteins compatible with matrix-assisted laser desorption/ionization and electrospray ionization-mass spectrometry. *Electrophoresis,* **21**, 3666–3672.

Yao, X., Freas, A., Ramirez, J., Demirev, P.A. and Fenselau, C. (2001) Proteolytic 18O labeling for comparative proteomics: model studies with two serotypes of adenovirus. *Analytical Chemistry,* **73**, 2836–2842.

Yates, J.R., III Eng, J.K. and McCormack, A.L. (1995) Mining genomes: correlating tandem mass spectra of modified and unmodified peptides to sequences in nucleotide databases. *Analytical Chemistry,* **67**, 3202–3210.

Yu, L.R., Conrads, T.P., Uo, T., Issaq, H.J., Morrison, R.S. and Veenstra, T.D. (2004) Evaluation of the acid-cleavable isotope-coded affinity tag reagents: application to camptothecin-treated cortical neurons. *Journal of Proteome Research,* **3**, 469–477.

3
Proteomic Technologies for the Analysis of Protein Complexes

Ming Zhou and Timothy D. Veenstra

3.1
Introduction

John Donne, writing in his *Devotions Upon Emergent Occasions* (Meditation XVII), stated that "No man is an island entire of itself .... " What is meant by this statement is that humans do not thrive when isolated from others. The same can be said for proteins. The ability of a protein to carry out its designed function is absolutely dependent on its ability to interact with other biomolecules, whether they are proteins, DNA, RNA, or small organic/inorganic molecules. Proteins interact with other proteins to provide structural integrity to the cell (e.g. actin filaments), transport molecules (e.g. hemoglobin), propagate signals (e.g. kinases), transcribe DNA, translate other proteins, and so on. There is no protein yet discovered that acts on its own without interacting with any other entity. Classical examples include the ribosomes and proteasomes, which are built up by multiprotein complexes consisting of more than 20 proteins. Recent studies have evidenced that interaction with multiple other proteins seem rather the rule than the exception (Ho *et al.*, 2002; Stelzl *et al.*, 2005; Gavin *et al.*, 2006). This notion holds especially true for the nervous system, where proteomic-based analyses have demonstrated huge protein complexes such as the NMDA receptor complex (Grant *et al.*, 2005) or the huntingtin protein (Goehler *et al.*, 2004).

Basic science has long recognized the importance of identifying the interactions that occur among proteins. The identification of specific proteins that interact with a targeted protein is still primarily accomplished through hypothesis-driven approaches. These studies rely heavily on antibodies as affinity-capture agents to extract a targeted protein and those that may interact with it. The isolated complex is then separated on a gel and the proteins blotted onto a membrane. This membrane is interrogated with antibodies directed towards proteins that are hypothesized to bind to the targeted protein. If the antibody recognizes a protein on the membrane then a positive interaction with the targeted protein is concluded. This popular technique, known as

Proteomics of the Nervous System. Edited by H.G. Nothwang and S.E. Pfeiffer
Copyright © 2008 WILEY-VCH Verlag GmbH & Co. KGaA, Weinheim
ISBN: 978-3-527-31716-5

Western blotting (Burnette, 1981), remains a cornerstone in the identification and validation of protein–protein interactions.

While hypothesis-driven approaches will continue to play a major role, the "omics"-era has brought with it technologies that allow the design of discovery-driven experiments for the identification of protein–protein interactions. Most of the technologies used in these discovery-driven approaches are designed to identify as many possible binding partners for a single targeted protein in the shortest time possible. While high-throughput techniques that scan the inventory of genomic (Brown, 1994) and proteome components (Liu *et al.*, 2002) are presently available, the next challenge will be to understand interactions at the proteome-wide level. In this chapter, we will discuss several of the technologies available for characterizing the components of protein complexes, as well as the benefits and drawbacks of each.

3.2
Methods for Isolating Protein Complexes

3.2.1
Immunoprecipitation

Isolating the protein complex is the most critical step in determining the success of the downstream proteomic analysis. The importance of this aspect should never be underestimated. While mass spectrometry analysis is often pictured as the crucial step in such studies, the greatest amount of effort should go into optimizing the isolation of the experimental sample. Extraction or enrichment (rather than isolation) of a protein complex may be the more correct term, because, presently, there is no technology that is capable of isolating a protein complex without the inclusion of non-specifically bound proteins. The most widely used method for protein complex isolation is antibody-based immunoprecipitation. Unlike regular immunoprecipitation whose intended use is for Western blotting, the isolation of a protein complex via immunoprecipitation requires mild cell lysis conditions to preserve the integrity of the protein complex. These conditions include, for example, up to 0.5% Triton X-100, PBS or Tris buffer at neutral pH, physiological ionic strength ($I = 150$ mM), 5–10% glycerol, and so on. To avoid protein degradation and dephosphorylation, protease inhibitors and phosphatase inhibitors should always be added during cell lysis. For best results, the antibody should be covalently conjugated to Protein G Sepharose beads (Ory *et al.*, 2003). There are two major advantages realized through the use of covalently coupled antibody beads. First, it increases the quantity of the protein complex that is isolated. Second, it ensures that the antibody does not interfere with protein separation during sodium dodecyl sulfate polyacrylamide gel electrophoresis (SDS-PAGE) and subsequent MS analysis. The protein complex that is extracted requires several washing steps before it should be eluted from the antibody-conjugated beads. The washing stringency, such as salt concentration, detergent concentration, and so on, must be optimized to reduce the background of unspecific binding of the antibody without interrupting the protein complex. Unfortunately, since different proteins have different binding characteristics, these washing steps require careful optimization for each target complex.

Another difference between conducting an immunoprecipitation procedure for protein complex characterization and for Western blotting is the amount of material required. Protein complex characterization (via MS, for example) requires significantly more material than is needed for a simple Western blot analysis and requires starting with cells that are transfected with an expression plasmid of the target protein. Like a regular immunoprecipitation, protein complex analysis requires comparison to a control sample, which can be cells that are not transfected with the target protein of interest or blank vector transfected cells. This control needs to be lysed and immunoprecipitated in the same manner as the cells that are transfected with an expression vector containing the protein target. Depending on the protein expression efficiency, for an overexpressed mammalian cell system several (e.g. 5–10) million cells are usually needed for liquid chromatography coupled with tandem MS (LC-MS/MS) analysis. In cases where endogenous protein is targeted, cells that are known not to express the protein of interest can be used as the negative control. As with transfected cells, the expression level of the endogenous protein will dictate the number of cells required for the analysis. The proteins observed in the control can be used to background subtract proteins from the experimental protein complex sample by two different methods. First, separation and visualization of the experimental and control samples by SDS-PAGE reveals proteins that are common to each and therefore not specific to the protein complex and do not require downstream MS identification. Second, peptides that are identified in a direct (no gel separation) analysis of the experimental and control samples by LC-MS/MS can be considered as non-specifically bound and not part of the targeted protein complex.

While antibodies that are specifically directed towards the protein of interest can be used, when utilizing transfected cells, the antibody is often targeted to an epitope expressed on a chimeric protein. Several popular epitope tags, such as, Myc, Flag, hemagglutinin, Pyo, and so on, are often inserted in either the N- or C-terminus of the recombinant target proteins that are transiently or stably expressed in cells. While it would seem that the use of such tags permits a standardized method for the isolation of the tagged protein and its complex, in practice the antibody specificity and affinity is still attenuated by the three-dimensional structure of the tagged proteins and nature of the protein complexes. Therefore, careful optimization of the isolation of the tagged protein complex is still necessary.

3.2.2
Oligoprecipitation

Often, proteins do not permanently execute their function. For example, phosphorylation of a specific site is commonly used to activate a protein. The binding partners of a protein in its active and inactive state are usually different. In a vast majority of cases it is the binding partners of the active protein that are of the greatest interest. Transcription factors are an obvious example of having both an inactive and active form of the protein within a cell. Most research is focused on measuring the active form of a transcription factor when it is bound to DNA. The use of an antibody-based immunoprecipitation to extract a targeted transcription factor will generally isolate the transcriptionally active and inactive forms of the protein and therefore it can be difficult to determine which binding partners are relevant to gene transcription. An alternative approach is to use an oligonucleotide that carries the consensus binding sequence to which the active form of the transcription factor binds (Meng *et al.*, 2006). Theoretically, oligoprecipitation only captures the "active form" of protein complexes because the interactions between transcriptors and their consensus DNA sequences are transient. In practice the oligonucleotide is coupled to streptavidin beads via a biotin group that is covalently attached to the double-stranded oligonucleotide (Figure 3.1). A nuclear extract prepared from the cells of interest is then passed over the column to capture the active transcriptional complex. As with immunoprecipitation, a negative control is critical to identify proteins that are non-specifically bound to the complex or other oligoprecipitation reagents (e.g. streptavidin, biotin, etc.). In the case of oligoprecipitation, the same oligonucleotide with a mutation(s) that abrogates binding of the transcription factor can be used as a control.

3.2.3
Tagged Protein Pull-Down

Another method to isolate protein complexes (a specific application in whole proteome screening will be discussed later in this chapter) is the use of a tagged recombinant protein as "bait." In this method, the target protein is expressed as a chimera with another protein or a short stretch of amino acids. The most commonly used tags are glutathione *S*-transferase (GST), maltose-binding protein (MBP), calmodulin-binding peptide (CBP), and hexahistidine (His$_6$) (Dougherty *et al.*, 2005; Olesky *et al.*, 2005; Lechward *et al.*, 2006). In some cases, these tags are combined with immuno-epitope tags (Yang *et al.*, 2006). The recombinant tagged proteins can be either expressed in the cell system studied or can be purified from other expression system and then incubated with the cell lysate. These recombinantly tagged proteins differ from those expressed with epitope tags in that non-antibody-based affinity methods (e.g. immobilized metal affinity chromatography for His$_6$-tagged proteins) are

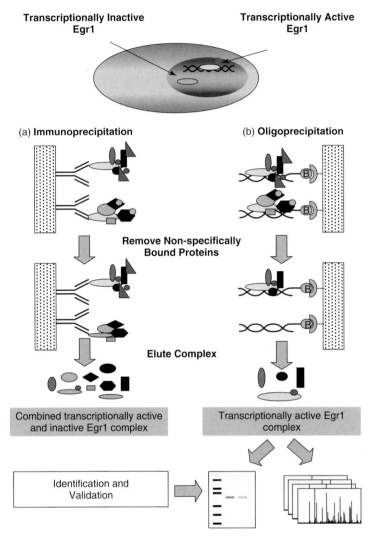

Transcriptionally Inactive Egr1

Transcriptionally Active Egr1

(a) **Immunoprecipitation**

(b) **Oligoprecipitation**

Remove Non-specifically Bound Proteins

Elute Complex

Combined transcriptionally active and inactive Egr1 complex

Transcriptionally active Egr1 complex

Identification and Validation

Figure 3.1 Comparison of oligoprecipitation of an active transcription factor protein to an immunoprecipitation of the same target protein. In this schematic using early growth response protein 1 (Egr1) as an example, the oligoprecipitation approach targets the transcriptionally active, phosphorylated version of Egr1. The immunoprecipitation method results in the isolation of protein complexes built around both the active and inactive forms of Egr1. (Please find a color version of this figure in the color plates.)

used to isolated the protein complex. As with immunoprecipitation isolation, the cell lysis condition and washing stringency varies due to the different nature of the protein complexes. These conditions must be optimized to preserve the intact protein complexes and to minimize the background. As a starting point, the buffers need to be close to the physiological pH and ionic strength. Isolating protein complex is one of the most critical steps for the proteomic analysis. The importance of this aspect should never be underestimated.

3.3
Techniques for Identifying Protein Complexes

3.3.1
Gel Electrophoresis and Mass Spectrometry

The standard procedure for identifying proteins in a complex is quite straightforward (Figure 3.2). Once a protein complex of interest is isolated (see Section 3.2), it is separated using SDS-PAGE (Laemmli, 1970) followed by staining with a colorimetric reagent such as Coomassie Blue or Silver stain (see Chapter 8). After digestion with a proteolytic enzyme, peptides are analyzed by MS.

Beyond sample preparation, the greatest challenge in these targeted studies is filtering the MS data to determine which potential protein interactions are biologically significant. While not often reported in published manuscripts, it is extremely rare that a single gel band provides a single protein identification (i.e. every peak seen in a peptide map or LC-MS/MS spectrum corresponds to the same protein). The best-case scenario is that one protein will be identified by a large number of peptide ions and any other protein is only represented by one or two. In many cases, however, no single protein stands "above the crowd," making it difficult to determine the relative contribution of any protein to the excised gel piece. For this reason, any novel protein–protein interaction that is discovered using SDS-PAGE and MS requires secondary validation to substantiate its relevance.

3.3.2
Whole Proteome Screening Using Tandem Affinity Purification and Mass Spectrometry

One of the major capabilities that the proteomics era has brought to protein science is the ability to conduct global scans of interactions occurring within the cell. The goal in such efforts is to produce a comprehensive map of protein–protein interactions that occur within an organism. Such information can be used to study any of the observed complexes in greater detail as well as provide the foundational data required to gain a "systems" view of cellular function. Two studies were recently published by Gavin *et al.* (2006) and Krogan *et al.* (2006) in which tandem affinity purification of tagged yeast proteins was used to purify protein complexes from *Saccharomyces cerevisiae*

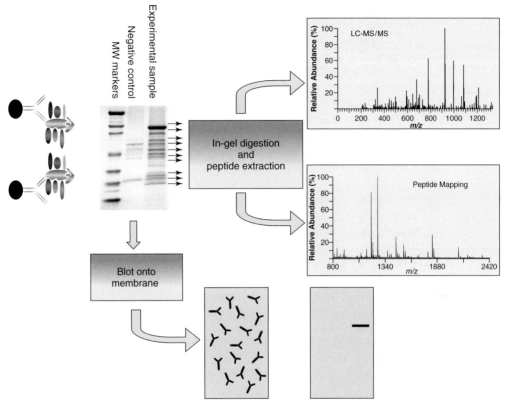

Figure 3.2 Discovery and hypothesis-driven methods of identifying interacting partners of target proteins. In a discovery-driven approach, a target protein and its binding partners are extracted from cells using a technique such as immunoprecipitation. The extracted proteins are separated by gel electrophoresis and stained bands are excised and processed for analysis by peptide mapping or liquid chromatography coupled on-line with tandem mass spectrometry (LC-MS/MS). In a hypothesis-driven approach, the proteins from the gel are blotted onto a membrane, which is interrogated with an antibody specific for a protein that is believed to interact with the target protein. (Please find a color version of this figure in the color plates.)

that were identified using MS. Both studies were able to successfully purify on the order of 2000 tagged proteins. Gavin *et al.*, was able to find 491 complexes composed of 1483 proteins, while the 547 complexes containing 2702 proteins were identified by Krogan *et al.* Combining the two datasets and removing redundancy reveals the identification of 3033 proteins (i.e. 47% of the *S. cerevisiae* proteome) involved in the identified complexes (Goll and Uetz, 2006). Only 1152 proteins, however, were found to be common to both datasets. In addition, only six complexes are identical between the two datasets. Almost 200 of the complexes reported by Krogan *et al.*, do not share a single protein found in any complex reported by Gavin *et al.* Conversely, only 20 complexes discovered by Gavin *et al.* do not share any proteins with any of the complexes reported by Krogan *et al.* Approximately 87% of the complexes found by Gavin *et al.* have less than 50% overlap with those shown by Krogan *et al.* Conversely, 77% of the complexes reported by Krogan *et al.*, have less than 50% overlap with those found by Gavin *et al.* Quite remarkably, 35% of the complexes reported by Krogan *et al.* had less than 5% overlap with those published by Gavin *et al.*

On the surface, the small overlap between these two studies appears "disconcerting." This result, however, is not without precedent. Approximately 5 years ago, two similar studies were published in which yeast protein complexes were characterized using affinity purification of tagged proteins followed by MS identification of the isolated components (Gavin *et al.*, 2002; Ho *et al.*, 2002). In one study TAP-tagging was used, while in the other the isolation was conducted via a FLAG (i.e. DYKDDDDK) epitope-tag, with both groups using similar sample preparation steps prior to MS identification. As with the more recent studies (Gavin *et al.*, 2006; Krogan *et al.*, 2006) these two datasets showed very little overlap. Since it is impossible to systematically validate all of the complexes characterized in any of the studies, it is difficult to assess the relative quality of the datasets. The studies by Gavin *et al.* (2006) and Krogan *et al.* (2006) used their own specific set of algorithms to determine correctly identified proteins and determine probabilistic measurements of the components of the reported complexes. An excellent collaborative study would constitute a swap of raw data between the two groups to enable a comparison of the effects of their respective software tools on the final results. Beyond the effects of different bioinformatic tools, the most likely source of dissimilarity between these two studies is in the purification of the TAP-tagged proteins. As described in studies presented in the following section, a huge percentage of the proteins identified in the analysis of extracted protein complexes that were analyzed by MS are classified as non-specifically bound (Selbach and Mann, 2006). As discussed in previous sections of this article, optimization of the isolation of the protein complex is critical in obtaining a sample that will provide accurate results that can stand the rigor of validation.

3.3.3
A QUICK LC-MS Method to Identify Specifically-Bound Proteins

One of the biggest conundrums of combining protein extraction methods such as immunoprecipitations and purification of target proteins is the presence of non-specifically bound proteins that are identified in the analysis. In the extract of a protein complex, many different classes of proteins can be isolated. These classes include the target protein itself, proteins specifically bound to the target protein, and proteins that non-specifically bind to any of the machinery (i.e. antibody, beads, tag portion of a chimera protein, etc.) used to isolate the target protein. In some cases, so many non-specifically bound proteins are identified that it is difficult to conclude which proteins truly interact with the targeted protein.

As described above, the prevailing method to discriminate between specific and non-specific interactions within an isolated protein complex is to compare proteins identified after isolation of a targeted protein with those proteins observed using a cell lysate that does not contain the protein of interest. Recently, the laboratory of Matthias Mann developed a rapid LC-MS/MS-based strategy to discriminate specifically and non-specifically bound members of an extracted protein complex (Figure 3.3). This strategy, termed QUICK (quantitative immunoprecipitation combined with knockdown; Selbach and Mann, 2006), combines stable-isotope labeling with amino acids in cell culture (SILAC; Ong *et al.*, 2002) with immunoprecipitation and RNA interference (RNAi) to knockdown protein expression (Gunsalus and Piano, 2005). The strategy is initiated by growing one of the cell cultures in medium containing a heavy isotope-substituted amino acid (e.g. $^{13}C_6$ lysine), so that each translated protein will contain the heavy version of that particular amino acid. The other culture is grown in normal isotopic abundance medium. RNAi is used in one of the cell cultures to knockdown the expression of the target protein of interest. Immunoprecipitation is then used to extract the protein complex of interest. At this stage, the two immunoprecipitation samples are combined, proteolytically digested, and analyzed by LC-MS/MS. In principle, peptides originating from proteins that interact with the antibody or beads should be represented in the mass spectra by doublets in a 1:1 ratio. Specifically bound members of the complex will be represented by a doublet in which the peptide peaks originating from the RNAi-treated culture will be of much lower intensity than their untreated counterparts.

The QUICK method was applied in two separate studies to discovering specific binding partners of β-catenin and Cbl (Selbach and Mann, 2006). Using β-catenin as the target protein, three proteins, T cell-specific transcription factor 4, α-catenin, and β-catenin interacting protein, were all found to have significantly increased abundance ratios, as calculated from the mass spectral data. In the Cbl study, three proteins that are known to interact with Cbl were identified, as well as sorting nexin 18, a protein that is involved in receptor-mediated endocytosis. While not every known interaction partner of the targeted proteins was observed, the QUICK strategy was able to eliminate, in the case of β-catenin, well over 100 non-specifically interacting proteins that were identified by LC-MS/MS. While the examples provided in the original manuscript are limited to immunoprecipitation extraction and RNAi treatment, the QUICK strategy is also amenable to monitoring changes in the composition of protein complexes extracted using different methods and as a result of different types of stress on the cell. The one obvious drawback to the overall method is the inability to use it with tissue samples. However, considering that a vast majority of protein complex discovery studies are conducted using cells in culture, this drawback is minor.

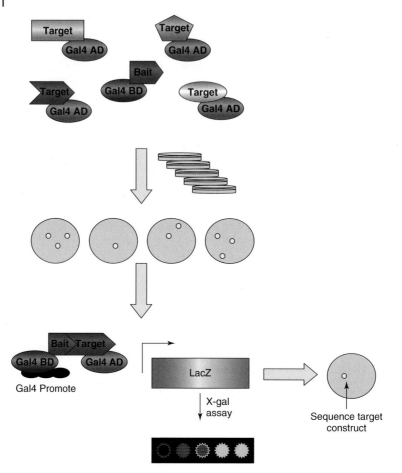

Figure 3.3 Schematic of the yeast two-hybrid method. In the yeast-two hybrid method, a plasmid containing a bait protein fused to the DNA-binding domain of a transcription factor (Gal4 in this example) is constructed. This construct is transformed into yeast cells containing a library of plasmids containing target proteins fused to the activation domain of the same transcription factor. The transformed cell population is cultured on a series of plates containing the appropriate growth medium. The interaction of the bait with a target protein brings the two domains of the transcription factor together, resulting in the expression of a reporter gene (i.e. LacZ). Colonies that have an activated reporter gene are selected and the plasmid inserts sequenced to identify the target protein that interacted with the bait protein. (Please find a color version of this figure in the color plates.)

3.4
Yeast Two-Hybrid Screening

All of the methods described up to this point measure protein interactions after the complexes have been removed from the cellular environment. While the perfect *in vivo* interaction study has yet to be designed, the yeast two-hybrid system at least provides a method to screen protein–protein interactions within living cells (Figure 3.4; Walhout *et al.*, 2000). In yeast two-hybrid screening, a "bait" protein (e.g. X) is expressed as a chimeric protein fused to the DNA-binding domain of a transcription factor (usually Gal4). The "target" proteins (i.e. Y) that the bait protein is to be screened against are expressed within the cell fused to the activation domain of the same transcription factor. If the bait binds to a target protein, the binding and activation domains of the transcription factor are brought into close enough proximity to physically interact and form an active transcriptional complex. The transcriptional complex is designed to activate the expression of a reporter gene that allows the yeast to grow on selection media. If the interaction does not occur, the reporter gene is not expressed and the yeast does not grow.

To generate interactomes for entire proteomes, individual bait proteins are transformed into cultures of yeast cells containing a library of target

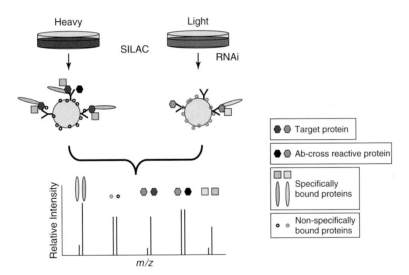

Figure 3.4 Principles of quantitative immunoprecipitation combined with knockdown (QUICK). Proteins are differentially labeled with stable isotopes by culturing cells in medium containing light or heavy amino acids (SILAC). The expression of the target protein is knocked down in one of the cultures using RNA interference (RNAi). After extraction of the target protein complex by immunoprecipitation, the samples are combined and analyzed by liquid chromatography coupled directly on-line with tandem mass spectrometry (LC-MS/MS). Proteins that non-specifically bind to components of the immunoprecipitation apparatus (i.e. beads, antibody) will be represented in the mass spectrum by peaks of equal intensity. Proteins that specifically interact with the target protein, as well as the target protein itself, will produce peaks of lesser relative intensity from the cells in which RNAi was used to knock down the expression of the target protein. (Please find a color version of this figure in the color plates.)

proteins. The liquid cultures are then spread onto a series of Petri dishes containing solid media that lacks the nutrient provided by reporter gene expressed by the activation of the transcription factor formed through a binding domain–activation domain interaction. Colonies in which the binding domain–activation domain interaction does not occur will not grow. Most two-hybrid screens use at least two selection criteria based on the activation of different reporter genes. Therefore, colonies passing the first nutrient-based selection criterion are tested in a colorimetric assay, generally based on the expression of LacZ, an *E. coli* gene that causes cells to turn blue (Sanchez-Ramos *et al.*, 2000). In this yeast system, the LacZ gene is inserted in the yeast DNA immediately after the Gal4 promoter so that an interaction between the bait and target proteins leads to expression of the protein.

Some of the obvious advantages of the yeast two-hybrid system are that DNA, not proteins, is manipulated to study protein–protein interactions, allowing the copious genomic resources that are available for a variety of different organisms to be utilized. Yeast two-hybrid screening is also high-throughput as illustrated by the large-scale interaction studies that have been completed for *S. cerevisiae* (Uetz *et al.*, 2000; Ito *et al.*, 2001), *Helicobacter pylori* (Rain *et al.*, 2001), *Caenorhabditis elegans* (Li *et al.*, 2004), *Drosophila melanogaster* (Giot *et al.*, 2003), and *Homo sapiens* (Rual *et al.*, 2005). These screens have produced over 4000 and 3000 potential interactions in *C. elegans* and *S. cerevisiae*, respectively. Ideally, a two-hybrid screen using all the proteins of a complex would yield all the binary interactions within that complex, but this is rarely the case. Generally, only a small percentage of the potential interactions are discovered (Walhout *et al.*, 2000). The greatest disadvantage of the yeast two-hybrid system is its false positive rate (Walhout *et al.*, 2000). This system detects a significant number of interactions of no biological significance. This challenge is illustrated by the comparison of data obtained by two independent groups that conducted two-hybrid screening for the same ∼6000 yeast bait proteins. These studies showed less than 15% overlap in the interaction pairs detected (Uetz *et al.*, 2000; Ito *et al.*, 2001). There have been many improvements recently to minimize the number of false positive identifications, however, as with most discovery-driven protein interaction studies, the results require independent validation before they can be considered as absolutely legitimate. In addition, two-hybrid screening produces only binary interactions, whereas other methods such as immunoprecipitation combined with MS identify multiple binding partners for each protein of interest. Therefore, it is not too surprising that comparisons of interactome data obtained in studies utilizing two-hybrid screening show very little correspondence to tandem affinity purification/MS-based studies. The reasons given for this discrepancy point primarily to the vast differences in the techniques and the fact that two-hybrid screening tends to detect transient interactions while protein purification methods identify stable interactions.

3.5
Fluorescence Microscopy

Most of the techniques used to characterize protein interactions acquire the data after the complex has been extracted from its cellular environment. Ideally, any putatively discovered protein association would be validated within its corresponding cellular milieu. Fortunately, improvements made in the fluorescent tagging of proteins and laser scanning confocal microscopy (LSCM) have made such studies possible (Miyashita, 2004; Hutter, 2006). Most approaches using LSCM use dual color images that are collected separately and then superimposed to detect the presence of co-localizing signals. To detect the location of a protein, the cell is irradiated with a laser corresponding to the specific absorption wavelength of the fluorophore of interest (Figure 3.5, upper panel). The wavelength at which the fluorophore emits is then detected. This process is repeated for a second fluorophoric compound that absorbs and emits light of a different wavelength. The images are then combined and if a "blending" of the signals is observed, a putative protein interaction is concluded. For example, images of proteins tagged with green and red fluorophores are commonly obtained. If the proteins co-localize within the cell, superimposition of these images will result in orange pixels being observed (Figure 3.5, lower panel; Conrads *et al.*, 2006). When signals from two proteins tagged with different fluorophores overlap, it suggests that the proteins occupy the same space within the cell and hence are interacting.

The development of various fluorescent tagging mechanisms has tremendously advanced the field of protein co-localization (Giepmans *et al.*, 2006). Proteins can be covalently modified with fluorophores such as Cy2, Cy3, and Cy5 or they can be expressed directly within transfected cells as a chimera containing a fluorescent tag such as green, red or yellow fluorescent protein (GFP, RFP, or YFP). Fluorescently tagged antibodies directed towards the proteins of interest can also be used. This method is known popularly as immunofluorescence. Regardless of which tagging method is used, the first step is to attach the cells of interest to a solid support, such as a microscope slide. Adherent cells may be grown directly on microscope slides while cells grown in suspension may be centrifuged onto slides or bound to a solid support using covalent linkers. If neither of these options is viable, these cells can be analyzed while in suspension. If immunofluorescence is used, the cells may also have to be fixed, either through the use of organic solvents such as alcohols and acetone or with paraformaldehyde. Paraformaldehyde cross-linking preserves the cellular architecture better than organic solvents but requires a permeabilization step (using digitonin, for example) to be added to the process to provide free access of the antibody to its antigen. Since the aim in using LSCM is to visualize a protein interaction in its native state, it is important that the cells are not perturbed prior to data acquisition. The process of fluorescence co-localization may require that the cells be chemically fixed (using paraformaldehyde, for example) onto microscope slides and then

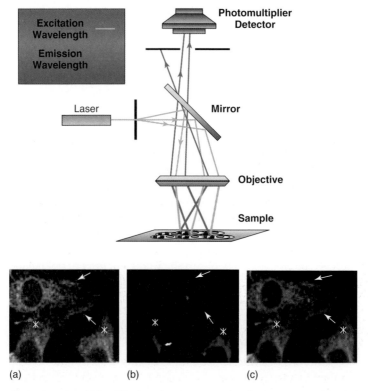

Figure 3.5 Principles of laser scanning confocal microscopy (LSCM). Top: In LSCM, the sample of interest is irradiated using a laser with a wavelength of light that causes excitation within a fluorophore that is associated with a protein of interest. The emission wavelength of the excited compound is then recorded. Bottom: To determine whether or not proteins co-localize, proteins are tagged with fluorophores that have different excitation and emission wavelengths. Overlaying of the two images results in a color combination that suggests the two proteins of interest occupy the same space within the cell. (Please find a color version of this figure in the color plates.)

permeabilized (with digitonin, for example) depending on the method of fluorescent tagging being used. Permeabilization may be required for introducing Cy-labeled proteins or fluorescent-labeled antibodies into the cell.

Once the cells of interest have been prepared and the fluorescent-tagging system is introduced into the cells, the process of determining whether two (or more) proteins co-localize can be started. The fluorescent tags on the proteins of interest are excited using lasers tuned to the excitation wavelengths of the tags and the fluorescent emission at a different wavelength is monitored. As described above, if the images obtained from the different fluorophores overlap, the proteins are believed to interact by virtue of occupying the same space within the cell. Currently, most applications of LSCM are used in hypothesis-driven studies to validate hypothetical protein interactions and are typically limited in the number of interactions that can be monitored within a given system.

3.5.1
Multi-Epitope-Ligand Cartography

In its present state, LSCM does not permit discovery-driven approaches since the proteins of interest must be targeted through covalent fluorophore incorporation or by antibody-specific detection. Recently, a method termed multi-epitope-ligand cartography (MELC) that is capable of mapping the location of tens of proteins within the same cell or tissue sample has been reported (Schubert *et al.*, 2006). This technology uses fluorescently labeled antibodies (or other affinity reagents) in a multiplexed mode to localize proteins of interest. Unlike typical LSCM studies, however, MELC introduces multiple rounds of introducing antibodies into the cell. After the introduction of a single antibody, its image is captured, the fluorescent signal is bleached, and the next fluorescently tagged antibody is introduced into the cell. This process is repeated multiple times to record the localization of tens of different proteins within the same system.

While the technology behind the procedure appears to be straightforward enough, interpretation and presentation of the data is anything but. In one of the simplest studies illustrating the utility of MELC, fluorescently tagged antibodies were used in tandem to map the location of eighteen cell surface receptors in peripheral blood mononuclear cells (PBMCs) (Schubert *et al.*, 2006). Pairs of antibodies were used in nine cycles comprising introduction of the fluorescently tagged antibodies to the cells, capture of the individual fluorescent images, bleaching to remove any residual signal, and then introduction of the next pair of tagged antibodies. The localization of each targeted protein, and the determination of any proteins that co-localized with it was visualized directly by superimposing the intensities of the signals obtained for all 18 fluorescently tagged antibodies. Unfortunately, this visualization method provides an overly complex image in which it is difficult to provide an estimate of the protein complexes that formed *in vivo*. To simplify the analysis, the data generated from each epitope were converted into a vector representing the intensity of the signal acquired using each antibody at each pixel recorded in the image. Collections of these vectors could be presented in a tabular view allowing numerical visualization of the fluorescence of each antibody at individual locations within the cell.

The ability to differentiate changes in protein complexes using MELC was also tested on skin biopsies obtained from patients with psoriasis, atopic dermatitis (a related but distinct condition) (Boguniewica and Leung, 2006), and healthy controls. The position of 49 different proteins was assayed in each of the clinical biopsies. The goal was to identify proteins that have diagnostic value or could act as a therapeutic target. Analysis of the results across the tissue sections revealed that protein levels at the measured pixels were generally similar in the psoriasis and atopic dermatitis samples. Compilation of all the results, however, revealed protein complex motifs that were unique to atopic dermatitis. Not only were components within these complexes able to discriminate psoriasis from atopic dermatitis, they could also distinguish both of these skin conditions from healthy controls. While this method still does not bring a truly discovery-driven approach to LSCM-based proteomics, if the author's claim that potentially hundreds of proteins can be co-localized using MELC is true, it definitely broadens the range of the hypotheses that can be tested.

3.6
Conclusions

The development of proteomics technology in the past decade has brought tremendous advances in how protein complex characterization experiments are conducted. While this review attempts to discuss many of the predominant proteomic methods for identifying protein interactions, it remains incomplete as the entire field of protein arrays was not discussed. For a comprehensive review on this topic, the reader is directed to an excellent article written by Michael Snyder, a leading researcher in this area (Kung and Snyder, 2006). While basic researchers used to be confined to confirming or refuting hypothetical interactions, tools that allow novel interactions to be discovered are now commonplace. The developments highlighted above span the entire range of complexity right from the characterization of proteins bound to a single protein target to entire proteome-wide scanning to measure entire interactomes. There are, however, many difficulties that state-of-the-art technology cannot yet overcome. For instance, MS is no different from any other "black-box" instrument and operates under the law of "garbage in, garbage out." The need for advanced sample preparation methods to limit the number of non-specific entities identified within protein complexes will be crucial for obtaining interaction maps that truly reflect cell physiology. The lack of congruence among large-scale interactome studies suggests that each analytic method only provides part of the truth. Whether repeated analysis or continued comparison amongst large interactome datasets will provide an accurate view of the protein circuitry within the cell remains to be seen. At this time, many of the discovery-based methods for identifying protein interactions provide "possibilities" that require further validation before any certain biological function can be established for a novel protein-protein interaction.

Acknowledgments

This project has been funded in whole or in part with federal funds from the National Cancer Institute, National Institutes of Health, under Contract N01-CO-12400. The content of this publication does not necessarily reflect the views or policies of the Department of Health and Human Services, nor does mention of trade names, commercial products, or organizations imply endorsement by the United States Government.

References

Boguniewicz, M. and Leung, D.Y. (2006) Atopic dermatitis. *Journal of Allergy and Clinical Immunology*, **117**, S475–S480.

Brown, P.O. (1994) Genome scanning methods. *Current Opinion in Genetics & Development*, **4**, 366–373.

Burnette, W.N. (1981) "Western blotting": electrophoretic transfer of proteins from sodium dodecyl sulfate–polyacrylamide gels to unmodified nitrocellulose and radiographic detection with antibody and radioiodinated protein A. *Analytical Biochemistry*, **112**, 195–203.

Conrads, T.P., Tocci, G.M., Hood, B.L., Zhang, C.O., Guo, L., Koch, K.R., Michejda, C.J., Veenstra, T.D. and Keay, S.K. (2006) CKAP4/p63 is a receptor for the frizzled-8 protein-related antiproliferative factor from interstitial cystitis patients. *Journal of Biological Chemistry*, **281**, 37836–37843.

Dougherty, M.K., Müller, J., Ritt, D.A., Zhou, M., Zhou, X.Z., Copeland, T.D., Conrads, T.P., Veenstra, T.D., Lu, K.P. and Morrison, D.K. (2005) Regulation of Raf-1 by direct feedback phosphorylation. *Molecules and Cells*, **17**, 215–224.

Gavin, A.C., Bösche, M., Krause, R., Grandi, P., Marzioch, M., Bauer, A., Schultz, J., Rick, J.M., Michon, A.M., Cruciat, C.M., Remor, M., Höfert, C., Schelder, M., Brajenovic, M., Ruffner, H., Merino, A., Klein, K., Hudak, M., Dickson, D., Rudi, T., Gnau, V., Bauch, A., Bastuck, S., Huhse, B., Leutwein, C., Heurtier, M.A., Copley, R.R., Edelmann, A., Querfurth, E., Rybin, V., Drewes, G., Raida, M., Bouwmeester, T., Bork, P., Seraphin, B., Kuster, B., Neubauer, G. and Superti-Furga, G. (2002) Functional organization of the yeast proteome by systematic analysis of protein complexes. *Nature*, **415**, 141–147.

Gavin, A.C., Aloy, P., Grandi, P., Krause, R., Boesche, M., Marzioch, M.,

Rau, C., Jensen, L.J., Bastuck, S., Dümpelfeld, B., Edelmann, A., Heurtier, M.A., Hoffman, V., Hoefert, C., Klein, K., Hudak, M., Michon, A.M., Schelder, M., Schirle, M., Remor, M., Rudi, T., Hooper, S., Bauer, A., Bouwmeester, T., Casari, G., Drewes, G., Neubauer, G., Rick, J.M., Kuster, B., Bork, P., Russell, R.B. and Superti-Furga, G. (2006) Proteome survey reveals modularity of the yeast cell machinery. *Nature*, **440**, 631–636.

Giepmans, B.N., Adams, S.R., Ellisman, M.H. and Tsien, R.Y. (2006) The fluorescent toolbox for assessing protein location and function. *Science*, **312**, 217–224.

Giot, L., Bader, J.S., Brouwer, C., Chaudhuri, A., Kuang, B., Li, Y., Hao, Y.L., Ooi, C.E., Godwin, B., Vitols, E., Vijayadamodar, G., Pochart, P., Machineni, H., Welsh, M., Kong, Y., Zerhusen, B., Malcolm, R., Varrone, Z., Collis, A., Minto, M., Burgess, S., McDaniel, L., Stimpson, E., Spriggs, F., Williams, J., Neurath, K., Ioime, N., Agee, M., Voss, E., Furtak, K., Renzulli, R., Aanensen, N., Carrolla, S., Bickelhaupt, E., Lazovatsky, Y., DaSilva, A., Zhong, J., Stanyon, C.A., Finley, R.L., Jr., White, K.P., Braverman, M., Jarvie, T., Gold, S., Leach, M., Knight, J., Shimkets, R.A., McKenna, M.P., Chant, J. and Rothberg, J.M. (2003) A protein interaction map of Drosophila melanogaster. *Science*, **302**, 1727–1736.

Goehler, H., Lalowski, M., Stelzl, U., Waelter, S., Stroedicke, M., Worm, U., Droege, A., Lindenberg, K.S., Knoblich, M., Haenig, C., Herbst, M., Suopanki, J., Scherzinger, E., Abraham, C., Bauer, B., Hasenbank, R., Fritzsche, A., Ludewig, A.H., Büssow, K., Coleman, S.H., Gutekunst, C.A., Landwehrmeyer, B.G., Lehrach, H. and

Wanker, E.E. (2004) A protein interaction network links GIT1, an enhancer of huntingtin aggregation, to Huntington's disease. *Molecules and Cells*, **15**, 853–865.

Goll, J. and Uetz, P. (2006) The elusive yeast interactome. *Genome Biology*, **7**, 223.

Grant, S.G.N., Marshall, M.C., Page, K.-L., Cumiskey, M.A. and Armstrong, J.D. (2005) Synapse proteomics of multiprotein complexes: en route from genes to nervous system diseases. *Human Molecular Genetics*, **14**, R225–R234.

Gunsalus, K.C. and Piano, F. (2005) RNAi as a tool to study cell biology; building the genome-phenome bridge. *Current Opinion in Cell Biology*, **17**, 3–8.

Ho, Y., Gruhler, A., Heilbut, A., Bader, G.D., Moore, L., Adams, S.L., Millar, A., Taylor, P., Bennett, K., Boutilier, K., Yang, L., Wolting, C., Donaldson, I., Schandorff, S., Shewnarane, J., Vo, M., Taggart, J., Goudreault, M., Muskat, B., Alfarano, C., Dewar, D., Lin, Z., Michalickova, K., Willems, A.R., Sassi, H., Nielsen, P.A., Rasmussen, K.J., Andersen, J.R., Johansen, L.E., Hansen, L.H., Jespersen, H., Podtelejnikov, A., Nielsen, E., Crawford, J., Poulsen, V., Sørensen, B.D., Matthiesen, J., Hendrickson, R.C., Gleeson, F., Pawson, T., Moran, M.F., Durocher, D., Mann, M., Hogue, C.W., Figeys, D. and Tyers, M. (2002) *Nature*, **415**, 180–183.

Hutter, H. (2006) Fluorescent reporter methods. *Methods in Molecular Biology*, **351**, 155–173.

Ito, T., Chiba, T., Ozawa, R., Yoshida, M., Hattori, M. and Sakaki, Y. (2001) A comprehensive two-hybrid analysis to explore the yeast protein interactome. *Proceedings of the National Academy of Sciences of the United States of America*, **98**, 4569–4574.

Krogan, N.J., Cagney, G., Yu, H., Zhong, G., Guo, X., Ignatchenko, A., Li, J., Pu, S., Datta, N., Tikuisis, A.P., Punna, T., Peregrín-Alvarez, J.M., Shales, M., Zhang, X., Davey, M., Robinson, M.D., Paccanaro, A., Bray, J.E., Sheung, A., Beattie, B., Richards, D.P., Canadien, V., Lalev, A., Mena, F., Wong, P., Starostine, A.,

Canete, M.M., Vlasblom, J., Wu, S., Orsi, C., Collins, S.R., Chandran, S., Haw, R., Rilstone, J.J., Gandi, K., Thompson, N.J., Musso, G., St Onge, P., Ghanny, S., Lam, M.H., Butland, G., Altaf-Ul, A.M., Kanaya, S., Shilatifard, A., O'Shea, E., Weissman, J.S., Ingles, C.J., Hughes, T.R., Parkinson, J., Gerstein, M., Wodak, S.J., Emili, A. and Greenblatt, J.R. (2006) Global landscape of protein complexes in the yeast *Saccharomyces cerevisiae*. *Nature*, **440**, 637–643.

Kung, L.A. and Snyder, M. (2006) Proteome chips for whole-organism assays. *Nature Reviews. Molecular Cell Biology*, **7**, 617–622.

Laemmli, U.K. (1970) Cleavage of structural proteins during the assembly of the head of bacteriophage T4. *Nature*, **227**, 680–685.

Lechward, K., Sugajska, E., de Baere, I., Goris, J., Hemmings, B.A. and Zolnierowicz, S. (2006) Interaction of nucleoredoxin with protein phosphatase 2A. *FEBS Letters*, **580**, 3631–3637.

Li, S., Armstrong, C.M., Bertin, N., Ge, H., Milstein, S., Boxem, M., Vidalain, P.O., Han, J.D., Chesneau, A., Hao, T., Goldberg, D.S., Li, N., Martinez, M., Rual, J.F., Lamesch, P., Xu, L., Tewari, M., Wong, S.L., Zhang, L.V., Berriz, G.F., Jacotot, L., Vaglio, P., Reboul, J., Hirozane-Kishikawa, T., Li, Q., Gabel, H.W., Elewa, A., Baumgartner, B., Rose, D.J., Yu, H., Bosak, S., Sequerra, R., Fraser, A., Mango, S.E., Saxton, W.M., Strome, S., Van Den Heuvel, S., Piano, F., Vandenhaute, J., Sardet, C., Gerstein, M., Doucette-Stamm, L., Gunsalus, K.C., Harper, J.W., Cusick, M.E., Roth, F.P., Hill, D.E. and Vidal, M. (2004) A map of the interactome network of the metazoan *C. elegans*. *Science*, **303**, 540–543.

Liu, H., Lin, D. and Yates, J.R. 3rd (2002) Multidimensional separations for protein/peptide analysis in the post-genomic era. *Biotechniques*, **32**, 898–902.

Meng, Z., Camalier, C.E., Lucas, D.A., Veenstra, T.D., Beck, G.R., Jr. and

Conrads, T.P. (2006) Probing early growth response 1 interacting proteins at the active promoter in osteoblast cells using oligoprecipitation and mass spectrometry. *Journal of Proteome Research*, **5**, 1931–1939.

Miyashita, T. (2004) Confocal microscopy for intracellular co-localization of proteins. *Methods in Molecular Biology*, **261**, 399–410.

Olesky, M., McNamee, E.E., Zhou, C., Taylor, T.J. and Knipe, D.M. (2005) Evidence for a direct interaction between HSV-1 ICP27 and ICP8 proteins. *Virology*, **331**, 94–105.

Ong, S.E., Blagoev, B., Kratchmarova, I., Kristensen, D.B., Steen, H., Pandey, A. and Mann, M. (2002) Stable isotope labeling by amino acids in cell culture, SILAC, as a simple and accurate approach to expression proteomics. *Molecular & Cellular Proteomics: MCP*, **1**, 376–386.

Ory, S., Zhou, M., Conrads, T.P., Veenstra, T.D. and Morrison, D.K. (2003) Protein phosphatase 2A positively regulated Ras signaling by dephosphorylating KSR1 and Raf-1 on critical 14-3-3 binding sites. *Current Biology: CB*, **13**, 1356–1364.

Rain, J.C., Selig, L., De Reuse, H., Battaglia, V., Reverdy, C., Simon, S., Lenzen, G., Petel, F., Wojcik, J., Schächter, V., Chemama, Y., Labigne, A. and Legrain, P. (2001) The protein–protein interaction map of *Helicobacter pylori*. *Nature*, **409**, 211–215.

Rual, J.F., Venkatesan, K., Hao, T., Hirozane-Kishikawa, T., Dricot, A., Li, N., Berriz, G.F., Gibbons, F.D., Dreze, M., Ayivi-Guedehoussou, N., Klitgord, N., Simon, C., Boxem, M., Milstein, S., Rosenberg, J., Goldberg, D.S., Zhang, L.V., Wong, S.L., Franklin, G., Li, S., Albala, J.S., Lim, J., Fraughton, C., Llamosas, E., Cevik, S., Bex, C., Lamesch, P., Sikorski, R.S., Vandenhaute, J., Zoghibi, H.Y., Smolyar, A., Bosak, S., Sequerra, R., Doucette-Stamm, L., Cusick, M.E., Hill, D.E., Roth, F.P. and Vidal, M. (2005) Towards a proteome-scale map of the human protein-protein interaction network. *Nature*, **437**, 1173–1178.

Sanchez-Ramos, J., Song, S., Dailey, M., Cardozo-Pelaez, F., Hazzi, C., Stedeford, T., Willing, A., Freeman, T.B., Saporta, S., Zigova, T., Sanberg, P.R. and Snyder, E.Y. (2000) The X-gal caution in neural transplantation studies. *Cell Transplantation*, **9**, 657–667.

Schubert, W., Bonnekoh, B., Pommer, A.J., Philipsen, L., Böckelmann, R., Malykh, Y., Gollnick, H., Friedenberger, M., Bode, M. and Dress, A.W. (2006) Analyzing proteome topology and function by automated multidimensional fluorescence microscopy. *Nature Biotechnology*, **24**, 1270–1278.

Selbach, M. and Mann, M. (2006) Protein interaction screening by quantitative immunoprecipitation combined with knockdown (QUICK). *Nature Methods*, **3**, 981–983.

Stelzl, U., Worm, U., Lalowski, M., Haenig, C., Brembeck, F.H., Goehler, H., Stroedicke, M., Zenkner, M., Schoenherr, A., Koeppen, S., Timm, J., Mintzlaff, S., Abraham, C., Bock, N., Kietzmann, S., Goedde, A., Toksöz, E., Droege, A., Krobitsch, S., Korn, B., Birchmeier, W., Lehrach, H. and Wanker, E.E. (2005) A human protein-protein interaction network: a resource for annotating the proteome. *Cell*, **122**, 957–968.

Uetz, P., Giot, L., Cagney, G., Mansfield, T.A., Judson, R.S., Knight, J.R., Lockshon, D., Narayan, V., Srinivasan, M., Pochart, P., Qureshi-Emili, A., Li, Y., Godwin, B., Conover, D., Kalbfleisch, T., Vijayadamodar, G., Yang, M., Johnston, M., Fields, S. and Rothberg, J.M. (2000) A comprehensive analysis of protein-protein interactions in Saccharomyces cerevisiae. *Nature*, **403**, 623–627.

Walhout, A.J., Boulton, S.J. and Vidal, M. (2000) Yeast two-hybrid systems and protein interaction mapping projects for yeast and worm. *Yeast*, **17**, 88–94.

Yang, P., Sampson, H.M. and Krause, H.M. (2006) A modified tandem affinity purification strategy identifies cofactors of the Drosophila nuclear receptor dHNF4. *Proteomics*, **6**, 927–935.

4
Analysis of Membrane Protein Complexes by Blue Native-PAGE

Veronika Reisinger and Lutz Andreas Eichacker

4.1
Introduction

4.1.1
Membrane Protein Complexes

About a third of all proteins encoded by the human genome are membrane proteins (Wallin and von Heijne, 1998). Membrane proteins play a decisive role in all living cells. They are involved in various processes such as biological energy conversion, material exchange between cellular compartments, antigen processing, exocytosis, or the recognition and processing of external stimuli. Furthermore, the majority of drug targets are membrane proteins and numerous human diseases result from malfunctions of membrane proteins (Hopkins and Groom, 2002). In general, membrane proteins can be divided into two groups (Santoni *et al.*, 2000). One group consists of the so-called integral membrane proteins, which have at least one transmembrane helix and are integral parts of the membrane lipid bilayer. The transmembrane helix is formed either by non-polar amino acids (α-helix) or by alternate polar and non-polar amino acids (β-barrel). Therefore, proteins comprising only α-helices are more hydrophobic than proteins comprising β-barrel structures. Furthermore, hydrophobicity of integral membrane proteins increases with the number of transmembrane helices.

The second group includes all membrane-associated proteins, which are linked to the membrane by, for example, covalent attachment to a fatty acid, to oligosaccharides or interaction with integral membrane proteins. They are collectively called peripheral membrane proteins. As peripheral membrane proteins do not cross the lipid bilayer, they are more hydrophilic than integral membrane proteins.

Due to the hydrophobic nature of transmembrane-spanning helices, integral membrane proteins represent a major challenge in proteomic research. Two main aims have to be achieved: first, integral membrane proteins have to be extracted from the membrane and second, aggregation of the

Proteomics of the Nervous System. Edited by H.G. Nothwang and S.E. Pfeiffer
Copyright © 2008 WILEY-VCH Verlag GmbH & Co. KGaA, Weinheim
ISBN: 978-3-527-31716-5

isolated membrane proteins has to be suppressed. Both problems can be solved by the use of detergents incorporating the membrane proteins into micelles (le Maire *et al.*, 2000; Seddon *et al.*, 2004). In a subsequent step, solubilized membrane proteins can be separated by electrophoretic or non-electrophoretic techniques. Classical two-dimensional polyacrylamide-based gel electrophoresis (2D-PAGE) is hardly compatible with integral membrane proteins (Santoni *et al.*, 2000). This incompatibility is caused by the low solubilization capacity of detergents used for isoelectric focusing (IEF)-PAGE, combined with the tendency of membrane proteins to aggregate at high concentrations especially around their isoelectric point (pI) (see Chapter 2). Therefore alternative methods have to be applied to analyze the protein composition of membrane compartments.

4.1.2
Separation Methods for Membrane Protein Complexes

Common non-electrophoretic methods for the analysis of single membrane proteins and membrane protein complexes include density gradient centrifugation and chromatographic separation using ion-exchange columns, affinity tagging, chromatofocussing and shotgun liquid chromatography/mass spectrometry (Wu and Yates, 2003; Kashino, 2003). All of these methods operate with large amounts of sample. But sample amount is often the limiting factor in membrane protein research. Therefore, analytical techniques that get by with small sample amounts are required. It turned out that gel-based electrophoresis represents a suitable alternative to separate single membrane proteins as well as native membrane protein complexes.

Since one-dimensional sodium dodecyl sulfate polyacrylamide-based gel electrophoresis (1D-SDS-PAGE) has a limited capacity to separate highly complex samples and two-dimensional isoelectric focusing (2D-IEF)/SDS-PAGE is restricted to hydrophilic proteins, alternative 2D approaches had to be developed for complex membrane protein samples (Williams *et al.*, 2006). In the last years, different denaturing 2D techniques for the separation of membrane proteins have been established. Due to the excellent solubilization power of SDS, all methods are combined with SDS-PAGE as second dimension. For the first dimension, different ionic detergents such as SDS, 16-benzyldimethyl-*n*-hexadecyl-ammonium chloride (BAC) or cetyltrimethylammoniumbromide (CTAB) are used (Braun *et al.*, 2007). Experiments have shown that the combination of different ionic detergents in the two dimensions leads to a noticeable increase in resolution. Specifically, SDS/SDS-PAGE approaches were found to be primarily advisable for separation of highly hydrophobic membrane proteins. In this approach, however, membrane protein complexes are destroyed.

Native complex separation is achieved by solubilization of membrane protein complexes by non-ionic detergents and separation of the solubilized complexes by colorless-native (CN)- or blue native (BN)-PAGE (Braun *et al.*, 2007). CN-PAGE separates complexes according to their internal negative charge, whereas in BN-PAGE, negative charges are externally provided to the complexes by Coomassie Blue. As a result of the standard electrophoretic setup with proteins loaded at the cathodic side, CN-PAGE is useful for protein complexes with a pI > 7 to yield negatively charged protein complexes at the neutral pH of the electrophoretic buffer system. The lowered charge state of protein complexes in CN-PAGE is known to lead to a lower resolution compared to separation in BN-PAGE. However, Coomassie binding to protein complexes also exerts some denaturing effect on protein complexes. Hence, the lack of Coomassie in CN-PAGE offers the possibility of separating labile supramolecular assemblies of membrane protein complexes, which would dissociate in BN-PAGE (Wittig and Schagger, 2005). Still, BN-PAGE has revealed to be a very robust method for most applications of native membrane protein complex separation, and should be the method of choice when you start to separate your protein complexes of interest by electrophoresis.

4.1.3
Blue Native PAGE

BN-PAGE was first described in 1991 for the separation of membrane protein complexes from the respiratory chain of human mitochondria (Schagger and von Jagow, 1991). Up to now, BN-PAGE has been shown to be a powerful method for the analysis of protein interactions in membranes of homogenates originating from tissues, cultured cells, or subcellular fractions. Many studies using BN-PAGE have dealt with the membrane intrinsic electron/proton transfer complexes of mitochondria and thylakoid membranes (Dencher *et al.*, 2006; Dudkina *et al.*, 2006; Granvogl *et al.*, 2006; Danielsson *et al.*, 2006; Yao *et al.*, 2007). Recently, BN-PAGE was extended to various protein complexes in the molecular mass range between 10 and 10 000 kDa. These analyses provided novel insights into the oligomeric state, the stoichiometry, the enzymatic activity, and the molecular structure of multi-enzyme complexes (Krause, 2006).

4.1.3.1 Separation Principle
In general, the term "electrophoresis" relates to the transport of charged particles along an electric field gradient. In a homogeneous electric field, particles will move at constant velocity when the electromotive force of the accelerating electric field is balanced by the constricting frictional resistance and ionic forces of the separation medium. The frictional resistance of the separation medium can be alleviated by performing electrophoresis in a medium containing a chemically inert matrix. Popular matrices are agarose and polyacrylamide. The latter turned out to be particularly suitable for the

separation of proteins and protein complexes. The gel is normally mounted between two buffer chambers and represents the only electrical connection between them. Most often, vertical slab gel systems are used as they have a direct liquid buffer connection allowing efficient use of the electric field. Because of the high frictional resistance of the gel, the gel should be cooled during electrophoresis. Empirically, the velocity of a particle and consequently its separation distance are directly proportional to the charge state and the field strength, and inversely proportional to the size and/or mass of the particle and the viscosity of the separation medium.

If the charge to molecular mass and/or size ratio is kept constant during separation, the mobility of all particles will be constant and separation will be a function of the molecular mass/size of a particle. This principle also forms the basis of separation of membrane protein complexes by BN-PAGE.

In BN-PAGE, Coomassie Blue G 250 is present during solubilization of protein complexes by a non-ionic detergent. This dye binds to the protein surface and thus provides negative charge to the protein complexes. Therefore all solubilized protein complexes are negatively charged and migrate to the anode during electrophoresis. To achieve high resolution in BN-PAGE, separation of protein complexes is carried out in gradient gels. By the decreasing pore size of the gel, the velocity is gradually decreased to zero when the protein complexes reach their pore size limit.

Casting of gradient gels requires a gradient-forming apparatus and can be carried out in two different ways: either the gradient maker can be positioned above the gel cassette to use gravity to form the gradient, or the gradient can be cast from the bottom of the casting stand by the use of a peristaltic pump. Formation of the gradient from the bottom of the gel cassette normally takes more time but results in more stable gradients. Both approaches lead to a higher concentration of acrylamide at the bottom than at the top of the gel. In either case, glycerol is added to the gel solution containing the higher acrylamide concentration to ensure proper formation of the gradient.

There are two types of gradient gels: linear and non-linear gradient gels which are generated by different geometries of the gradient maker. For BN-PAGE applications, mostly linear gradient gels are used. For this kind of gel, the gradient maker has to have two identical chambers connected by a small tube (Figure 4.1). One of the chambers (chamber 1) has to have an additional outlet to the casting stand. Formation of the gradient takes place in this second chamber due to the hydrodynamic pressure, which keeps the levels of gel solution equal in both chambers. As the solution in chamber 1 is constantly stirred, it is progressively mixed and, consequently, a linear gradient is formed.

4.1.3.2 Membrane Solubilization

For optimal results, solubilization of the membrane protein complexes is the most critical step. As mentioned before, the aim of BN-PAGE is to separate membrane protein complexes in a native state. Membrane complexes are

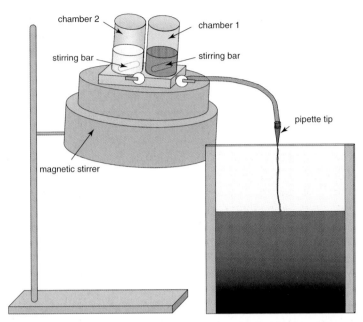

Figure 4.1 Schematic setup for casting of gradient gels from the top. The gradient mixer is placed in such a way that chamber 1 is positioned at the center of a magnetic stirrer which shows a moderate decline towards the casting stand. This will ensure the directed flow of the gel solutions. Chamber 1 is filled with the heavy acrylamide solution, chamber 2 with the light acrylamide solution. Both chambers contain a stirring bar. The gradient mixer is connected to the glass plate sandwich by a cut pipette tip. To start gradient formation, all ports are closed and the magnetic stirrer is switched on. The port between the chambers is opened and after liquid connection between both chambers, the port connecting the chamber 1 to the glass plate sandwich is opened. (Please find a color version of this figure in the color plates.)

identified as "native," when they are able to catalyze at least one specific biochemical reaction in the isolated state or when their cellular structure can be identified by biochemical or genetic methods (Nelson and Yocum, 2006). In summary, a protein complex is the minimal unit of a cellular compartment composed of genuine subunits (proteins and cofactors) that is able to carry out a biological activity.

Native protein complexes are normally extracted from the membrane bilayer by amphiphilic detergents. They are composed of a polar head group (hydrophilic) and a hydrocarbon tail (hydrophobic), resulting in the formation of thermodynamically stable micelles above a critical monomer concentration (CMC) of the detergent in aqueous media. The CMC is dependent on the temperature, pH, ionic strength, and purity of the detergent. The lower the CMC, the more stable the micelles and the more slowly the molecules are incorporated into the micelle. Besides physical parameters, the lipid composition of the membrane bilayer affects its solubilization properties (Garavito and Ferguson-Miller, 2001). Therefore detergent concentration and detergent type have to be determined experimentally for each kind of membrane individually in order to maintain protein complexes in their native state and to solubilize one kind of complex per micelle. It should also be noted that the formation of micelles is dependent on the detergent concentration. Here, the detergent-to-lipid and detergent-to-protein ratios should be considered carefully.

As mentioned before, SDS was found to be most effective for complete solubilization of membrane protein complexes. But its strong denaturing activity precludes solubilization of native protein complexes by SDS. In general, non-ionic detergents are more suitable for native electrophoresis than anionic, cationic, and zwitterionic detergents because ionic detergents (e.g. SDS) normally modify protein structures to a greater extent. Most non-ionic detergents are non-denaturing but less effective in disrupting lipid bilayer and protein aggregation. The most frequently used non-ionic detergents are digitonin and n-dodecyl-β-D-maltoside, as they yield the best results in BN-PAGE applications (Krause, 2006).

4.1.3.3 Combination of Blue Native PAGE (First Dimension) with other Electrophoretic Techniques as Second Dimension

Depending on the experimental aim, BN-PAGE can be combined with different electrophoretic techniques. The standard combination is the use of BN-PAGE as first dimension and SDS-PAGE as second dimension. This combination allows subunit composition to be analyzed and the assembly stages of different protein complexes to be characterized (Reisinger and Eichacker, 2007). Vertical analysis of the position of protein spots released from the protein complexes in the second dimension gel are particularly useful in allowing determination of the subunit composition of the protein complexes. Furthermore, horizontal analysis of the protein spots makes it possible to study the molecular mass increase of protein complexes containing the one specific protein of interest. Analysis of protein fractions from selected time points of a cell culture system in the first and second dimension gels then allows determination of the assembly of protein subunits in time. A protocol for BN/SDS-PAGE is given in this chapter (Section 4.2).

In contrast, BN/BN-PAGE approaches give insights into the subcomplex composition of so-called "supercomplexes" (Schagger and Pfeiffer, 2000; Eubel *et al.*, 2004). Here, membrane complexes are gently solubilized with one non-ionic detergent (e.g. digitonin) prior to the first dimension. After the first dimension, one lane of the BN-PAGE is cut and incubated in another non-ionic detergent which is known to be less mild (e.g. DM). Fragmentation of the supercomplexes into protein subcomplexes can then be analyzed by vertical analysis of the protein pattern in the second dimension.

Another approach is the combination of BN-PAGE in the first dimension with IEF-PAGE in the second dimension. Here, single complex bands, separated by BN-PAGE, are cut out of the gel, eluted from the gel matrix (e.g. by electroelution), denatured, and the single proteins separated by IEF-PAGE. This method offers the possibility to determine whether individual proteins of a given complex are modified under certain experimental conditions. This approach was successfully used for the analysis of outer mitochondrial membranes (Werhahn and Braun, 2002). Interestingly, highly hydrophobic membrane-anchored proteins were shown to be well separated during isoelectric focussing following BN-PAGE.

Finally, BN/BN-PAGE and BN/IEF-PAGE can both be combined with SDS-PAGE as third dimension. This allows determination of the molecular mass and subunit composition of complex protein assemblies, and characterization of the isoelectric points plus molecular masses of the corresponding denatured protein subunits.

4.1.3.4 Complex Visualization and Identification

Visualization can occur at the stage of native protein complexes or single protein subunits by all known staining methods (Coomassie, silver, fluorescence). The only limitation relates to fluorescent dyes directly applied to BN-PAGE. Bound Coomassie quenches the fluorescence emission, leading to a decreased sensitivity of fluorescence detection. In contrast, fluorescence detection after second dimension SDS-PAGE works well, as Coomassie is released from protein complexes during the denaturing step between the first and second dimensions.

An attractive feature of native gel systems is the detection of proteins by their enzymatic activity (Sabar *et al.*, 2005; Yan *et al.*, 2007; Bisetto *et al.*, 2007). Enzymatic assays often deliver a colored product which allows detection and identification directly in a single step. However, one has to be aware that this kind of experiment will often not be able to identify one specific enzyme due to the low specificity of the available enzymatic tests. For definite identification of a protein, immunodetection or mass spectrometry has to be performed.

Immunodetection was carried out successfully after BN-PAGE or BN/SDS-PAGE (Camacho-Carvajal *et al.*, 2004; Di Pancrazio *et al.*, 2006; Faye *et al.*, 2007). It should be noted that Coomassie blocks hydrophobic binding sites on gel-blots and therefore impairs antigen detection. Hence, the blue cathode buffer should be exchanged with a colorless buffer after the blue buffer front reaches half of the separating gel.

Direct identification of protein complexes can be achieved by mass spectrometry of peptides released from either the protein complexes or the isolated single protein species by tryptic in-gel digestion. The method can also be applied to proteins after the first or the second dimension gel electrophoresis. Since protein complexes will release a high number of peptides, a combination of in-gel digestion with approaches to separate the peptide species by high-performance liquid chromatography (HPLC) is useful. The peptide separation

Table 4.1 Detection methods after first and second dimension BN/SDS-PAGE.

Detection method	BN-PAGE	BN/SDS-PAGE
	First dimension	Second dimension
Radioactive isotopes	+	+
Fluorescent dyes	−	+
Organic dyes	±	+
Enzymatic activity	+	−
Antibodies	±	+
Online ESI	+	+
Offline ESI/MALDI	±	+

Different detection methods are rated in terms of their usability after BN-PAGE or BN/SDS-PAGE. Some methods yield optimal results (+) after the first dimension but not after the second dimension (±) and vice versa. Some methods are not compatible with BN- or BN/SDS-PAGE (−).

step is then coupled online with mass measurements which drastically improves the exact determination of the peptide quality and quantity and hence leads to a higher number of identified proteins.

Table 4.1 summarizes the methods utilized for visualization and identification of proteins and protein complexes after electrophoresis and estimates their utility regarding BN-PAGE and BN/SDS-PAGE separation of proteins.

4.2
Protocols

4.2.1
Blue Native PAGE (First Dimension)

4.2.1.1   Casting of Gradient Gels

Requirements
BN gel buffer: 3 M ε-amino caproic acid, 0.3 M Bis-Tris-HCl pH 7.0; 30% (w/v) acrylamide solution (acrylamide/bis acrylamide solution (30 : 0.8; 2.6%C)); glycerol; N, N, N, N'-tetramethyl-ethylenediamine (TEMED); 10% (w/v) ammonium persulfate (APS) solution; water-saturated isobutanol; denatured ethanol; glass plate sandwich (18 × 24 × 0.75 cm); 10-well-comb; casting stand; gradient mixer; magnetic stirrer.
   1. Clean both glass plates and spacers with denatured ethanol and assemble all parts on the casting stand. Ensure a perpendicular position of the casting stand.

2. Prepare the gradient gel solutions for the separating gel:

	12%	6%
Acrylamide	4.60 mL	2.30 mL
BN gel buffer	1.92 mL	1.92 mL
Glycerol	2.30 g	—
ddH$_2$O	3.29 mL	7.28 mL
Total	11.5 mL	11.5 mL

3. Place the gradient mixer on the magnetic stirrer and place a stirring rod in each chamber.
4. Close all ports and fill the 12% gradient gel solution in chamber 1 (Figure 4.1).
5. Open the valve between both chambers of the gradient mixer shortly to fill the valve between the two chambers with gel solution.
6. Fill the 6% gradient gel solution in chamber 2 of the gradient mixer (Figure 4.1).
7. Start stirring. Ensure uniform stirring in chamber 1 for correct settling of a linear gradient. Uniform stirring in chamber 2 is not important (stirring rod is only used for balancing the solution levels in both chambers).
8. Connect the pipette tip with the casting stand (Figure 4.1).
9. Add 5.5 µL TEMED and 22 µL APS to each chamber.
10. First open the valve between the both chambers and afterwards the front port. The solution will rinse between the glass plate sandwich.
11. Overlay the cast separating gel with isobutanol.
12. After polymerization of the separating gel remove the isobutanol by dH$_2$O.
13. Dry the area above the separating gel with blotting paper.
14. Place the comb between the glass plates.
15. Prepare the stacking gel solution:

	4%
Acrylamide (30/0.8)	1.35 mL
BN gel buffer	1.67 mL
ddH$_2$O	6.98 mL
Total	10.00 mL

16. Add 10 µL TEMED and 100 µL APS and cast the stacking gel.
17. After polymerization of the stacking gel, remove the comb.

4.2.1.2 Membrane Complex Isolation

All steps of sample preparation have to be carried out on ice to maintain the native state of the protein complexes and to minimize the activity of proteases. As mentioned above, there is no universal rule for protein complex solubilization, as it depends on the membrane. The given detergent amount presents a useful starting point for your experiments but you will have to perform a dilution series to find the optimal detergent concentration for your protein complexes.

Requirements

Sample buffer: 750 mM ε-amino caproic acid, 50 mM Bis-Tris-HCl pH 7.0, 0.5 mM EDTA-Na$_2$; detergent solution: 10% (w/v) DM.

1. Pellet an aliquot corresponding to 400 µg of protein of the isolated membrane fraction by centrifugation at 4 °C.
2. Resuspend the membrane pellet in 70 µL sample buffer.
3. Add 10 µL detergent solution and mix gently.
4. Incubate the sample at least for 10 min on ice.
5. Remove all unsolubilized material by centrifugation at maximum speed for 10 min.
6. Transfer the supernatant to a new 1.5-mL centrifuge tube.

4.2.1.3 Native Electrophoresis

Requirements

Loading buffer: 750 mM ε-amino caproic acid, 5% (w/v) Coomassie G 250; blue cathode buffer: 50 mM Tricine, 15 mM Bis-Tris-HCl pH 7.0, 0.02% Coomassie G 250; colorless cathode buffer: 50 mM Tricine, 15 mM Bis-Tris-HCl pH 7.0; anode buffer: 50 mM Bis-Tris-HCl pH 7.0.

1. Add 5 µL of loading buffer to the supernatant containing the solubilized membrane complexes and keep the samples on ice.
2. Assemble the electrophoretic apparatus and fill the blue cathode buffer into the cathode buffer chamber.
3. Underlay the samples with a microsyringe completely in the wells. Rinse the microsyringe thoroughly with buffer if you apply different samples.
4. Pour the anode buffer in the anode buffer tank and complete the assembly of the electrophoresis unit.
5. Set the electrophoretic parameters to 12 mA, 1200 V and 24 W and start the electrophoresis. Electrophoresis is carried out at 4 °C.
6. When the blue cathode buffer front has reached half of the separating gel, replace the blue cathode buffer by the colorless cathode buffer.
7. Continue the electrophoresis until the blue buffer front has reached the bottom of the separating gel.

8. After the end of the electrophoretic run disassemble the electrophoretic unit and divide the gel into single lanes by using the spacer. Each lane has to correspond to one single sample.

4.2.2
SDS-PAGE (Second Dimension)

4.2.2.1 Casting of Uniform Gels

Requirements
8 × separating gel buffer: 3 M Tris pH 8.8; urea; 2 × stacking gel buffer: 250 mM Tris pH 6.8; 30% (w/v) acrylamide solution (acrylamide/bis acrylamide solution (30 : 0.8; 2.6%C)); TEMED; 10% (w/v) APS solution; water-saturated isobutanol; denatured ethanol; glass plate sandwich (18 × 24 × 1 cm); casting stand.

1. Clean the glass plates and spacers with denatured ethanol and assemble all parts on the casting stand.
2. Prepare the separating gel solution:

	12.5%
Urea	7.21 g
Acrylamide (30/0.8)	12.50 mL
8× separating gel buffer	3.75 mL
ddH$_2$O	9.00 mL
Total	30 mL

3. Dissolve the urea.
4. Add 15 μL TEMED and 50 μL APS and mix the solution.
5. Cast the separation gel and overlay the cast gel with isobutanol.
6. After polymerization of the separating gel remove the isobutanol by dH$_2$O.
7. Dry the area above the separating gel with blotting paper.
8. Prepare the stacking gel solution:

	4%
Acrylamide (30/0.8)	0.82 mL
2 × stacking gel buffer	2.54 mL
ddH$_2$O	1.64 mL
Total	5.00 mL

9. Add 5 μL TEMED and 50 μL APS and mix the solution.

10. Pour the stacking gel solution on top of the separating gel up to approximately 3 cm under the upper edge of the glass plate.
11. Overlay the cast gel with isobutanol.
12. After polymerization of the separating gel, remove the isobutanol by rinsing with dH_2O.

4.2.2.2 Complex Denaturation

Requirements
Solubilization buffer: 2% (w/v) SDS, 66 mM Na_2CO_3; 2% β-mercaptoethanol; overlay solution: 0.5% (w/v) agarose in SDS running buffer.

1. Transfer a cut lane in a 50-mL centrifuge tube containing about 20 mL of the solubilization buffer.
2. Shake the tube gently for 20 min at room temperature.
3. After 20 min position the strip between the glass plates of the SDS gel touching the surface of the stacking gel (Figure 4.2). Avoid air bubbles between the gels.
4. Place a piece of blotting paper soaked with 10 μL of SDS protein marker on the surface of the SDS stacking gel next to the first dimension strip (Figure 4.2).
5. Overlay the first dimension strip and the marker piece with overlay solution.

4.2.2.3 Denaturing Electrophoresis

Requirements
SDS running buffer: 25 mM Tris, 192 mM glycine, 0.1% (w/v) SDS.

1. Assemble the electrophoretic unit and fill the SDS running buffer both in the cathode and the anode tank.
2. Start the electrophoresis (5 mA constant) overnight.
3. Stop the electrophoresis and disassemble the electrophoresis unit, when the blue front reached the bottom of the separating gel.
4. Visualize protein subunits by staining (Coomassie, silver, fluorescence) or by immunodetection.

4.3
Outlook

BN-PAGE is a microscale method that allows the analysis of membrane protein complexes in a short time. A sample of 400 μg of protein is sufficient as starting material to obtain Coomassie-stainable bands. Protein solubilization and first-dimension electrophoresis can be performed within 5 h on a standard gel

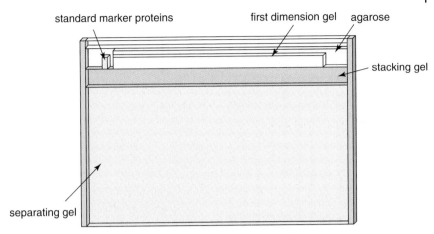

standard marker proteins   first dimension gel   agarose

stacking gel

separating gel

Figure 4.2 Transfer of the first dimension BN-PAGE strip to the second dimension SDS-PAGE. After solubilization, a strip of the first dimension gel is transferred onto a second dimension stacking gel. The strip is positioned centrally on top of the second dimension. A piece of Whatman filter paper soaked with SDS-PAGE standard marker proteins is positioned next to the first dimension strip onto the stacking gel. The gel strip and the SDS size marker are fixed with agarose. (Please find a color version of this figure in the color plates.)

system (18 × 24 × 0.75 cm). Separation time can be further reduced to a total of 2 h for solubilization and electrophoresis by the use of mini-gels. They also require smaller sample amounts (~100 µg of protein), as the band width is decreased. However, as the separating distance is limited, the resolution of complexes is lower. Mini-gels are easy to set up and enable solubilization conditions and sample amounts to be optimized before high-resolution gels are run.

In general, BN-PAGE is an appropriate method for the separation of native membrane protein complexes according to their molecular mass. However, there are two limitations for BN applications. The Coomassie dye used in BN-PAGE interferes with in-gel fluorescence detection and some in-gel catalytic activity assays. For this reason, alternative electrophoretic methods have been developed. Besides CN-PAGE, which suffers from enhanced protein aggregation and broadening of protein bands during electrophoresis, high-resolution clear native (hrCN) electrophoresis has been developed (Wittig *et al.*, 2007). HrCN-PAGE combines the advantage of CN-PAGE (fluorescence and catalytic activity detection in the absence of Coomassie) and BN-PAGE (high-resolution separation) but results obtained by hrCN-PAGE differ from those obtained by BN-PAGE. Up to now, hrCN-PAGE has only been used for the analysis of mitochondrial protein complexes. If its adaptability for other types of membranes can be proven, it would be an alternative solution for the analysis of membrane protein complexes.

References

Bisetto, E., Di Pancrazio, F., Simula, M.P., Mavelli, I. and Lippe, G. (2007) Mammalian ATP synthase monomer versus dimer profiled by blue native PAGE and activity stain. *Electrophoresis,* **28**, 3178–3185.

Braun, R.J., Kinkl, N., Beer, M. and Ueffing, M. (2007) Two-dimensional electrophoresis of membrane proteins. *Analytical and Bioanalytical Chemistry,* **389**, 1033–1045.

Camacho-Carvajal, M.M., Wollscheid, B., Aebersold, R., Steimle, V. and Schamel, W.W. (2004) Two-dimensional Blue native/SDS gel electrophoresis of multi-protein complexes from whole cellular lysates: a proteomics approach. *Molecular & Cellular Proteomics: MCP,* **3**, 176–182.

Danielsson, R., Suorsa, M., Paakkarinen, V., Albertsson, P.A., Styring, S., Aro, E.M. and Mamedov, F. (2006) Dimeric and monomeric organization of photosystem II. Distribution of five distinct complexes in the different domains of the thylakoid membrane. *Journal of Biological Chemistry,* **281**, 14241–14249.

Dencher, N.A., Goto, S., Reifschneider, N.H., Sugawa, M. and Krause, F. (2006) Unraveling age-dependent variation of the mitochondrial proteome. *Annals of the New York Academy of Sciences,* **1067**, 116–119.

Di Pancrazio, F., Bisetto, E., Alverdi, V., Mavelli, I., Esposito, G. and Lippe, G. (2006) Differential steady-state tyrosine phosphorylation of two oligomeric forms of mitochondrial F0F1ATPsynthase: a structural proteomic analysis. *Proteomics,* **6**, 921–926.

Dudkina, N.V., Heinemeyer, J., Sunderhaus, S., Boekema, E.J. and Braun, H.P. (2006) Respiratory chain supercomplexes in the plant mitochondrial membrane. *Trends in Plant Science,* **11**, 232–240.

Eubel, H., Heinemeyer, J. and Braun, H.P. (2004) Identification and characterization of respirasomes in potato mitochondria. *Plant Physiology,* **134**, 1450–1459.

Faye, A., Esnous, C., Price, N.T., Onfray, M.A., Girard, J. and Prip-Buus, C. (2007) Rat liver carnitine palmitoyltransferase 1 forms an oligomeric complex within the outer mitochondrial membrane. *Journal of Biological Chemistry,* **282**, 26908–26916.

Garavito, R.M. and Ferguson-Miller, S. (2001) Detergents as tools in membrane biochemistry. *Journal of Biological Chemistry,* **276**, 32403–32406.

Granvogl, B., Reisinger, V. and Eichacker, L.A. (2006) Mapping the proteome of thylakoid membranes by de novo sequencing of intermembrane peptide domains. *Proteomics,* **6**, 3681–3695.

Hopkins, A.L. and Groom, C.R. (2002) The druggable genome. *Nature Reviews. Drug discovery,* **1**, 727–730.

Kashino, Y. (2003) Separation methods in the analysis of protein membrane complexes. *Journal of Chromatography. B, Analytical Technologies in the Biomedical and Life Sciences,* **797**, 191–216.

Krause, F. (2006) Detection and analysis of protein-protein interactions in organellar and prokaryotic proteomes by native gel electrophoresis: (Membrane) protein complexes and supercomplexes. *Electrophoresis,* **27**, 2759–2781.

le Maire, M., Champeil, P. and Moller, J.V. (2000) Interaction of membrane proteins and lipids with solubilizing detergents. *Biochimica et Biophysica Acta,* **1508**, 86–111.

Nelson, N. and Yocum, C.F. (2006) Structure and function of photosystems I and II. *Annual Review of Plant Biology,* **57**, 521–565.

Reisinger, V. and Eichacker, L.A. (2007) How to analyze protein complexes by 2D Blue Native SDS-PAGE. *Proteomics,* **7**, Suppl 1, 6–16.

Sabar, M., Balk, J. and Leaver, C.J. (2005) Histochemical staining and quantification of plant mitochondrial respiratory chain complexes using blue-native polyacrylamide gel electrophoresis. *Plant Journal,* **44**, 893–901.

Santoni, V., Molloy, M. and Rabilloud, T. (2000) Membrane proteins and proteomics: un amour impossible? *Electrophoresis*, **21**, 1054–1070.

Schagger, H. and Pfeiffer, K. (2000) Supercomplexes in the respiratory chains of yeast and mammalian mitochondria. *EMBO Journal*, **19**, 1777–1783.

Schagger, H. and von Jagow, G. (1991) Blue native electrophoresis for isolation of membrane protein complexes in enzymatically active form. *Analytical Biochemistry*, **199**, 223–231.

Seddon, A.M., Curnow, P. and Booth, P.J. (2004) Membrane proteins, lipids and detergents: not just a soap opera. *Biochimica et Biophysica Acta*, **1666**, 105–117.

Wallin, E. and von Heijne, G. (1998) Genome-wide analysis of integral membrane proteins from eubacterial, archaean, and eukaryotic organisms. *Protein Science*, **7**, 1029–1038.

Werhahn, W. and Braun, H.P. (2002) Biochemical dissection of the mitochondrial proteome from *Arabidopsis thaliana* by three-dimensional gel electrophoresis. *Electrophoresis*, **23**, 640–646.

Williams, T.I., Combs, J.C., Thakur, A.P., Strobel, H.J. and Lynn, B.C. (2006) A novel Bicine running buffer system for doubled sodium dodecyl sulfate—polyacrylamide gel electrophoresis of membrane proteins. *Electrophoresis*, **27**, 2984–2995.

Wittig, I. and Schagger, H. (2005) Advantages and limitations of clear-native PAGE. *Proteomics*, **5**, 4338–4346.

Wittig, I., Karas, M. and Schagger, H. (2007) High resolution clear native electrophoresis for in-gel functional assays and fluorescence studies of membrane protein complexes. *Molecular & Cellular Proteomics: MCP*, **6**, 1215–1225.

Wu, C.C. and Yates, J.R. 3rd (2003) The application of mass spectrometry to membrane proteomics. *Nature Biotechnology*, **21**, 262–267.

Yan, L.J., Yang, S.H., Shu, H., Prokai, L. and Forster, M.J. (2007) Histochemical staining and quantification of dihydrolipoamide dehydrogenase diaphorase activity using blue native PAGE. *Electrophoresis*, **28**, 1036–1045.

Yao, D., Kieselbach, T., Komenda, J., Promnares, K., Prieto, M.A., Tichy, M., Vermaas, W. and Funk, C. (2007) Localization of the small CAB-like proteins in photosystem II. *Journal of Biological Chemistry*, **282**, 267–276.

5
Current Approaches to Protein Structure Analysis

Andrew P. Turnbull and Udo Heinemann

5.1
Bioinformatics

Primary sequence analysis, such as similarity searches against protein sequence databases, protein domain architecture determination, identification of specialized local structural motifs, and prediction of protein structure are possible with a variety of homology-based modeling methods (Figure 5.1) (Sanchez *et al.*, 2000; del Val *et al.*, 2004). Sequence database searches are particularly useful in selecting targets for protein structure analysis and, where possible, generating homologous probes for determining structures by the molecular replacement method (Brenner, 2000; Watson *et al.*, 2003; Linial and Yona, 2000). For example, the Web-based program 3D-PSSM (http://www.sbg.bio.ic.ac.uk/~3dpssm/) (Kelley *et al.*, 2000) is a fast method for predicting the protein fold from the primary amino acid sequence, and SWISS-MODEL (http://swissmodel.expasy.org/) (Schwede *et al.*, 2003) is a fully automated protein structure homology-modeling server.

5.1.1
Structure-to-Function Approaches

There are a number of bioinformatics resources available that are aimed at identifying a protein's biochemical function from its three-dimensional structure (Figure 5.2) (Laskowski *et al.*, 2003). For example, Dali (http://www2.ebi.ac.uk/dali) (Holm and Sander, 1993) and VAST (Vector Alignment Search Tool; http://www.ncbi.nlm.nih.gov:80/Structure/VAST/vastsearch.html) (Madej *et al.*, 1995) offer Web-based servers for automatically comparing the fold of a newly determined structure against known folds, as represented by the protein structures in the PDB (Novotny *et al.*, 2004). Such comparisons can often reveal striking similarities between proteins that are not evident from sequence analysis alone, and that

Proteomics of the Nervous System. Edited by H.G. Nothwang and S.E. Pfeiffer
Copyright © 2008 WILEY-VCH Verlag GmbH & Co. KGaA, Weinheim
ISBN: 978-3-527-31716-5

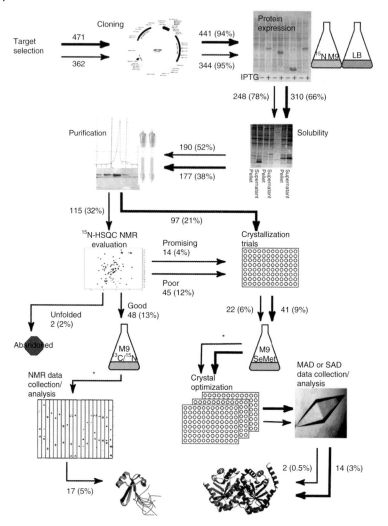

Figure 5.1 Schematic flow diagram of the strategies employed in structural genomics initiatives, using *Methanobacterium thermoautotrophicum* as an example. The number of protein targets after each step and the percentage relative to the number of starting targets are indicated in brackets. Thin arrows and italicized numbers are for smaller molecular weight proteins, and wide arrows and bold numbers are for larger molecular weight proteins. (Diagram taken from Yee *et al.*, 2003.) (Please find a color version of this figure in the color plates.)

can provide important insights into biological function even in the absence of any other biochemical or functional data. However, computer-based approaches fail to assign functions to proteins that adopt novel folds. Enzymes are a notable exception to this rule, because the arrangement of residues

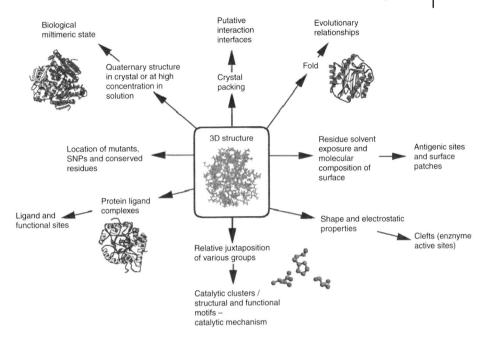

Figure 5.2 Summary of the information deriving from the three-dimensional structure of a protein relating to its biological function. (Taken from Thornton *et al.*, 2000.) (Please find a color version of this figure in the color plates.)

constituting their active sites tend to be highly conserved in their spatial disposition even in cases where there is no overall similarity in sequence or fold. For example, the relative positioning of the Ser-His-Asp catalytic triad of the serine proteases is highly conserved even when found in protein structures adopting different folds. Hence, screening a new protein structure against a database of enzyme active-site templates such as PROCAT (http://www.biochem.ucl.ac.uk/bsm/PROCAT/PROCAT.html) can reveal key functional residues. The spatial patterns of residues can be automatically generated using various techniques including graph theory (ASSAM) (Spriggs *et al.*, 2003) and "fuzzy pattern matching" (RIGOR) (Kleywegt, 1999). Alternative approaches to identifying enzymes on the basis of their three-dimensional structure and predicting their functions have recently been reported. Here, a vector machine-learning algorithm is used, based on the secondary structure of proteins the propensities of amino acids, and surface properties, in order to discriminate enzymes from non-enzymes (Dobson and Doig, 2003). Another approach analyzes protein surface charges to identify conserved residues that can serve as catalytic sites (Bate and Warwicker, 2004). Once a general class of biochemical function of a protein has been proposed, experimental screening of enzymatic activity can be used to derive the precise biochemical function.

For example, after the structure determination of BioH (an enzyme involved in biotin biosynthesis in *E. coli*) the protein structure was screened against a library of enzyme active sites, a Ser-His-Asp catalytic triad was identified, and subsequent hydrolase assays showed BioH to be a carboxylesterase (Sanishvili *et al.*, 2003).

5.1.2
Identification of Disordered Regions in a Protein

The occurrence of regions in proteins that lack any fixed tertiary structure is increasingly being observed in structural studies (Pandey *et al.*, 2004). These disordered regions or "random coils" are inherently flexible and are involved in a variety of functions, including the modulation of the specificity/affinity of protein-binding interactions, activation by cleavage, and DNA recognition. During the target selection process, it is important to consider any intrinsic protein disorder, because it can often lead to problems with the expression of protein-coding genes, protein stability, purification, and crystallization (Li *et al.*, 1999, 2000). PONDR, DisEMBL, and GlobPlot are useful tools for predicting potential disordered regions within a protein sequence that can be used to help design constructs corresponding to globular proteins or domains. PONDR (Predictor of Naturally Disordered Regions; www.pondr.com) (Garner *et al.*, 1998, 1999) and DisEMBL (Linding *et al.*, 2003a) use methods based on artificial neural networks, whereas GlobPlot (http://globplot.embl.de) relies on a novel, propensity-based disorder-prediction algorithm (Linding *et al.*, 2003b). These methods can also be used to predict inherently flexible regions in protein sequences. For example, PONDR predicted that the linker between the DNA operator-binding central domain of the transcriptional regulator KorB (KorB-O) and the KorB dimerization domain (KorB-C) is flexible, which was indeed observed in crystal structures and is thought to facilitate complex formation on circular plasmids (Figure 5.3) (Delbrück *et al.*, 2002; Khare *et al.*, 2004).

5.1.3
Protein–Ligand Complexes

Protein–ligand complexes are the most useful in terms of providing functional information because they reveal the nature of the ligand, the site at which it is bound to the protein, the location of the active site, and of the catalytic machinery (if the protein is an enzyme). There are several examples of structural analyses in which an unexpected protein-bound ligand or cofactor derived from the cloning organism was discovered. For example, the structure of the trimeric human protein p14.5 was found to have picked up benzoate molecules from the crystallization buffer at its inter-subunit tunnels, which most likely mark a hydrolytic active site (Figure 5.4) (Manjasetty *et al.*, 2004). When such data are available at high resolution, proposing a biological function

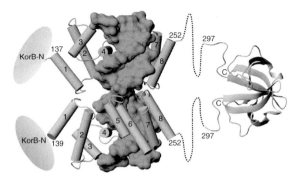

Figure 5.3 Natively disordered regions in the bacterial trancriptional regulator and partitioning protein KorB. The KorB DNA-binding domains (KorB-O, center) are connected by flexible linkers to N-terminal domains of unknown structure and function (KorB-N, left), and the KorB dimerization domains (KorB-C, right). (Picture taken from Khare et al., 2004.) (Please find a color version of this figure in the color plates.)

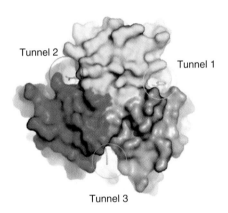

Figure 5.4 Crystal structure of the trimeric human protein, hp14.5. Benzoate molecules picked up from the crystallization buffer bind in the inter-subunit tunnels and mark putative hydrolytic active sites (Manjasetty et al., 2004). (Picture with permission from Dr B.A. Manjasetty.) (Please find a color version of this figure in the color plates.)

for the protein can be relatively straightforward, because these data identify the nature of the ligand, the ligand-binding site, and the arrangement of catalytic residues from which a catalytic mechanism can be postulated.

5.2
Protein Production

Protein expression and purification play a central role in high-throughput protein structure analysis. Cloning using restriction enzymes is impractical for high-throughput approaches because of the complications of selecting compatible and appropriate restriction enzymes for each cloning procedure, and the multiple steps of experimental refinement and treatment that must be performed. Therefore, high-throughput cloning requires procedures based on the polymerase chain reaction (PCR). High-throughput cloning and expression methods are now being developed in many laboratories, enabling the generation and testing of up to hundreds of DNA constructs for high-level expression in parallel, using rapid and generic protocols. To generate expression vector clones, generic cloning systems can be used; the Gibco/Life Technologies GATEWAY system is one such example, streamlining the expression and cloning process by alleviating recloning steps and avoiding the use of restriction enzymes in the cloning and subcloning processes. In addition, vectors for the co-expression of two or more protein-coding genes have been designed (Alexandrov *et al.*, 2004; Romier *et al.*, 2006; Scheich *et al.*, 2007).

High-throughput approaches may rely on both prokaryotic and eukaryotic hosts. *Escherichia coli* expression systems are advantageous for many reasons, most notably because the overproduced protein is usually obtained without any posttranslational modification heterogeneity, and protein expression is cheaper and faster than with eukaryotic systems. However, it is not always possible to obtain soluble protein for many eukaryotic proteins, in particular, human proteins, by using the heterologous expression of eukaryotic genes, in which the codon usage for a cDNA could be suboptimal in *E. coli*. Furthermore, eukaryotic systems are necessary for the expression of proteins that require posttranslational modifications for their correct folding and activity. In situations in which a protein cannot be synthesized in *E. coli*, the eukaryotic yeasts (*Saccharomyces cerevisiae* and *Pichia pastoris*), baculovirus-infected insect cells, *Leishmania tarentolae*, and the cell-free wheat germ systems that have been developed for high-throughput approaches can be used. Furthermore, in these and other eukaryotic expression systems, the codon usage is closer to that in humans. The various merits of each system are discussed below.

5.2.1
Yeast

The yeasts *S. cerevisiae* and *P. pastoris* can be used for the routine production of recombinant proteins (Prinz *et al.*, 2004). More recently, *P. pastoris* has emerged as the preferred yeast because of its strong, highly inducible promoter system resulting in higher yields of recombinant protein, stable genomic integration and posttranslational modifications, such as phosphorylation, which may be important for both the structure and function of some human proteins (Cereghino and Cregg, 2000). In comparison with *S. cerevisiae*, the distribution and chain length of *N*-linked oligosaccharides are significantly shorter, and therefore this system represents a suitable alternative for the extracellular expression of human proteins (Grinna and Tschopp, 1989). An additional advantage of the methylotrophic *P. pastoris* expression system is that it makes it possible to introduce ^{13}C label into recombinant proteins (by feeding ^{13}C-labeled methanol) for nuclear magnetic resonance (NMR) structural analyses.

5.2.2
Baculovirus–Insect Cell

The recombinant baculovirus–insect cell expression system accomplishes most posttranslational modifications, including phosphorylation, N- and O-linked glycosylation, acylation, disulfide cross-linking, oligomeric assembly, and subcellular targeting, which may all be critical for the accurate production and function of human proteins (Albala et al., 2000). In contrast to bacterial expression systems, the recombinant baculovirus expression system usually produces soluble proteins without the need for induction or specific temperature conditions.

5.2.3
Leishmania tarentolae (Trypanosomatidae)

The use of the parasitic Trypanosomatidae species L. tarentolae, as the host for in vitro protein production has recently been reported, and can achieve high levels of protein expression (Breitling et al., 2002). The Trypanosomatidae species of parasites naturally produce large amounts of glycoproteins, which is an advantage in the production of sialylated heterologous glycosylated proteins. Furthermore, given the natural auxotrophy of L. tarentolae for methionine, it has been suggested that such a system could prove to be useful for the production of selenomethionine-labeled proteins, for high-throughput X-ray crystallographic structure determination using single-wavelength anomalous diffraction (SAD) or multiple-wavelength anomalous diffraction (MAD) phasing techniques.

5.2.4
Cell-free Expression Systems

Cell-free systems facilitate the parallel expression of many protein-coding genes, and are therefore suitable for high-throughput protein production. Obtaining the protein directly in a form suitable for X-ray crystallography or NMR spectroscopy is another prerequisite for high-throughput structure analysis. For the purpose of X-ray analysis, anomalous diffraction techniques (SAD or MAD) necessitate the substitution of methionine residues with selenomethionine. Additionally, NMR structure analysis often requires the labeling of proteins with ^{13}C and/or ^{15}N, which can be introduced through cell growth on media containing these isotopes in the form of ^{13}C-glucose and $^{15}NH_4Cl$. In this respect, the *E. coli* cell-free protein synthesis system of Kigawa *et al.* (1999) permits the straightforward incorporation of isotopes for NMR analysis. However, this system is not always suitable for the expression of some eukaryotic proteins and can result in aggregation, formation of insoluble inclusion bodies, and degradation of the expression product. Furthermore, in the case of multidomain proteins, which are found more often in eukaryotes, correct folding occurs more frequently in eukaryotic than in prokaryotic translation systems (Netzer and Hartl, 1997; Kolb *et al.*, 2000). Another limitation with the use of *E. coli* systems for high-throughput cell-free expression is that PCR-generated fragments are not transcribed and translated efficiently in these systems: contamination by the mRNA- and DNA-degradation enzymes originating from the cell decreases the stability of the templates and reduces yields. By contrast, in eukaryotic cell-free systems, the added mRNAs are stable for long periods of time, and therefore these systems overcome many of the limitations associated with *E. coli* cell-free systems. Furthermore, cell-free systems can produce high yields of correctly folded proteins and, unlike *in vivo* systems, facilitate the expression of proteins that would otherwise interfere with the host cell physiology. Recently, the synthesis and screening of gene products based on the cell-free system prepared from eukaryotic wheat embryos has been reported; this method bypasses many of the time-consuming cloning steps involved in conventional expression systems and lends itself to the high-throughput expression of proteins, using automated robotic systems (Sawasaki *et al.*, 2002; Endo and Sawasaki, 2004).

5.3
Purification

Protein purification has also seen significant improvements because of the use of affinity tags fused to the protein of interest, so that it can be separated from the host cell proteins rapidly by using standardized purification schemes. N-terminal tags range from large tags, such as glutathione-*S*-transferase (GST), maltose-binding protein (MBP), thioreductase, and the chitin-binding protein, to fairly small tags such as His_6, and various epitope tags (Stevens, 2000). In some systems, the use of large tags can lead to the production of fusion products that are too large for high-level expression, but the use of such tags can improve the correct folding and stability of the overexpressed protein. His_6 is the most commonly used purification tag, because it is easier to incorporate into expression constructs and it allows a generic one-step purification using automated methods based on nickel-nitrilotriacetic acid (Ni-NTA) or other immobilized metal-affinity chromatography resins (Bruel *et al.*, 2000). The use of an additional C-terminal StrepII tag enables dual-affinity column purification, which ensures that only full-length gene products are separated (Voss and Skerra, 1997). For crystallization to occur, it is generally agreed that the fusion tags must be removed because they can introduce flexible regions into the protein, which can interfere with crystallization or lead to various forms of microheterogeneity. In a recent study, the compatibility of small peptide affinity tags with protein crystallization was assessed, in which the N-terminus of the chicken spectrin SH3 domain was labeled with a His_6 tag and a StrepII tag, fused to the N- and C-termini, respectively. The resulting protein, His_6-SH3-StrepII, comprised 83 amino acid residues, 23 of which originated from the tags (accounting for 23% of the total fusion protein mass). In contrast to the general consensus that the presence of affinity tags is detrimental in structural studies, this study demonstrated that the fused affinity tags did not interfere with crystallization or structure analysis, and did not change the protein structure. This suggests that, in some cases, protein constructs utilizing both N- and C-terminal peptide tags may lend themselves to structural investigations in high-throughput regimes (Mueller *et al.*, 2003).

5.4
Structure Determination by X-Ray Crystallography

5.4.1
Crystallization

Crystallization is regarded as a major bottleneck in structure determination by X-ray crystallography and can be divided into two stages: coarse screening for initial crystallization conditions, followed by optimization of the conditions in order to produce diffraction-quality single crystals. The field of crystallization has recently been revolutionized by significant developments in automation, miniaturization, and process integration. These developments have led to the availability of robotic liquid-handling systems that are capable of rapidly and efficiently screening thousands of crystallization conditions, in which different parameters such as ionic strength, precipitant concentration, additives, pH, and temperature are altered. High-throughput screening begins with the automated preparation and/or reformatting of precipitant solutions into crystallization microplates. The latest nanoliter robotic liquid-dispensing systems are capable of dispensing very small drops (typically containing between 25 and 100 nL of protein), which reduces the amount of protein required for screening conditions and the overhead on protein production (Brown *et al.*, 2003; Walter *et al.*, 2003). Furthermore, smaller drops equilibrate faster than larger drops, leading to a more rapid appearance of crystals. The crystallization experiments are then regularly monitored using an imaging robot, and the collected images can either be analyzed visually or by using automatic crystal recognition systems.

   A recent development in protein crystallization has been the use of a microfluidic system for crystallizing proteins, using the free-interface diffusion method at the nanoliter scale. This system is capable of screening hundreds of crystallization conditions in which droplets, each containing solutions of

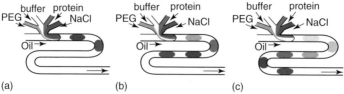

(a)   (b)   (c)

Figure 5.5 Droplet-based microfluidic system for protein crystallization. (a–c) A schematic illustration: As the flow rate of the NaCl stream is decreased and the flow rate of the buffer stream is increased, the volume of NaCl solution injected into each droplet decreases, and the concentration of NaCl in each droplet decreases. The shade of the droplets represents NaCl concentration. Each successive droplet represents a trial that tests a different ratio of stock solutions. (Taken from Zheng *et al.*, 2003.) (Please find a color version of this figure in the color plates.)

protein, precipitants, and additives in various ratios, are formed in the flow of immiscible fluids inside a polydimethylsiloxane (PDMS)/glass capillary composite microfluidic device (Figure 5.5) (Zheng *et al.*, 2003, 2004). The system is capable of performing multidimensional screening (mixing 5–10 solutions) and therefore explores more of the crystallization space than the conventional method of vapor diffusion, increasing the likelihood of obtaining crystals. Furthermore, the capillary containing protein crystals can be directly exposed to the synchrotron X-ray beam, eliminating the need to manually manipulate the crystal. These features also mean that it has the potential to serve as the basis for future high-throughput automated crystallization systems.

Membrane proteins represent the most persistent bottleneck for all preparatory procedures and analytical methods, because they are water soluble only in the presence of detergents, and are difficult to overproduce in the quantities required for structural studies (Heinemann *et al.*, 2003). Membrane proteins, which constitute up to 30% of the protein repertoire of an organism, represent the targets for more than 50% of the drugs that are being currently used and tested (Stewart *et al.*, 2002). An adapted robotic system has recently been reported that enables high-throughput crystallization of membrane proteins using lipidic mesophases (Cherezov *et al.*, 2004). Recently, the first crystal structures of a ligand-regulated G protein-coupled receptor, the β_2-adrenergic receptor have been reported (Cherezov *et al.*, 2007; Rasmussen *et al.*, 2007).

5.4.2
Data Collection

X-ray data collection has been revolutionized over the past decade, with the development of improved X-ray sources and detectors and the universal adoption of flash-freezing techniques that greatly reduce crystal radiation damage (Garman, 1999). New third-generation synchrotrons are now available across the world, which provide more intense and stable X-ray beams and, combined with new, faster, larger, and more sensitive X-ray detectors, allow higher quality data to be collected much more rapidly, leading to a dramatic increase in the success rate of structure determination (Abola *et al.*, 2000; Jhoti, 2001). Furthermore, specialized, highly collimated microfocus beamlines, such as ID13 at the ESRF (Grenoble, France; http://www.esrf.fr/exp_facilities/ID13/index.html) and the protein crystallography beamline at the Swiss Light Source (SLS), are specifically tailored to study biological crystals with small physical dimensions (microcrystals from 5 to 50 μm in size) or very large unit cell dimensions. Future developments in detector design, such as the large quantum-limited area X-ray detector Pilatus (Eikenberry *et al.*, 2003) operational at the SLS, promise larger continuous active areas, higher spatial resolution, very low noise, and fast readout times (~1 s). High-throughput X-ray data collection has also led to the development of automated robotic sample changers that store and mount crystals sequentially while maintaining the samples at liquid-nitrogen temperatures (100 K). A novel system has recently been described, using a proprietary crystallization plate that facilitates the preliminary investigation of the diffraction properties of crystals *in situ* in the drop, by direct exposure to the X-ray beam (Watanabe *et al.*, 2002). The BIOXHIT project (Biocrystallography (X) on a Highly Integrated Technology Platform for European Structural Genomics; www.bioxhit.org), comprising more than 20 research groups from all over Europe, aims to develop an integrated technology platform for synchrotron beamlines by promoting new approaches to crystallization, and fully automating diffraction data collection and structure determination.

Recent developments in technology have not been limited exclusively to synchrotron sources. The latest generation of high-intensity X-ray generators has revolutionized X-ray sources to such an extent that the latest "in-house" systems from Rigaku/MSC (e.g. the FR-E SuperBright; www.rigakumsc.com/) and Bruker AXS (www.bruker-axs.com) are comparable in intensity to first-generation synchrotron sources and, coupled with automated sample changers, make high-throughput crystallography possible in the laboratory. Furthermore, the development of the Compact Light Source (Lyncean Technologies Inc., Palo Alto, CA, USA) promises to have a huge impact on protein structure determination, offering the possibility of a "synchrotron beamline" for home laboratory applications. This tunable, tabletop X-ray source combines an electron beam with a laser beam to generate an intense X-ray beam and, as a next-generation X-ray source, directly addresses the increasing demand for high-throughput protein crystallography.

5.4.3
Phasing

The central problem in X-ray crystallography is the determination of the protein phases. X-ray data collected from a crystal consist of structure factor amplitudes, but there is no way of directly measuring the phase associated with each amplitude. Recent advances in macromolecular phasing have simplified and further automated this crucial stage of X-ray structure determination to such an extent that the eventual success of a project is usually assured, if well-diffracting crystals are available (Dauter, 2002). The techniques of isomorphous replacement, anomalous scattering, molecular replacement, and single- (SAD) and multiple-wavelength (MAD) anomalous dispersion are commonly used to solve the phase problem. However, phase determination has been dramatically facilitated by the widespread adoption of SAD and MAD phasing techniques by the crystallographic community, primarily as a consequence of the availability of stable and tunable synchrotron sources. These allow the optimal exploitation of the anomalous effect as a source of phase information by delivering X-ray energies corresponding to absorption maxima of the anomalous scatterers, very often selenium introduced as selenomethionine through substitution of methionine. Additionally, heavy-atom labels (mercury, platinum, and others) may be bound to crystalline proteins by soaking to yield phase information by anomalous diffraction techniques.

Modern phasing techniques, such as fast halide soaks and sulfur SAD, hold promise of simpler and faster protein structure determination than traditional methods. Fast halide soaks using bromide and iodide that diffuse rapidly into the crystal and display significant anomalous scattering signals can be used to quickly derivatize protein crystals (Dauter *et al.*, 2000). Heavy-atom reagents can also be incorporated into the crystal in a relatively short time if a concentration greater than 10 mM is used. These derivatives then display better isomorphism and diffraction qualities than those obtained after a standard, prolonged soak (Sun and Radaev, 2002; Sun *et al.*, 2002). The availability of stable synchrotron beamlines and improvements in data-processing programs make it possible to collect extremely accurate diffraction data, and to determine structures using the very weak anomalous signals from atoms such as sulfur and phosphorus that are inherently present in macromolecules or nucleic acids; several novel structures have been determined by using sulfur-SAD phasing.

5.4.4
Automated Structure Determination

High-throughput crystallographic structure determination requires software that is automated and designed for minimum user intervention (Lamzin and Perrakis, 2000). There has been considerable development in the direct-method programs, SHELXD and SnB (Xu *et al.*, 2002), which can automatically determine heavy-atom substructures from a very small signal. HKL2MAP connects several programs from the SHELX suite to guide the user from analyzing scaled diffraction data (SHELXC), through substructure solution (SHELXD) and phasing (SHELXE), to displaying an electron density map (Xfit) (Schneider and Sheldrick, 2002; Pape and Schneider, 2004).

There are a number of other automated software systems, such as ACrS (automated crystallographic system) (Brunzelle *et al.*, 2003) and PHENIX (Python-based hierarchical environment for integrated Xtallography) (Adams *et al.*, 2004) that are currently being developed to meet the requirements of high-throughput structure determination by combining multiple structure-determination software packages into one intuitive interface.

Finally, new algorithms for interpreting electron density maps and for automated model building, such as, SOLVE/RESOLVE (Terwilliger and Berendzen, 1999; Terwilliger, 2000), AUTOSHARP/SHARP (de la Fortelle and Bricogne, 1997), and ARP/wARP (Perrakis *et al.*, 1999), enable rapid construction of protein models without the need for significant manual intervention. At present, the success rates for these programs are dependent on the resolution of the diffraction data (typically, 2.5 Å resolution or higher is necessary for automatic chain fitting).

5.4.5
Molecular Replacement

When an approximate structural model of a protein under investigation is available, either from NMR, a homologous X-ray structure, or from homology modeling, initial phases can be obtained using molecular replacement where the homologous probe structure is fitted to the experimental data using three rotational and three translational parameters. The programs AMoRe (Navaza, 2001) and MolRep (Vagin and Teplyakov, 1997) that are integrated into the CCP4i GUI (Collaborative Computational Project No. 4, 1994; Potterton *et al.*, 2003) simplify the problem of positioning a molecule in the asymmetric unit by running sequential rotational and translational searches. Advances in molecular replacement include the implementation of the maximum likelihood-based algorithms in BEAST (Read, 2001), and the six-dimensional evolutionary search algorithm in EPMR (Kissinger *et al.*, 1999). As the number of protein structures increases, it is anticipated that molecular replacement will become the standard method for structure determination, using a generalized search of all unique protein domains present in the Protein Data Bank (PDB).

5.5
Structure-Based Drug Design

Knowledge of the three-dimensional structure of proteins can play a key role in the development of small-molecule drugs because being able to verify how lead compounds bind to their targets accelerates drug development and is more cost-effective. Notable drugs that have been successfully designed using protein three-dimensional structure information include the HIV protease inhibitors Viracept (Agouron, USA and Eli Lilly, USA) (Kim *et al.*, 1995; Kaldor *et al.*, 1997) and Agenerase (Vertex, USA; Kissei, Japan; Glaxo Wellcome,

UK) (Kim *et al.*, 1995). However, it is usually necessary to screen a large number of protein–ligand complex structures in the iterative process of rational structure-based drug design. Hence, high-throughput protein X-ray crystallography offers an unprecedented opportunity for facilitating drug discovery. Recent advances in rapid binding-site analysis of de novo targets using virtual ligand (in silico) screening and small-molecule co-crystallization methodologies, in combination with the miniaturization and automation of structural biology, enable more rapid lead compound identification and faster optimization, providing a framework for direct integration into the drug discovery process (Goodwill *et al.*, 2001; Kuhn *et al.*, 2002; Stewart *et al.*, 2002; Tickle *et al.*, 2004). In the high-throughput structure determination of protein–ligand complexes, it is desirable to use tools that can locate, build, and refine the structure of the bound ligand with minimal human intervention. One such tool is X-LIGAND, part of the QUANTA software package (Accelrys, San Diego, CA, USA) that automatically searches for unoccupied regions of electron density in the structure of the protein–ligand complex in which it tries to fit the ligand (Oldfield, 2001).

5.6
Structure Determination by NMR

Solution-state NMR spectroscopy can serve as a technique complementary to X-ray crystallography in protein structure analysis, particularly in the context of structural genomics initiatives (Montelione *et al.*, 2000), where many protein targets either do not crystallize or do not form crystals suitable for crystallographic studies (owing to small crystal size or poor diffraction quality). NMR measurements are performed in aqueous solution, obviating the need to grow crystals. This technique is applicable primarily to small proteins (<30 kDa) that are highly soluble (millimolar concentrations), and is particularly useful in the study of proteins that are partially unfolded in the absence of their appropriate binding partners. The additional technique of solid-state NMR is useful in providing structural information for some integral membrane proteins that may not be accessible using crystallographic methods. Furthermore, chemical shift perturbation studies can be used to validate proposed biochemical functions, to map ligand-binding epitopes, and to screen for small-molecule ligands in drug development.

High-throughput, NMR-based structure determination requires rapid and automated data acquisition and analysis methods. The major challenges in realizing this have been those of increasing instrumentation sensitivity (signal-to-noise ratio) and reducing the time required for data collection. These technical issues have been addressed by constructing new high-field magnets and by the recent introduction of cryogenic probes that operate at low temperatures ($\sim$25 K), permitting the investigation of proteins that have either low solubility or low yields from purification. Additionally, the application of TROSY (transverse relaxed optimized spectroscopy), a novel spectroscopic concept based on the selection of slowly relaxing NMR transitions, has provided significant sensitivity enhancements for large proteins.

The most time-consuming aspects of structure determination by NMR are the long data collection times necessary for independently sampling three or more indirect dimensions along with the time taken to interpret the correspondingly large number of spectra from $^{13}C/^{15}N$-isotope-labeled samples. Rapid resonance assignment is a prerequisite for high-throughput NMR structure determination; techniques such as reduced-dimensionality ^{13}C, ^{15}N, ^{1}H-triple resonance NMR also avoid the sampling limited regime through the simultaneous frequency-labeling of two spin types in a single indirect dimension (Szyperski *et al.*, 2002). Heteronuclear multidimensional data reduce complications arising from interspectral variations by maximizing the dimensionality of the spectra and decrease signal overlap of data sets sufficiently for the data to be analyzed automatically. Recent approaches to automated structure elucidation from NMR spectra include NOESY-Jigsaw (Bailey-Kellogg *et al.*, 2000), in which sparse and unassigned NMR data can be used to reasonably and accurately assess secondary structure and align it. The information thus retrieved is useful for quick structural assays for assessing folds before full structural determination and can therefore assist in fold prediction. Additionally, the program ATNOS (automated NOESY peak picking) enables automated peak picking and nuclear Overhauser effect (NOE) signal identification in homonuclear 2D and heteronuclear 3D [^{1}H, ^{1}H]-NOESY spectra during de novo protein structure determination (Herrmann *et al.*, 2002).

References

Abola, E., Kuhn, P., Earnest, T. and Stevens, R.C. (2000) Automation of X-ray crystallography. *Nature Structural Biology*, **7**, 973–977.

Adams, P., Gopal, K., Grossekunstleve, R.W., Hung, L.-W., Ioerger, T.R., McCoy, A.J., Moriarty, N.W., Pai, R.K., Read, R.J., Romo, T.D., Sacchettini, J.C., Sauter, N.K., Storoni, L.C. and Terwilliger, T.C. (2004) Recent developments in the PHENIX software for automated crystallographic structure determination. *Journal of Synchrotron Radiation*, **11**, 53–55.

Albala, J.S., Franke, K., McConnell, I.R., Pak, K.L., Folta, P.A., Rubinfeld, B., Davies, A.H., Lennon, G.G. and Clark, R. (2000) From genes to proteins: high-throughput expression and purification of the human proteome. *Journal of Cellular Biochemistry*, **80**, 187–191.

Alexandrov, A., Vignali, M., LaCount, D.J., Quartley, E., de Vriest, C., De Rosa, D., Babulski, J., Mitchell, S.F., Scheonfeld, L.W., Fields, S., Hol, W.G., Dumont, M.E., Phizicky, E.M. and Grayhack, E.J. (2004) A facile method for high-throughput co-expression of protein pairs. *Molecular & Cellular Proteomics: MCP*, **3**, 934–938.

Bailey-Kellogg, C., Widge, A., Kelley, J.J., Berardi, M.J., Bushweller, J.H. and Donald, B.R. (2000) The NOESY jigsaw: automated protein secondary structure and main-chain assignment from sparse, unassigned NMR data. *Journal of Computational Biology*, **7**, 537–558.

Bate, P. and Warwicker, J. (2004) Enzyme/non-enzyme discrimination and prediction of enzyme active site location using charge-based methods. *Journal of Molecular Biology*, **340**, 263–276.

Breitling, R., Klingner, S., Callewaert, N., Pietrucha, R., Geyer, A., Ehrlich, G., Hartung, R., Muller, A., Contreras, R., Beverley, S.M. and Alexandrov, K. (2002) Non-pathogenic trypanosomatid protozoa as a platform for protein research and production. *Protein Expression and Purification*, **25**, 209–218.

Brenner, S.E. (2000) Target selection for structural genomics. *Nature Structural Biology*, **7**(Suppl.), 967–969.

Brown, J., Walter, T.S., Carter, L., Abrescia, G.A., Aricescu, A.R., Batuwangala, T.D., Bird, L.E., Brown, N., Chamberlain, P.P., Davis, S.J., Dubinina, E., Endicott, J., Fennelly, J.A., Gilbert, R.J.C., Harkiolaki, M., Hon, W.-C., Kimberley, F., Love, C.A., Mancini, E.J., Manso-Sancho, R., Nichols, C.E., Robinson, R.A., Sutton, G.C., Schueller, N., Sleeman, M.C., Stewart-Jones, G.B., Vuong, M., Welburn, J., Zhang, Z., Stammers, D.K., Owens, R.J., Jones, E.Y., Harlos, K. and Stuart, D.I. (2003) A procedure for setting up high-throughput nanoliter crystallization experiments. II. Crystallization results. *Journal of Applied Crystallography*, **36**, 315–318.

Bruel, C., Cha, K., Reeves, P.J., Getmanova, E. and Khorana, H.G. (2000) Rhodopsin kinase: expression in mammalian cells and a two-step purification. *Proceedings of the National Academy of Sciences of the United States of America*, **97**, 3004–3009.

Brunzelle, J.S., Shafaee, P., Yang, X., Weigand, S., Ren, Z. and Anderson, W.F. (2003) Automated crystallographic system for high-throughput protein structure determination. *Acta Crystallographica*, **D59**, 1138–1144.

Cereghino, J.L. and Cregg, J.M. (2000) Heterologous protein expression in the methylotrophic yeast Pichia pastoris. *FEMS Microbiology Reviews*, **24**, 45–66.

Cherezov, V., Peddi, A., Muthusubramaniam, L., Zheng, Y.F.

and Caffrey, M. (2004) A robotic system for crystallizing membrane and soluble proteins in lipidic mesophases. *Acta Crystallographica*, **D60**, 1795–1807.

Cherezov, V., Rosenbaum, D.M., Hanson, M.A., Rasmussen, S.G.F., Thian, F.S., Kobilka, T.S., Choi, H.-J., Kuhn, P., Weis, W.I., Kobilka, B.K. and Stevens, R.C. (2007) High-resolution crystal structure of an engineered human β_2-adrenergic G protein-coupled receptor. *Science*, **318**, 1258–1265.

Collaborative Computational Project, No. 4 (1994) The CCP4 suite: Programs for protein crystallography. *Acta Crystallographica*, **D50**, 760–763.

Dauter, Z. (2002) New approaches to high-throughput phasing. *Current Opinion in Structural Biology*, **12**, 674–678.

Dauter, Z., Dauter, M. and Rajashankar, K.R. (2000) Novel approach to phasing proteins: Derivatization by short cryo-soaking with halides. *Acta Crystallographica*, **D56**, 232–237.

de la Fortelle, E. and Bricogne, G. (1997) Maximum-likelihood heavy-atom parameter refinement for multiple isomorphous replacement and multiwavelength anomalous diffraction methods. *Methods in Enzymology*, **276**, 472–494.

del Val, C., Mehrle, A., Falkenhahn, M., Seiler, M., Glatting, K.H., Poustka, A., Suhai, S. and Wiemann, S. (2004) High-throughput protein analysis integrating bioinformatics and experimental assays. *Nucleic Acids Research*, **32**, 742–748.

Delbrück, H., Ziegelin, G., Lanka, E. and Heinemann, U. (2002) An Src homology 3-like domain is responsible for dimerization of the repressor protein KorB encoded by the promiscuous IncP plasmid RP4. *Journal of Biological Chemistry*, **277**, 4191–4198.

Dobson, P.D. and Doig, A.J. (2003) Distinguishing enzyme structures from non-enzymes without alignments. *Journal of Molecular Biology*, **330**, 771–783.

Eikenberry, E.F., Bronnimann, C., Hulsen, G., Toyokawa, H., Horisberger, R., Schmitt, B.,

Schulze-Briese, C. and Tomizaki, T. (2003) PILATUS: A two-dimensional X-ray detector for macromolecular crystallography. *Nuclear Instruments and Methods in Physics Research A*, **501**, 260–266.

Endo, Y. and Sawasaki, T. (2004) High-throughput, genome-scale protein production method based on the wheat germ cell-free expression system. *Journal of Structural and Functional Genomics*, **5**, 45–57.

Garman, E. (1999) Cool data: quantity AND quality. *Acta Crystallographica*, **D55**, 1641–1653.

Garner, E., Cannon, P., Romero, P., Obradovic, Z. and Dunker, A.K. (1998) Predicting disordered regions from amino acid sequence: common themes despite differing structural characterization. *Genome Informatics. Series: Workshop on Genome Informatics*, **9**, 201–213.

Garner, E., Romero, P., Dunker, A.K., Brown, C. and Obradovic, Z. (1999) Predicting binding regions within disordered proteins. *Genome Informatics. Series: Workshop on Genome Informatics*, **10**, 41–50.

Goodwill, K.E., Tennant, M.G. and Stevens, R.C. (2001) High-throughput x-ray crystallography for structure-based drug design. *Drug Discovery Today*, **15**(Suppl.), 113–118.

Grinna, L.S. and Tschopp, J.F. (1989) Size distribution and general structural features of N-linked oligosaccharides from the methylotrophic yeast, Pichia pastoris. *Yeast*, **5**, 107–115.

Heinemann, U., Büssow, K., Mueller, U. and Umbach, P. (2003) Facilities and methods for the high-throughput crystal structure analysis of human proteins. *Accounts of Chemical Research*, **36**, 157–163.

Herrmann, T., Guntert, P. and Wuthrich, K. (2002) Protein NMR structure determination with automated NOE-identification in the NOESY spectra using the new software ATNOS. *Journal of Biomolecular NMR*, **24**, 171–189.

Holm, L. and Sander, C. (1993) Protein structure comparison by alignment of distance matrices. *Journal of Molecular Biology*, **233**, 123–138.

Jhoti, H. (2001) High-throughput structural proteomics using X-rays. *Trends in Biotechnology*, **19**, S67–S71.

Kaldor, S.W., Kalish, V.J., Davies, J.F., II, Shetty, B.V., Fritz, J.E., Appelt, K., Burgess, J.A., Campanale, K.M., Chirgadze, N.Y., Clawson, D.K., Dressman, B.A., Hatch, S.D., Khalil, D.A., Kosa, M.B., Lubbehusen, P.P., Muesing, M.A., Patick, A.K., Reich, S.H., Su, K.S. and Tatlock, J.H. (1997) Viracept (nelfinavir mesylate, AG1343): a potent, orally bioavailable inhibitor of HIV-1 protease. *Journal of Medicinal Chemistry*, **40**, 3979–3985.

Kelley, L.A., MacCallum, R.M. and Sternberg, M.J. (2000) Enhanced genome annotation using structural profiles in the program 3D-PSSM. *Journal of Molecular Biology*, **299**, 499–520.

Khare, D., Ziegelin, G., Lanka, E. and Heinemann, U. (2004) Sequence-specific DNA binding determined by contacts outside the helix-turn-helix motif of the ParB homolog KorB. *Nature Structural & Molecular Biology*, **11**, 656–663.

Kigawa, T., Yabuki, T., Yoshida, Y., Tsutsui, M., Ito, Y., Shibata, T. and Yokoyama, S. (1999) Cell-free production and stable isotope labeling of milligram quantities of proteins. *FEBS Letters*, **442**, 15–19.

Kim, E.E., Baker, C.T., Dwyer, M.D., Murcko, M.A., Rao, B.G., Tung, R.D. and Navia, M.A. (1995) Crystal structure of HIV-1 protease in complex with VX-478, a potent and orally bioavailable inhibitor of the enzyme. *Journal of the American Chemical Society*, **117**, 1181–1182.

Kissinger, C.R., Gehlhaar, D.K. and Fogel, D.B. (1999) Rapid automated molecular replacement by evolutionary search. *Acta Crystallographica*, **D55**, 484–491.

Kleywegt, G.J. (1999) Recognition of spatial motifs in protein structures. *Journal of Molecular Biology*, **285**, 1887–1897.

Kolb, V.A., Makeyev, E.V. and Spirin, A.S. (2000) Co-translational folding of an eukaryotic multidomain protein in a prokaryotic translation system. *Journal of Biological Chemistry*, **275**, 16597–16601.

Kuhn, P., Wilson, K., Patch, M.G. and Stevens, R.C. (2002) The genesis of high-throughput structure-based drug discovery using protein crystallography. *Current Opinion in Chemical Biology*, **6**, 704–710.

Lamzin, V.S. and Perrakis, A. (2000) Current state of automated crystallographic data analysis. *Nature Structural Biology*, **7**(Suppl.), 978–981.

Laskowski, R.A., Watson, J.D. and Thornton, J.M. (2003) From protein structure to biochemical function? *Journal of Structural and Functional Genomics*, **4**, 167–177.

Li, X., Romero, P., Rani, M., Dunker, A.K. and Obradovic, Z. (1999) Predicting protein disorder for N-, C-, and internal regions. *Genome Informatics. Series: Workshop on Genome Informatics*, **10**, 30–40.

Li, X., Obradovic, Z., Brown, C.J., Garner, E.C. and Dunker, A.K. (2000) Comparing predictors of disordered protein. *Genome Informatics. Series: Workshop on Genome Informatics*, **11**, 172–184.

Linding, R., Russell, R.B., Neduva, V. and Gibson, T.J. (2003a) GlobPlot: exploring protein sequences for globularity and disorder. *Nucleic Acids Research*, **31**, 3701–3708.

Linding, R., Jensen, L.J., Diella, F., Bork, P., Gibson, T.J. and Russell, R.B. (2003b) Protein disorder prediction: implications for structural proteomics. *Structure*, **11**, 1453–1459.

Linial, M. and Yona, G. (2000) Methodologies for target selection in structural genomics. *Progress in Biophysics and Molecular Biology*, **73**, 297–320.

Madej, T., Gibrat, J.F. and Bryant, S.H. (1995) Threading a database of protein cores. *Proteins*, **23**, 356–369.

Manjasetty, B.A., Delbruck, H., Pham, D.T., Mueller, U., Fieber-Erdmann, M., Scheich, C., Sievert, V., Bussow, K., Niesen, F.H., Weihofen, W., Loll, B., Saenger, W., Heinemann, U. and Niesen, F.H. (2004)

Crystal structure of Homo sapiens protein hp14.5 *Proteins*, **54**, 797–800.

Montelione, G.T., Zheng, D., Huang, Y.J., Gunsalus, K.C. and Szyperski, T. (2000) Protein NMR spectroscopy in structural genomics. *Nature Structural Biology*, **7**(Suppl.), 982–985.

Mueller, U., Büssow, K., Diehl, A., Bartl, F.J., Niesen, F.H., Nyarsik, L. and Heinemann, U. (2003) Rapid purification and crystal structure analysis of a small protein carrying two terminal affinity tags. *Journal of Structural and Functional Genomics*, **4**, 217–225.

Navaza, J. (2001) Implementation of molecular replacement in AMoRe. *Acta Crystallographica*, **D57**, 1367–1372.

Netzer, W.J. and Hartl, F.U. (1997) Recombination of protein domains facilitated by co-translational folding in eukaryotes. *Nature*, **388**, 343–349.

Novotny, M., Madsen, D. and Kleywegt, G.J. (2004) Evaluation of protein fold comparison servers. *Proteins*, **54**, 260–270.

Oldfield, T.J. (2001) X-LIGAND: an application for the automated addition of flexible ligands into electron density. *Acta Crystallographica*, **D57**, 696–705.

Pandey, N., Ganapathi, M., Kumar, K., Dasgupta, D., Das Sutar, S.K. and Dash, D. (2004) Comparative analysis of protein unfoldedness in human housekeeping and non-housekeeping proteins. *Bioinformatics*, **20**, 2904–2910.

Pape, T. and Schneider, T.R. (2004) HKL2MAP: a graphical user interface for phasing with SHELX programs. *Journal of Applied Crystallography*, **37**, 843–844.

Perrakis, A., Morris, R. and Lamzin, V.S. (1999) Automated protein model building combined with iterative structure refinement. *Nature Structural Biology*, **6**, 458–463.

Potterton, E., Briggs, P., Turkenburg, M. and Dodson, E. (2003) A graphical user interface to the CCP4 program suite. *Acta Crystallographica*, **D59**, 1131–1137.

Prinz, B., Schultchen, J., Rydzewski, R., Holz, C., Boettner, M., Stahl, U. and Lang, C. (2004) Establishing a versatile fermentation and purification procedure for human proteins expressed in the yeasts Saccharomyces cerevisiae and

Pichia pastoris for structural genomics. *Journal of Structural and Functional Genomics*, **5**, 29–44.

Rasmussen, S.G.F., Choi, H.-J., Rosenbaum, D.M., Kobilka, T.S., Thian, F.S., Edwards, P.C., Burghammer, M., Ratnala, V.R.P., Sanishvili, R., Fischetti, R.F., Schertler, G.F.X., Weis, W.I. and Kobilka, B.K. (2007) Crystal structure of the human β_2 adrenergic G-protein-coupled receptor. *Nature*, **450**, 383–387.

Read, R.J. (2001) Pushing the boundaries of molecular replacement with maximum likelihood. *Acta Crystallographica*, **D57**, 1373–1382.

Romier, C., Ben Jelloul, M., Albeck, S., Buchwald, G., Busso, D., Celie, P.H.N., Christodoulou, E., De Marco, V., van Gerwen, S., Knipscheer, P., Lebbink, J.H., Notenboom, V., Poterszman, A., Rochel, N., Cohen, S.X., Unger, T., Sussman, J.L., Moras, D., Sixma, T.K. and Perrakis, A. (2006) Co-expression of protein complexes in prokaryotic and eukaryotic hosts: Experimental procedures, database tracking and case studies. *Acta Crystallographica*, **D62**, 1232–1242.

Sanchez, R., Pieper, U., Melo, F., Eswar, N., Marti-Renom, M.A., Madhusudhan, M.S., Mirkovic, N. and Sali, A. (2000) Protein structure modeling for structural genomics. *Nature Structural Biology*, **7**(Suppl.), 986–990.

Sanishvili, R., Yakunin, A.F., Laskowski, R.A., Skarina, T., Evdokimova, E., Doherty-Kirby, A., Lajoie, G.A., Thornton, J.M., Arrowsmith, C.H., Savchenko, A., Joachimiak, A. and Edwards, A.M. (2003) Integrating structure, bioinformatics, and enzymology to discover function: BioH, a new carboxylesterase from Escherichia coli. *Journal of Biological Chemistry*, **278**, 26039–26045.

Sawasaki, T., Ogasawara, T., Morishita, R. and Endo, Y. (2002) A cell-free protein synthesis system for high-throughput proteomics. *Proceedings of the National Academy of Sciences of the United States of America*, **99**, 14652–14657.

Scheich, C., Kümmel, D., Soumailakakis, D., Heinemann, U. and Büssow, K. (2007) Vectors for co-expression of an unrestricted number of proteins. *Nucleic Acids Research*, **35**(e43), 1–7.

Schneider, T.R. and Sheldrick, G.M. (2002) Substructure solution with SHELXD. *Acta Crystallographica*, **D58**, 1772–1779.

Schwede, T., Kopp, J., Guex, N. and Peitsch, M.C. (2003) SWISS-MODEL: an automated protein homology-modeling server. *Nucleic Acids Research*, **31**, 3381–3385.

Spriggs, R.V., Artymiuk, P.J. and Willett, P. (2003) Searching for patterns of amino acids in 3D protein structures. *Journal of Chemical Information and Computer Sciences*, **43**, 412–421.

Stevens, R.C. (2000) Design of high-throughput methods of protein production for structural biology. *Structure Folding and Design*, **8**, R177–R185.

Stewart, L., Clark, R. and Behnke, C. (2002) High-throughput crystallization and structure determination in drug discovery. *Drug Discovery Today*, **7**, 187–196.

Sun, P.D. and Radaev, S. (2002) Generating isomorphous heavy-atom derivatives by a quick-soak method. Part II: phasing of new structures. *Acta Crystallographica*, **D58**, 1099–1103.

Sun, P.D., Radaev, S. and Kattah, M. (2002) Generating isomorphous heavy-atom derivatives by a quick-soak method. Part I: test cases. *Acta Crystallographica*, **D58**, 1092–1098.

Szyperski, T., Yeh, D.C., Sukumaran, D.K., Moseley, H.N. and Montelione, G.T. (2002) Reduced-dimensionality NMR spectroscopy for high-throughput protein resonance assignment. *Proceedings of the National Academy of Sciences of the United States of America*, **99**, 8009–8014.

Terwilliger, T.C. (2000) Maximum-likelihood density modification. *Acta Crystallographica*, **D56**, 965–972.

Terwilliger, T.C. and Berendzen, J. (1999) Automated MAD and MIR structure solution. *Acta Crystallographica*, **D55**, 849–861.

Thornton, J.M., Todd, A.E., Milburn, D., Borkakoti, N. and Orengo, C.A. (2000) From structure to function: approaches and limitations. *Nature Structural Biology*, **7**(Suppl.), 991–994.

Tickle, I., Sharff, A., Vinkovic, M., Yon, J. and Jhoti, H. (2004) High-throughput protein crystallography and drug discovery. *Chemical Society Reviews*, **33**, 558–565.

Vagin, A. and Teplyakov, A. (1997) MOLREP: an automated program for molecular replacement. *Journal of Applied Crystallography*, **30**, 1022–1025.

Voss, S. and Skerra, A. (1997) Mutagenesis of a flexible loop in streptavidin leads to higher affinity for the Strep-tag II peptide and improved performance in recombinant protein purification. *Protein Engineering*, **10**, 975–982.

Walter, T.S., Diprose, J., Brown, J., Pickford, M., Owens, R.J., Stuart, D.I. and Harlos, K. (2003) A procedure for setting up high-throughput nanoliter crystallization experiments. I. Protocol design and validation. *Journal of Applied Crystallography*, **36**, 308–314.

Watanabe, N., Murai, H. and Tanaka, I. (2002) Semi-automatic protein crystallization system that allows in situ observation of X-ray diffraction from crystals in the drop. *Acta Crystallographica*, **D58**, 1527–1530.

Watson, J.D., Todd, A.E., Bray, J., Laskowski, R.A., Edwards, A., Joachimiak, A., Orengo, C.A. and Thornton, J.M. (2003) Target selection and determination of function in structural genomics. *IUBMB Life*, **55**, 249–255.

Xu, H., Hauptman, H. and Weeks, C.M. (2002) Sine-enhanced shake-and-bake: the theoretical basis for applications to Se-atom substructures. *Acta Crystallographica*, **D58**, 90–96.

Yee, A., Pardee, K., Christendat, D., Savchenko, A., Edwards, A.M. and Arrowsmith, C.H. (2003) Structural proteomics: toward high-throughput structural biology as a tool in functional genomics. *Accounts of Chemical Research*, **36**, 183–189.

Zheng, B., Roach, L.S. and Ismagilov, R.F. (2003) Screening of protein crystallization conditions on a microfluidic chip using nanoliter-size droplets. *Journal of the American Chemical Society*, **125**, 11170–11171.

Zheng, B., Tice, J.D., Roach, L.S. and Ismagilov, R.F. (2004) A droplet-based, composite PDMS/glass capillary microfluidic system for evaluating protein crystallization conditions by microbatch and vapor-diffusion methods with on-chip X-ray diffraction. *Angewandte Chemie-International Edition in English*, **43**, 2508–2511.

6

Primer to Proteins Underlying Cellular Complexity and Function in the Nervous System

Kojiro Yano

6.1
Molecular Complexity in Neurons

The nervous system displays an immense complexity in many different ways. Because the tasks it can perform are so sophisticated and unique, it would be natural to assume that the nervous system must incorporate specific proteins that somehow drive these specific functions. Moore and co-workers first identified the brain-specific proteins 14-3-2 protein and S-100 (Moore, 1969) by comparing two-dimensional patterns of brain and liver proteins fractionated by chromatography and electrophoresis. Their work was followed by the discovery of other brain-specific proteins such as neuron-specific enolase (ENO2) (Zomzely-Neurath and Walker, 1980) and glial fibrillary acidic protein (GFAP) (Eng, 1980). However, it became apparent that nervous system-specific proteins cannot turn non-neural tissue into neural tissue on its own. It is rather the combination and the interaction of proteins that create the structural and functional complexities within the nervous system. Therefore, the study of the complexity of the nervous system will inevitably require accurate pictures of protein expressions on a global scale and these have become attainable only after development of proteomic techniques integrating electrophoresis, chromatography, mass spectrometry, and bioinformatics to identify a large number of proteins from a sample.

Proteomic studies of the mammalian nervous system have allowed us to identify a wide variety of known and unknown proteins in different brain areas or subcellular compartments, such as plasma membrane, mitochondria, and synaptic membranes. The identified proteins can be studied further to characterize their distributions and functions in specific cell types of the nervous system.

Publicly available data for the proteome of the nervous system are not as abundant as the transcriptomic profiles, but recent quantitative proteomic studies have provided useful information that can give us some insights into the protein composition of the nervous system (Ong and Mann, 2005). Ishihama *et al.* (2005) obtained absolute quantification for over a hundred proteins in

Proteomics of the Nervous System. Edited by H.G. Nothwang and S.E. Pfeiffer
Copyright © 2008 WILEY-VCH Verlag GmbH & Co. KGaA, Weinheim
ISBN: 978-3-527-31716-5

mouse whole brain by using culture-derived isotope tags, which can accurately monitor the amount of each identified protein. Kislinger *et al.* (2006), on the other hand, profiled protein expression in subcellular fractions of brain (and other organs) and provided information on the relative protein abundance for >2000 proteins based on the number of spectral matches for each protein. Finally, Yu *et al.* (2004) obtained proteins from primary cultures of cortical neurons and semi-quantified their relative amounts from the number of unique peptides identified for each protein. Although these three studies were based on different sample preparation and quantification methods, it is possible to observe a consistent pattern (Table 6.1) with cytoskeletal proteins, molecular motors, chaperones, and metabolic proteins being among the most abundant proteins. These protein functional groups were also dominant in terms of the number of member proteins found in whole-protein expression profiles obtained by conventional qualitative proteomics (Shin *et al.*, 2005; Pollak *et al.*, 2006).

In the following sections, I will review the proteins that are frequently found in proteomic analyses of central nervous systems, both from cytosol and subcellular compartments. Rather than providing general descriptions of the proteins, I have concentrated on giving details about how they are expressed in the developing and adult brains, particularly in cerebral cortex and the particular roles they play in neurons.

6.1.1
Cytosolic Proteins

6.1.1.1 Cytoskeletons
Cytoskeletons are found ubiquitously in eukaryotic cells and are involved in fundamental cellular processes, including cell division, intracellular transport, and the maintenance of cellular structure. They are made up of three classes of proteins: microtubules, microfilaments, and intermediate filaments, and all classes are found abundantly in the nervous system.

Protofilaments are the core structure in microtubules. They are built up from dimers of α- and β-tubulins, polymerized end to end, and they assemble with each other to form a hollow tube. There are at least six isotypes known to both α- and β-tubulins and they have distinct spatial and temporal expression patterns, though the functional significance of having so many isoforms is yet to be fully understood (Ludueña, 1993). The brain has two major isotypes of α-tubulin; α1B (Tuba1B) and α1A (Tuba1A) (Sullivan, 1988). Tuba1B is one of the most abundant proteins in both embryonic and adult brain and its expression level shows little change during development, whereas the expression of Tuba1A is high in the embryonic brain, particularly in the cortical plate, and then decreases significantly in the adult brain (Miller *et al.*, 1987; Gloster *et al.*, 1994; Gloster *et al.*, 1999; Ishihama *et al.*, 2005). Moreover it has been shown that a disruption of the Tuba1A gene caused

Table 6.1 Three studies of brain proteomes and biological process gene ontologies which were over-represented.[a]

Studies	Ishihama *et al.* (2005)	Yu *et al.* (2004)	Kislinger *et al.* (2006)
Origin of the samples	Whole brains	Cultured cortical neurons	Cytosolic fractions of whole brains
Over-represented biological process gene ontologies	**Glycolysis** (ATP5O ATP5A1 ALDOA GAPDH PGAM1 ATP5B PKM2 ENO1)	**Cytoskeleton organization and biogenesis** (KIF5C SPNA2 ACTN4 MACF1 DYNC1H1 MYH9 MYH10 MYO5A RTN4 NBEA MTAP1B SPNB2 MTAP2 OPA1)	**Glycolysis** (GPI1 PKM2 PGK1 ENO2 ALDOA PGAM1 ENO1 UCHL1 ATP6V1A)
	Intracellular transport (VIM CALR ARBP YWHAZ SLC25A5 TUBA2 CFL1 RAN RPS8 RPS16 HSPA9 PRDX1 TUBB5)	**Cell motility** (KIF5C ACTN4 RTN4 MACF1 ATP1A1 MYH9 MYH10 ATP1A3)	**Cytoskeleton organization and biogenesis** (SPNA2 DYNC1H1 CFL1 TUBB3 TUBB2C TUBA1A UCHL1 MTAP2)
	Protein folding (HSPA8 HSPA9 CALR CCT8 HSP90AA1);	**Response to unfolded protein** (HSPA8 HSP90B1 HSPA5 HSP90AB1 HSPA4)	

[a] Calculated for 30 most strongly expressed genes using GOstat (http://gostat.wehi.edu.au/). Gene ontologies with the same members or only one member difference were clustered and only one representative gene ontology from each cluster is mentioned here for simplicity. Cluster members are listed in brackets. Gene ontology data were obtained from MGI.

aberrant neuronal migration in mice and lissencephaly in humans (Keays *et al.*, 2007). There are three major isotypes of β-tubulin: class I, II, and III. Class I and II are expressed in both neuronal and non-neuronal tissues, whereas class III is specifically expressed in neurons (Sullivan *et al.*, 1986; Burgoyne *et al.*, 1988). In general, their expression in the nervous system is higher during neuronal development (Joshi and Cleveland, 1989; Jiang and Oblinger, 1992) and class II and III (but not class I) β-tubulins are also upregulated during axonal regeneration (Hoffman, 1989; Moskowitz and Oblinger, 1995; Fournier and McKerracher, 1997). Moreover, class II β-tubulin is expressed in nestin- and vimentin-positive radial fibers in embryonic brain and neural stem cells as well as in outgrowing axons and dendrites, while class III β-tubulin is expressed at a later developmental stage, namely in postmitotic neuronal precursors (Lee *et al.*, 1990; Menezes and Luskin, 1994).

Microfilaments are actin-based thin filaments involved in intracellular transport and cell movement. Multiple actin genes exist in mammalian genomes and β- and γ-actins are present in the nervous system. In neurons, actin microfilaments are predominantly found in presynaptic terminals, dendritic spines, and growth cones, where they are directly involved in their formation, maintenance, and restructuring (Luo, 2002; Dillon and Goda, 2005). The actin genes are expressed throughout development, but they are strongly upregulated in the first postnatal week in rodents when synaptogenesis occurs, and then settle down to adult levels (Lazarini *et al.*, 1991; Poddar *et al.*, 1996). In the cytosol, actin exists either as F-actin (filament) or as G-actin (monomer) and transitions between the two states are fundamental for remodeling of actin filaments. The transitions are controlled by a number of actin-binding proteins which help to shape the actin filament networks designed for different purposes (Winder and Ayscough, 2005). For example, cofilin, a ubiquitous and abundant actin binding protein (Yonezawa *et al.*, 1987), promotes dissociation of actin from F-actin and cofilin activation by neurodegenerative stimuli disrupt distal neurite function in Alzheimer's disease (Minamide *et al.*, 2000).

Finally, intermediate filaments are cytosolic filaments with diameters between those of microfilaments and microtubules. They include a wide variety of proteins in both neuronal and non-neuronal tissues and constitute a protein family of five classes (types I–V). Vimentin (Carmo-Fonseca and David-Ferreira, 1990) is a highly abundant intermediate filament found in glia cells and early differentiating neurons (Bignami *et al.*, 1982). During axonal injury, vimentin forms a complex with importin-β as well as phosphorylated Erks and mediates the binding of Erks, via the importin, to dyneins. This results in translocation of Erks into lesioned nerves. Accordingly, in vimentin knockout mice, this process is disrupted and the mice showed significant delays in neuronal regeneration (Perlson *et al.*, 2005).

Neurofilaments are another major class of intermediate filament found predominantly in axons. They are composed of three subunits: light (NFL), medium (NFM), and heavy (NFH), which are named according to the C-terminal tail sizes. Neurofilaments are characterized by unusually high levels of phosphorylation which seems to affect association of neurofilaments to dynein (Motil *et al.*, 2006) and kinesin (Jung *et al.*, 2005). In neurodegenerative diseases, including amyotropic lateral sclerosis (ALS) (Lobsiger *et al.*, 2005), neurofilaments are often found to be disorganized and it has been suggested that abnormal neurofilaments can directly cause selective neuronal death (Julien, 1999). In NFH-null mice, reductions in motor axon growth were relatively small, perhaps because of compensatory changes in NFL and NFM, while disruptions of NFM or NFL resulted in significant axonal atrophy. On the other hand, overexpression of NFL caused its aggregation and resulted in neuronal dysfunctions similar to motor neuron diseases (Xu *et al.*, 1993). Moreover, mutations which are linked to Charcot-Marie-Tooth disease 2E ("axonal type") disrupted neurofilament assembly and promoted neurofilament aggregation in neurons (Sasaki *et al.*, 2006). These results suggest that abnormal accumulation of neurofilaments, rather than lack of them, is one of the key mechanisms of axonal degeneration in neurodegenerative diseases.

6.1.1.2 Protein Quality Control

Proteins produced by cells need to be folded into their characteristic shapes and to associate with correct partners to be fully functional in cells. Misfolded proteins can accumulate in a cell or in the extracellular space and will form cytotoxic aggregates which have been linked to disorders such as Alzheimer's disease, Creutzfeldt–Jakob disease and systemic amyloidosis (Selkoe, 2003). In order to facilitate protein production, molecular chaperones bind unstable proteins and help correct protein folding and complex formation. Since neurons need to produce a wide variety of proteins for complex subcellular compartments, such as axons or dendritic arbors, it is not surprising that molecular chaperones are abundant in the nervous system.

Major cytosolic chaperones in the nervous system include Hsp90-α and the highly homologous Hsp90-β as well as the Hsc70 (Aquino *et al.*, 1993). Both Hsp90-β and Hsc70 are expressed from E9.5 on, whereas Hsp90-α starts to be seen from E15.5 on (D'Souza and Brown, 1998; Loones *et al.*, 2000). In addition to their role as chaperones, hsp90s and hsc70 have more specific functions for neurons. Hsc70 is present in postsynaptic terminals (Suzuki *et al.*, 1999) and is involved in clathrin-uncoating in receptor-mediated endocytosis (Ungewickell, 1985; Morgan *et al.*, 2001) as well as in axonal vesicle transport (Tsai *et al.*, 2000). Hsp90, on the other hand, was found to be essential for retrieving Rab1 from the membrane and perhaps for other processes in Rab GTPase recycling in intracellular trafficking pathways (Chen and Balch, 2006).

6.1.1.3 Metabolic Enzymes

The brain exhibits the highest energy demand among all organs and uses glucose as the main energy source. As would be expected, the brain maintains high concentrations of proteins related to glucose metabolism, including glyceraldehyde-3-phosphate dehydrogenase (GAPDH), pyruvate kinase, enolase, phosphoglycerate mutase (PGAM), fluctose-bisphosphate aldolase, glucose-6-phosphate isomerase (G6PI), phosphoglycerate kinase 1 (PGK1), and lactate dehydrogenase (Ishihama *et al.*, 2005; Kislinger *et al.*, 2006). In addition to their classical roles, these enzymes have functions outside glycolysis and gluconeogenesis and influence various physiological and pathological processes in neurons. For example, GAPDH binds to several proteins related to neurodegenerative diseases, including β-amyloid, huntingtin, α-synuclein, parkin, atrophin, and ataxin-1 (Mazzola and Sirover,

2002) and the interactions can happen in the cytosol, the plasma membrane or the nucleus. The expression of GAPDH is upregulated by p53 and in apoptotic stimulus, and then GAPDH accumulates in the nucleus where it suppresses the transcription of pro-survival proteins Bcl-2 and Bcl-XL (Tatton *et al.*, 2003). On the other hand, G6PI, also known as neuroleukin, is a neurotrophic factor for spinal and sensory neurons (Gurney *et al.*, 1986) and its inhibition sensitizes neuronal cells to caspase-dependent apoptosis (Romagnoli *et al.*, 2003).

6.1.2
Molecular Organizations in Subcellular Neuronal Compartments

6.1.2.1 Plasma Membrane

As can be expected from the physiological functions of neurons, many of the abundant plasma membrane proteins are related to transmission of action potentials. The generation and propagation of action potentials are mainly mediated by inward Na^+ currents and outward K^+ currents, and the fluxes of these two ions across the membrane are driven in part by their concentration gradients, which are maintained by the Na^+/K^+ ATPase. Arrival of an action potential at the presynaptic terminal results in Ca^{2+} influx, which triggers the exocytosis of synaptic vesicles, which contain glutamate in excitatory synapses, and GABA or glycine in inhibitory synapses. An activation of ionotropic glutamate receptors triggers non-selective cation fluxes, resulting in membrane depolarization and, if sufficiently strong, initiation of action potentials. On the other hand, an activation of GABA or glycine receptors triggers Cl^- influx, which causes hyperpolarization of the postsynaptic neuron, thereby inhibiting the generation of action potentials.

Both α and β chains of the Na^+/K^+ pump are frequently found in the nervous system and so are the K^+/Cl^- cotransporters (KCC) which counteract the Na^+/K^+ pump by extruding K^+ and Cl^- from the cell. KCCs are believed to regulate cell volume and GABA receptor-mediated Cl^- flux by altering the Cl^- concentration gradient across the plasma membrane. The modulation of Cl^- flux by KCC2 is perhaps one of the mechanisms for spike time-dependent plasticity in inhibitory synapses (Stell and Mody, 2003). Proteins for cytosolic Ca^{2+} signaling, namely Ca^{2+} channels, Ca^{2+} pumps, Ca^{2+}-binding proteins and two types of endoplasmic Ca^{2+} release channels, namely IP_3 receptors and ryanodine receptors, are also frequently found in the plasma membrane. While it is possible that some are indeed present as integral proteins in the plasma membrane (Dellis *et al.*, 2006), the majority of the endoplasmic Ca^{2+} channels are probably present in the membrane of the endoplasmatic reticulum, which is in close contact with the plasma membrane (see below). Plasma membrane-bound Ca^{2+} ATPases (PMCA) and sarcoplasmic/endoplasmic Ca^{2+} ATPases (SERCA) terminate cytosolic Ca^{2+} signals by transporting Ca^{2+} into the extracellular space and into the ER, respectively. Their high abundance may underline their importance in limiting the time and spatial extents of Ca^{2+} microdomains (Berridge, 2006).

Plasma membrane proteins furthermore mediate attachment of cells to the extracellular space and are involved in cell movements. Both functions require subplasmalemmal cytoskeletons associated with large linker proteins. Spectrin is a large structural protein found abundantly in the nervous system (approximately 3% of the total lipid-soluble proteins). It forms a mesh-like protein complex with actin beneath the plasma membrane (Bennett and Gilligan, 1993) and its mutation causes spinocerebellar ataxia (Ikeda *et al.*, 2006). Spectrin can interact either directly or through the adaptor molecule ankyrin, to ion channels and cell adhesion molecules (e.g. NCAM-180) in the plasma membrane (Dubreuil, 2006). The interaction between spectrin and ankyrin is often found in specific cellular subdomains where it can affect distribution and function of membrane proteins. For example, a loss of spectrin at the neuromuscular junction will cause disorganization and elimination of essential synaptic cell-adhesion molecules and finally result in synaptic disassembly (Pielage *et al.*, 2005). The subplasmalemma spectrin–ankyrin complex also binds to plectin, which interacts with cytoskeletons as well as with proteins in intracellular membrane structures. While the function of its interaction with plectin in the nervous system remains to be elucidated, a result from MDCK (Madin-Darby canine kidney) cells suggests that it may be involved in polarized distribution of membrane proteins (Eger *et al.*, 1997).

Notably, subfractioned plasma membrane contains many proteins which are referred to as "contaminants." For example, Schindler *et al.* (2006) identified 197 plasma membrane proteins as well as proteins thought to be present in mitochondria (37 proteins) and in the ER (24 proteins). Olsen *et al.* (2007) identified the same number of plasma membrane proteins but also 102 mitochondrial proteins and 35 ER proteins in enriched plasma membrane fractions. While some of these proteins may represent contaminations, many of them are probably in direct contact with the plasma membrane.

Close alignments between the plasma membrane and the mitochondrial and ER membrane have been shown by immunoprecipitation (Lencesova *et al.*, 2004), electron microscopy of ER and mitochondrial membrane (Johnson *et al.*, 2003) as well as by the observation that Ca^{2+} entry through the plasma membrane rapidly increased Ca^{2+} levels in mitochondria or the ER (Mogami *et al.*, 1997).

6.1.2.2 Synaptic Vesicles

Chemical transmission of action potentials at the synapse occurs by the release of neurotransmitters from the presynaptic plasma membrane via exocytosis of synaptic vesicles (see Chapter 8). Synaptic vesicles are high in proton and zinc, which are maintained by vacuolar proton pumps (vATPases) and zinc transporters (ZnT), respectively. The proton gradient across the vesicular membrane drives transport of neurotransmitters such as glutamate (Shigeri *et al.*, 2004) and GABA (Gasnier, 2004) by proton exchangers while the vesicular zinc seems to be involved in synaptic plasticity (Kodirov *et al.*, 2006). Synaptic vesicles are associated with glycolytic enzymes, including aldolase, GAPDH, and lactate dehydrogenase, which may supply energy for ion transports in the vesicular membrane (Wu *et al.*, 1997). Furthermore, synaptic vesicles contain abundant Ca^{2+} which stabilizes vesicular proteins. The precise mechanism of maintaining intravesicular Ca^{2+} is not known, but it may partly be mediated by SV2 transporters.

Synaptic vesicles are often found to be clustered in front of the presynaptic plasma membrane, perhaps representing the reserve pool, and then move to the presynaptic plasma membrane ("docking") before undergoing exocytosis. Synaptic vesicles contain a considerable amount of neuronal phosphoproteins called synapsins. These proteins interact with cytoskeletal structures which are mainly composed of actin filaments, microtubules, and spectrins (Hilfiker *et al.*, 1999), and the interaction seems to influence localization of synaptic vesicles. Deletions of synapsin I and II genes increased vesicle release (Lonart and Simsek-Duran, 2006) but decreased the number of synaptic vesicles (Bogen *et al.*, 2006). This effect can partly be explained by a disrupted interaction between vesicles and actin filaments. These filaments are known to work as a scaffold for the vesicles in the terminals (Sankaranarayanan *et al.*, 2003) and disrupted interaction of synaptic vesicles with actin increases the probablity that vesicles will be released (Morales *et al.*, 2000).

Other synaptic proteins with a crucial role in vesicle trafficking are Rab proteins. Rab proteins are GTP-binding proteins, of which there are a number of subfamilies. Rab3 is the most abundant (about 25% of total Rab GTP binding in the brain is Rab3A) (Sudhof, 2004). In synaptic vesicles, Rab3A is in the GTP-bound form but hydrolyzes to GDP upon synaptic vesicle fusion and dissociates from synaptic vesicles in a Ca^{2+}-dependent manner (Ghijsen and Leenders, 2005). It is then recycled to other synaptic vesicles. According to studies in knockout mice, Rab3A is crucial for recruiting synaptic vesicles after depolarization (Leenders *et al.*, 2001) and lack of Rab3A results in impaired spatial learning (D'Adamo *et al.*, 2004). The GTP-bound form of Rab3A is associated with Rab3 effectors, which are released upon GTP hydrolysis. A genetic disruption of rabphilin, one of the Rab effectors, did not directly alter exocytosis, but recent evidence suggests that the protein regulates recovery of depleted synaptic vesicles (Deák *et al.*, 2006) and probably vesicular docking through interaction with SNAP-25 (see below) (Tsuboi and Fukuda, 2005).

During exocytosis, the synaptic vesicle membrane fuses tightly with the presynaptic plasma membrane. The proteins involved in this process are known as core complex or SNARE complex and are characterized by an amino acid sequence called the SNARE motif (Sudhof, 2004). The SNARE proteins involved in synaptic exocytosis are synaptobrevin (also called as vesicle-associated membrane protein or VAMP) on the vesicular membrane, and syntaxin 1 and SNAP-25 on the presynaptic plasma membrane. Association of synaptobrevin to the SNARE complex is regulated by synaptophysin (Valtorta *et al.*, 2004), which directly binds to synaptobrevin and regulates its availability to the complex. Inhibition of synaptophysin results in a marked decrease in frequency of neurotransmitter release but not in amplitude, a finding consistent with the idea that this molecule is involved in the final step of exocytosis rather than determining the quantal size of the transmitter release (Alder *et al.*, 1992, 1995). The SNARE complex is also likely to be involved in Ca^{2+} sensitivity of vesicular exocytosis. The complex itself does not contain Ca^{2+}-sensing domains, but can associate with synaptotagmins which then confer Ca^{2+} sensitivity to the vesicles. Synaptotagmin 1 and its less characterized isoform 2 have a transmembrane region and two cytoplasmic domains with five Ca^{2+}-binding sites in total. The Ca^{2+} binding occurs with a high cooperativity, resulting in a steep dependency of exocytosis on Ca^{2+} concentration. The exact molecular mechanism of synaptotagmin action is not resolved, but it has been proposed that synaptotagmins first bind to the SNARE complex in a Ca^{2+}-independent manner and an increase of Ca^{2+} concentration causes them to switch to the phospholipid membrane. This switch may then generate some mechanical stress to the fusion intermediate, forcing it to open the fusion pore.

6.1.2.3 Mitochondria

Mitochondria take centerstage in cellular ATP synthesis. The energy to produce ATP through ATP synthase originates from NADH and FADH, the majority of which is generated by the tricarboxylic acid cycle. Since the cycle depends heavily on glycolysis-derived products, mitochondria are often physically associated with some cytosolic glycolytic enzymes such as hexokinase (Kabir and Nelson, 1991), aldolase (Sáez and Slebe, 2000), and GAPDH (Tarze *et al.*, 2007), probably to improve the efficiency of the supply. In line with these findings, several cytosolic glycolytic enzymes (enolase, GAPDH, pyruvate kinase, and aldolase A) have been found to be abundant in brain mitochondria (Kislinger *et al.*, 2006).

Mitochondria require import of nuclear-encoded proteins. They therefore contain several chaperone proteins which, rather than responding to stress conditions, have important functions in this transport process (Voos and Röttgers, 2002). In the matrix of mitochondria, mitochondrial Hsp70 receives and stabilizes unfolded proteins from the cytosol coming through import channels which span across the outer and the inner membrane of mitochondria. The proteins are then passed to a complex formed by Hsp60 and Hsp10, which facilitates folding reactions: Finally, folded proteins are released into the matrix as mature proteins. Those which are not folded properly will be processed by proteases and hsp70 which facilitates degradation by unfolding the misfolded proteins (Savel'ev *et al.*, 1998).

In living cells, mitochondria often assume web-like shapes around the nucleus overwrapping with the ER. Sometimes they cluster below the plasma membrane or around secretory vesicles, and their shapes and distributions change continuously. Such changes require a network of cytoskeletal proteins to control movement and tethering of mitochondria (Anesti and Scorrano, 2006). In the brain, mitochondria are bound to tubulin, actin, and their associated proteins (cofilin and spectrin) as well as those related to intracellular vesicle targeting (synapsin and syntaxin) (Sudhof, 2004). While microtubules are primarily employed for long-distance transport of mitochondria (Hollenbeck and Saxton, 2005), short-distance transport and tethering of mitochondria at the cell surface as well as mitochondrial fission require actin cytoskeleton (De Vos *et al.*, 2005; Boldogh and Pon, 2006).

Cytoskeleton may also play significant roles in mitochondria-mediated apoptotic processes. This has been suggested from the observations that mitochondria tend to redistribute and aggregate around the nucleus in cells undergoing apoptosis (De Vos *et al.*, 1998). β-Actin is required for this change, and reduction of actin turnover (Li *et al.*, 2004) or stabilization of actin filaments by jasplakinolide induce cell death (Posey and Bierer, 1999).

6.2
Cellular Complexity in the Nervous System and Neuronal Cell Types

6.2.1
Basic Classification of Neuronal Cell Types

Neuronal cell types are classified according to a combination of criteria based on morphological, electrophysiological, and neurochemical characteristics. In the cerebral cortex, for example, neurons can be classified according to morphology as pyramidal and non-pyramidal cells (Table 6.2). Pyramidal cells have a characteristic triangular "pyramidal" morphology with a long apical dendrite, while "non-pyramidal" cells have thin dendrites spreading from small, round-shaped soma. While pyramidal cells are concentrated in particular cortical layers, non-pyramidal cells tend to have a more diffused distribution, showing less layer specificity. Electrophysiologically, pyramidal cells and non-pyramidal cells can be distinguished by spiking patterns during step-current injections, the former having wider spikes with lower maximum firing frequency than the latter (Figure 6.1). And finally, cortical pyramidal cells are excitatory neurons using glutamate as a neurotransmitter, while the majority of non-pyramidal cells are GABAergic inhibitory neurons. Although none of these criteria are perfectly specific to a particular cell type (e.g. some non-pyramidal cells have "pyramidal"-like spiking patterns), a combination of them gives us enough to define a neuronal cell type. Since the study of neuronal cell types has a long history, there are excellent reviews available for their general characteristics, some of which are listed in Table 6.2. These reviews are supplemented here by information which will be useful particularly for proteomic study of neuronal subtypes, namely their protein markers. It should be noted, however, that most of these markers are expressed in more

Table 6.2 Some interneurons in cerebral cortex.

Cell type	Morphological feature	Known marker	Reference
Basket cells	Dendrites go all directions, horizontal axons	Parvalbumin, NPY	(Markram *et al.*, 2004) (Kisvarday, 1993)
Bipolar cells	Vertically oriented oval soma with ascending and descending processes from the top and bottom ends	VIP	(Peters, 1990)
Double bouquet cells	Long vertical branching axons forming narrow bundles	Calbindin	(DeFelipe and Jones, 1992)
Martinotti cells	Multipolar, vertical axons going towards layer I and the pia	Somatostatin	(Xu *et al.*, 2006)
Chandelier cells	Extensive axons which synapse on the initial segments of pyramidal cell axons	Parvalbumin	(Howard *et al.*, 2005)

than one cell type and their distribution changes continuously during prenatal and postnatal development.

6.2.2
Molecular Markers and Neuronal Cell Types

From a proteomic point of view, molecular markers would be very useful to identify and isolate specific neuronal populations. These markers work most effectively when they are expressed in transgenic animals as fluorescent-tagged proteins. Particular neuronal subtypes can hence be easily identified and isolated by fluorescent microscopy or flow cytometry. Molecular markers for the subtypes include neuropeptides and the proteins which produce or transport neurochemical markers such as glutamate, GABA, or histamine. Other important cell type markers are calcium-binding proteins, such as parvalbumin, calbindin, and calretinin. While calcium-binding proteins have been used to identify subsets of non-pyramidal cells for some time, their physiological roles in specific cell types are still not fully understood.

More recently, efforts have been focused on discovering new sets of markers, such as transcription factors, using microarrays (Arlotta *et al.*, 2005; Sugino *et al.*, 2006) and single-cell reverse transcriptase polymerase chain reaction (RT-PCR) (Cauli *et al.*, 2000; Toledo-Rodriguez *et al.*, 2004). Microarray-based profiling is very effective when an anatomically or physiologically

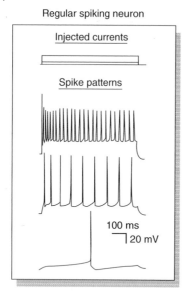
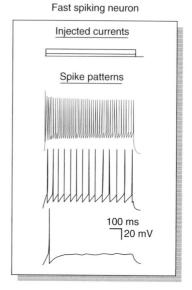

Figure 6.1 Spiking patterns of regular and fast spiking neurons during current injections. (Modified from Tateno *et al.*, 2004.)

homogeneous population can be directly isolated as a cell suspension. In one successful example (Arlotta *et al.*, 2005), groups of projecting neurons were retrogradely labeled and subsequently isolated by fluorescence-activated cell sorting (FACS). This approach resulted in enough cells to carry out microarray analysis. Single-cell RT-PCR is valuable when a technique to characterize a particular cell type, such as patch-clamping, has to be applied to individual living cells. The benefit of this approach is that it can be applied to poorly characterized or totally unknown groups of neurons to discover new cell types. It is also useful to validate the data from microarray analysis and possibly discover subclasses within the population investigated in the microarray experiment. Unfortunately, recovery of mRNAs from single cells is poor and amplifying them without distorting the relative abundance of each gene product is very challenging (Yano *et al.*, 2006). Consequently, most successful examples of this approach are limited to expression profiling of well-known neuronal genes (e.g. ion channels and calcium-binding proteins) in single cells.

Another possibility of discovering markers for neuronal cell types is to use a gene expression atlas. Currently two databases are available for spatial patterns of gene expression in the brain. The Gene Expression Nervous System Atlas (GENSAT) Project (www.gensat.org) is based on transgenic mice harboring bacterial artificial chromosomes (BACs) in which endogenous protein-coding sequences have been replaced by the EGFP reporter gene sequence. Cells expressing the gene of interest can therefore be detected by EGFP fluorescence or by an anti-EGFP antibody. Histological data in GENSAT

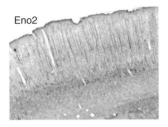 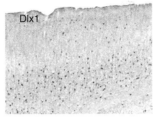

Figure 6.2 GENSAT images of neuron-specific enolase (ENO2)- and distal-less homeobox 1 (Dlx1)-expressing cells in cerebral cortex. (Please find a color version of this figure in the color plates.)

are available for mice at embryonic (E15.5) and postnatal development (P7) stages as well as adult animals. Currently, the database contains images of about 650 genes (as of March 2007). An advantage of this database is that it shows morphological details of cells expressing the gene of interest. For example, cortical cells expressing the protein ENO2 can be identified as pyramidal neurons because of their characteristic triangular soma and long apical dendrites, while those expressing the interneuron marker distal-less homeobox 1 (Dlx1) can be identified as interneurons from their oval soma and fine dendrites (Figure 6.2). Allen's Brain Atlas (www.brainatlas.org/aba/) is another depository of gene expression in the nervous system. This atlas contains *in situ* hybridization images of adult mouse brains for about 20 000 genes in two orientations (sagittal and coronal sections), side by side with Nissl-stained sections. Unfortunately, identification of cell types in the images in this atlas is more difficult than in the GENSAT images because of the nature of its staining method. For example, ENO2 seems to have strong expression across the cerebral cortex in Allen's Brain Atlas, but it is not possible to say in which cells it was expressed, while vasoactive intestinal peptide (VIP)-expressing cells display a typical distribution of interneurons, namely a sparse distribution with little layer dependency (Figure 6.3). The latest version (as of March 2007) provides a summary of gene expression density and level for each brain subregion as well as a search tool called Neuroblast, which lists genes with similar spatial expression patterns to the gene of interest.

While these technical developments are opening a new horizon for discovering and characterizing molecular markers, there is still a lot to be done to understand more classical makers for neuronal cell types. In the rest of this section, some of well-characterized markers for neuronal cell types and their physiological roles in the brain are described.

6.2.2.1 Vesicular Glutamate Transporters (vGLUTs)

Three vesicular glutamate transporter (VGLUT) isoforms, VGLUT1, 2, and 3, are known in mammals and all of them are expressed in the nervous

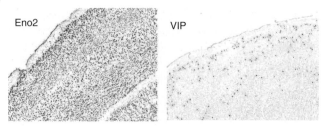

Figure 6.3 Images of neuron-specific enolase (ENO2)- and (VIP)-expressing cells in cerebral cortex from Allen's Brain Atlas. (Please find a color version of this figure in the color plates.)

system. VGLUT1 and 2 are exclusively present in glutaminergic neurons but show a largely non-overlapping distribution in the nervous system. The cerebral cortex, the hippocampus and the cerebellum express mainly VGLUT1, whereas VGLUT2 is mainly observed in the brainstem and the thalamus (Boulland *et al.*, 2004). VGLUT3 is expressed in similar brain areas as VGLUT2, but in more diverse cell types (e.g. GABAergic, serotogenic, and cholinergic neurons) than VGLUT2 (Takamori, 2006). Interestingly, the ion-transport properties of the three VGLUTs are not significantly different and the physiological significance of having the three isotypes is unclear. Neurological phenotypes observed in VGLUT transgenic mice reflect the difference in regional distributions. VGLUT1-heterozygous mice (Tordera *et al.*, 2007) display cognitive deficits such as increased anxiety and depression as well as impaired long-term memory, while decreased VGLUT2 expression resulted in impaired acquisition of neuropathic pain as well as lack of respiratory rhythms (Moechars *et al.*, 2006; Wallén-Mackenzie *et al.*, 2006). In line with these findings, neurophysiological studies revealed that loss of VGLUT1 resulted in a decreased reserve pool of synaptic vesicles in hippocampus and cerebellum (Tordera *et al.*, 2007; Fremeau *et al.*, 2004) while the quantal size in glutaminergic terminal in thalamic neurons was significantly decreased in VGLUT2-knockout mice (Moechars *et al.*, 2006).

6.2.2.2 Glutamate Decarboxylases (GADs)

Glutamate decarboxylases (GADs) are enzymes that catalyze the final reaction to produce GABA, that is, decarboxylation of glutamate. They are hence frequently used as markers for GABAergic neurons. GAD-positive neurons are found in the intermediate zone at E18 in rats and then gradually spread upward during the first 3 weeks of postnatal development (Wolff *et al.*, 1984). While at birth, the GABA concentration in the brain is already more than half the concentration of the adult brain, GAD activity at birth is only about 10% of that measured in the adult animal and it takes more than a month of postnatal period to reach 50% of the adult activity. This indicates significant differences in GABA metabolic processes between neonatal and adult brains (Coyle and Enna, 1976). There are two GAD isoforms in mammals encoded by separate genes: *Gad1* (GAD67) and *Gad2* (GAD65). Both are composed of two domains, a relatively well-conserved (73% identity) catalytic C-terminal domain and a less-conserved (23% identity) N-terminal domain (Soghomonian and Martin, 1998). Multiple parts of the N-terminal domain of GAD65 can be palmitoylated and this posttranslational modification acts as a sorting signal for post-Golgi trafficking to presynaptic sites (Kiser *et al.*, 1998). According to GAD65-GFP mice, cells which express the protein mainly originate from caudal ganglionic eminence and migrate to layers II–III of the cerebral cortex. In adults, these cells express calretinin and neuropeptide Y, and the majority of cholecystokinin (CCK)-positive neurons are also GAD65-positive (López-Bendito *et al.*, 2004). GAD65-knockout mice are born with no apparent abnormalities but gradually develop epileptic seizures (Asada *et al.*, 1996; Kash *et al.*, 1997), which are presumably related to decreased activities in inhibitory circuits. In adult GAD67-GFP mice, fluorescent signals can be observed across the cortex in almost all parvalbumin-, calretinin-, and somatostatin-positive neurons (Tamamaki *et al.*, 2003). During development, GAD67 expression is, unlike GAD65, not correlated with synaptic maturation during postnatal development and GAD67-knockout mice have major physical defects including cleft palate but no clear neurological abnormalities (Kash *et al.*, 1997; Asada *et al.*, 1996). This observation suggests that essential GAD67 functions outside the nervous system.

6.2.2.3 Somatostatin (SST)

Somatostatin (SST) is an inhibitory hormone which suppresses the release of gastrointestinal and pancreatic hormones (e.g. gastrin, cholecystokinin, and insulin) and acts as an inhibitory neurotransmitter in a subset of GABAergic interneurons. However, the net effect of SST on cortical networks is complex, because it can inhibit both GABA and glutamate releases from presynaptic terminals (Momiyama and Zaborszky, 2006). SST-immunoreactive cells are already found in layer VI of the visual cortex at birth and then spread to superficial layers mainly during the first 2 weeks of the postnatal period (McDonald *et al.*, 1982b). Recent studies with knockout mice suggested that the development of SST-positive neurons in the cortex depends on the Dlx1 homeobox transcription factor and the brain-derived neurotrophic factor (BDNF) (Cobos *et al.*, 2005; Grosse *et al.*, 2005). It is yet to be shown, however, at what stage of development these factors affect the production of SST neurons. Morphologically, SST is expressed in the majority of Martinotti cells and in some other GABAergic neurons (Toledo-Rodriguez *et al.*, 2005). Martinotti cells can be distinguished from other cells by the fact that they rarely express other protein markers such as parvalbumin or vasoactive intestinal peptide. Electrophysiologically, SST hyperpolarizes cells by increasing a muscarine-sensitive potassium current (M-current) (Moore *et al.*, 1988) and a voltage-insensitive potassium leak current (Schweitzer *et al.*,

1998). In an animal model of temporal lobe epilepsy, SST-positive neurons in hippocampus were more prone to be damaged than other interneurons (Sun et al., 2007) but it is unclear if the loss of SST-positive neurons is directly responsible for seizures in temporal lobe epilepsy (Buckmaster et al., 2002).

6.2.2.4 Cholecystokinin (CCK)

CCK is best known as a gastrointestinal hormone and stimulates bile production, gallbladder contraction and secretion from exocrine pancreas. In the CNS, CCK acts as a neuropeptide with complex effects on behavior such as feeding (Moran and Bi, 2006) and anxiety (Wang et al., 2005). CCK is expressed in almost all subtypes of interneurons as well as in some pyramidal neurons, and CCK-positive neurons are found more frequently in superficial cortical layers (layer I–III) than in deeper layers (Peters et al., 1983). In the cortex, CCK-positive interneurons often express VGLUT3 (Somogyi et al., 2004). While the distribution of CCK- and VIP-positive neurons overlaps in the cerebral cortex, CCK terminals are concentrated in deeper layers (layer II–V) than VIP terminals, suggesting distinct functions in the cortex. CCK increases the excitability of both pyramidal cells (Gallopin et al., 2006; Shinohara and Kawasaki, 1997) and interneurons (Miller et al., 1987), probably through the CCK-B receptor because blockage of the receptor by antagonists abolishes the effect of CCK in pyramidal cells. Moreover, CCK-positive basket cells express in presynaptic terminals a receptor (CB1) for endocannabinoids which are released from postsynaptic pyramidal cells, so that GABA release from the basket cells can be suppressed in a retrograde manner (Wilson and Nicoll, 2001; Földy et al., 2006; Neu et al., 2007). This suggests that the effect of endocannabinoids on emotions, such as stress response and anxiety (Viveros et al., 2005), may be mediated in part through CCK-expressing interneurons.

6.2.2.5 Vasoactive Intestinal Peptide (VIP)

VIP is another neuropeptide which is also expressed in the digestive system, where it stimulates fluid secretion from intestine and relaxes its smooth muscle. In the cerebral cortex, VIP is expressed in a relatively small set of GABAergic neurons, namely in bipolar cells, which comprise 1% of total cortical neurons (Morrison et al., 1984; Porter et al., 1998; Toledo-Rodriguez et al., 2005). They are mainly found in layers II–IV of the adult cerebral cortex and their terminals extend vertically across layer I–IV. VIP-positive neurons are first seen at P4 in deep cortical layers and it is not until postnatal week 4 that their number and distribution become adult-like (McDonald et al., 1982a; McGregor et al., 1982). Electrophysiologically, VIP-positive bipolar neurons in the cortex have characteristic irregular spiking patterns (Cauli et al., 1997) when a constant step current is injected. They are innervated by both pyramidal and interneurons (Staiger et al., 1997; Porter et al., 1998; Staiger et al., 2002) while their axons terminate at dendrites and cell bodies of interneurons in layers I–II and pyramidal neurons in most of the cortical layers (Hajós et al., 1988; Peters, 1990). VIP increases synaptic transmission to hippocampal pyramidal cells (Ciranna and Cavallaro, 2003) by activating the VIP receptors VIPR1 and VIPR2, which exert their effect through protein kinases C and A, respectively (Cunha-Reis et al., 2005). The same receptors are expressed in glial cells (Joo et al., 2004) and VIP exhibits a wide variety of effects on glial function, such as glycogenolysis (Sorg and Magistretti, 1992) and chemokine release (Delgado et al., 2002). Both VIP (Card et al., 1981) and VIPR2 (Cagampang et al., 1998) are highly expressed in neurons of the suprachiasmatic nucleus (SCN) which acts as a pacemaker for circadian rhythms. A null mutation of VIPR2 caused disruption in normal circadian rhythms, such as rest/activity behavior, circadian expression of clock genes and clock-controlled genes (Harmar et al., 2002) as well as rhythmic and synchronous firing of rhythmic neurons (Aton et al., 2005). Another notable function of VIP in the brain is the regulation of muscular tones of blood vessels in the brain. Stimulation of VIP or nitric oxide—positive interneurons or direct application of these molecules induced vascular dilation while somatostatin-positive neurons did the opposite (Cauli et al., 2004). In the lung (Said et al., 2007), deletion of VIP caused moderate arterial hypertension, but it is unclear whether there exist similar effects on cerebral circulation.

6.2.2.6 Neuropeptide Y (NPY)

Neuropeptide (NPY) is involved in a wide variety of biological processes, such as phagocytosis (Bedoui et al., 2007), angiogenesis (Zukowska-Grojec et al., 1998), bone remodeling (Allison et al., 2007), and tumor growth (Kitlinska et al., 2005) as well as processes such as food intake (Bi, 2007), ethanol dependency (Thorsell, 2007), cerebral circulation (Cauli et al., 2004), and epilepsy (Dubé, 2007). NPY is an abundant inhibitory neuropeptide in the brain and in the autonomic nervous system and frequently found in large-basket cells and nest basket cells (Toledo-Rodriguez et al., 2005). At birth, it is expressed in some SST-positive neurons in the subcortical plate, which postnatally migrate to superficial cortical layers. NPY potentiates the amplitude of inhibitory postsynaptic currents by increasing GABA release to pyramidal neurons (Bacci et al., 2002). However, NPY-knockout mice behave normally unless kainic acid is given to cause seizures, which progress much more aggressively in knockout mice than in wild-type animals (Baraban et al., 1997), suggesting that NPY release may occur only during electrical hyperactivity.

6.2.2.7 Parvalbumin

Parvalbumin is a cytosolic calcium-binding protein found in inhibitory neurons and other cell types outside the nervous system, such as muscle cells, ameloblasts, and Leydig cells (Berchtold *et al.*, 1984). It has been shown that parvalbumin-positive interneurons originate from the medial ganglionic eminence (Xu *et al.*, 2004) and migrate into the cerebral cortex. They appear in cortical layer IV at the end of the first postnatal week, and then extend across the cortex (except for layer I) during the following two weeks (Sánchez *et al.*, 1992). In the adult cerebral cortex, parvalbumin immunoreactivity is denser in deep layers where parvalbumin is found in basket cells, while in layer II and III, the protein is often expressed in chandelier cells (DeFelipe *et al.*, 1989; Kawaguchi and Kubota, 1997). Both parvalbumin-positive subtypes are characterized by their ability to fire at very fast rate ("fast-spiking") when a step current is injected, and this property is often used to identify these neurons electrophysiologically (Kawaguchi and Kubota, 1997). Because of its calcium-buffering capacity, parvalbumin affects the time course of Ca^{2+} transients in synaptic terminals after arrival of the action potential (Schmidt *et al.*, 2003; Collin *et al.*, 2005) and modulate short-term synaptic plasticity (Caillard *et al.*, 2000; Müller *et al.*, 2007). Moreover, parvalbumin-containing interneurons are electrically coupled through gap junctions and form a dense electrical network, suggesting that they may regulate synchronization or spatial smoothing of neuronal activities (Fukuda *et al.*, 2006). This may be related to the observation that parvalbumin-knockout mice have increased susceptibility to epileptic seizures (Schwaller *et al.*, 2004).

6.2.2.8 Calbindin-28k

Calbindin-28k was first identified as a vitamin-D-dependent calcium-binding protein in avian intestine (Wasserman *et al.*, 1968) and then later identified in rodent brain (Wood *et al.*, 1988). Calbindin-28k is detected in cortical plate neurons from embryonic day 18, which is much earlier than is the case for many other interneuron markers. At birth, calbindin-28k-positive cells are observed across the cortex, but as development proceeds, superficial layers (layer II–III) have denser cell density than the layers below (Sánchez *et al.*, 1992). Calbindin-28k-expressing cells have a highly heterogeneous morphology which resembles double-bouquet cells (Hendry *et al.*, 1989), Martinotti cells, neurogliaform cells (Gabbott *et al.*, 1997), and pyramidal cells (Sun *et al.*, 2002). There are some phenotypical characteristics that have been observed in calbindin-28k-deficient mice but they are less dramatic than expected from the high protein capacity (approx 160 μM) to bind calcium (Müller *et al.*, 2005). Although the effects of decreased cytosolic calcium-binding capacity can be seen as larger action potential-evoked Ca^{2+} transients in presynaptic terminals (Schmidt *et al.*, 2003), phenotypes which were expected from increased Ca^{2+} loads, such as compensatory upregulation of mitochondrial volume (Chen *et al.*, 2006) and increased cell death have been inconclusive (Klapstein *et al.*, 1998; Airaksinen *et al.*, 2000; Gary *et al.*, 2000).

6.2.2.9 **Calretinin**

Calretinin is a calcium-binding protein originally found in the retina, as its name suggests (Rogers, 1987). The protein is 58% homologous to calbindin-28k, but the two proteins display a very distinct tissue distribution. Most notably, calretinin expression is restricted to the nervous system and found abundantly in the metencephalon where there is little calbindin-28k expression. In contrast cerebellar purkinje cells, which have high levels of calbindin-28k, lack calretinin (Kadowaki *et al.*, 1993). In the cerebral cortex, calretinin can be seen in the marginal zone as early as E14, and at birth in all cortical layers of the cortex (Fonseca *et al.*, 1995). As the development progresses, calretinin-positive cells disappear from layer I and layer VI and are found more predominantly in layers II–III. In the cerebellum, calretinin is expressed in granule cells, and its loss significantly changes motor coordination (Gall *et al.*, 2003), which can be reversed by restoring calretinin (Bearzatto *et al.*, 2006). Calretinin-knockout mice showed impaired long-term potentiation in the dentate gyrus (Schurmans *et al.*, 1997), which was observed even in heterozygous animals. However, they did not show impairments in spatial memory and learning tasks (Gurden *et al.*, 1998).

6.3
Conclusion

It is clear that elucidating molecular and cellular complexity in the brain is imperative to gain a mechanistic understanding of how the nervous system works, and proteomics and other high-throughput techniques will be more and more important for neuroscientists who are tackling this problem. Knowledge of molecular architectures of neuronal subtypes will facilitate identification, characterization, and manipulation of neural circuits. It will also help us to uncover the molecular mechanisms underlying disorders of the nervous system, which are often caused by abnormalities in specific subsets of neurons. Needless to say, simply making a catalogue of neuronal cells and the molecules they express will not be enough to grasp the whole universe of the nervous system, but it will dramatically change all areas of neuroscience, just as genome sequencing did to molecular biology. The following chapters will show you how that might happen.

References

Airaksinen, L., Virkkala, J., Aarnisalo, A., Meyer, M., Ylikoski, J. and Airaksinen, M.S. (2000) Lack of calbindin-D28k does not affect hearing level or survival of hair cells in acoustic trauma. *ORL Journal for Otorhinolaryngol and its related specialities*, **62**, 9–12.

Alder, J., Xie, Z.P., Valtorta, F., Greengard, P. and Poo, M.M. (1992) Antibodies to synaptophysin interfere with transmitter secretion at neuromuscular synapses. *Neuron*, **9**, 759–768.

Alder, J., Kanki, H., Valtorta, F., Greengard, P. and Poo, M.M. (1995) Overexpression of synaptophysin enhances neurotransmitter secretion at Xenopus neuromuscular synapses. *The Journal of Neuroscience*, **15**, 511–519.

Allison, S.J., Baldock, P.A. and Herzog, H. (2007) The control of bone remodeling by neuropeptide Y receptors. *Peptides*, **28**, 320–325.

Anesti, V. and Scorrano, L. (2006) The relationship between mitochondrial shape and function and the cytoskeleton. *Biochimica et Biophysica Acta*, **1757**, 692–699.

Aquino, D.A., Klipfel, A.A., Brosnan, C.F. and Norton, W.T. (1993) The 70-kDa heat shock cognate protein (HSC70) is a major constituent of the central nervous system and is up-regulated only at the mRNA level in acute experimental autoimmune encephalomyelitis. *Journal of Neurochemistry*, **61**, 1340–1348.

Arlotta, P., Molyneaux, B.J., Chen, J., Inoue, J., Kominami, R. and Macklis, J.D. (2005) Neuronal subtype-specific genes that control corticospinal motor neuron development *in vivo*. *Neuron*, **45**, 207–221.

Asada, H., Kawamura, Y., Maruyama, K., Kume, H., Ding, R., Ji, F.Y., Kanbara, N., Kuzume, H., Sanbo, M., Yagi, T. and Obata, K. (1996) Mice lacking the 65 kDa isoform of glutamic acid decarboxylase (GAD65) maintain normal levels of GAD67 and GABA in their brains but are susceptible to seizures. *Biochemical and Biophysical Research Communications*, **229**, 891–895.

Aton, S.J., Colwell, C.S., Harmar, A.J., Waschek, J. and Herzog, E.D. (2005) Vasoactive intestinal polypeptide mediates circadian rhythmicity and synchrony in mammalian clock neurons. *Nature Neuroscience*, **8**, 476–483.

Bacci, A., Huguenard, J.R. and Prince, D.A. (2002) Differential modulation of synaptic transmission by neuropeptide Y in rat neocortical neurons. *Proceedings of the National Academy of Sciences of the United States of America*, **99**, 17125–17130.

Baraban, S.C., Hollopeter, G., Erickson, J.C., Schwartzkroin, P.A. and Palmiter, R.D. (1997) Knock-out mice reveal a critical antiepileptic role for neuropeptide Y. *The Journal of Neuroscience*, **17**, 8927–8936.

Bearzatto, B., Servais, L., Roussel, C., Gall, D., Baba-Aïssa, F., Schurmans, S., de Kerchove d'Exaerde, A., Cheron, G. and Schiffmann, S.N. (2006) Targeted calretinin expression in granule cells of calretinin-null mice restores normal cerebellar functions. *The FASEB Journal: Official Publication of the Federation of American Societies for Experimental Biology*, **20**, 380–382.

Bedoui, S., von Hörsten, S. and Gebhardt, T. (2007) A role for neuropeptide Y (NPY) in phagocytosis: implications for innate and adaptive immunity. *Peptides*, **28**, 373–376.

Bennett, V. and Gilligan, D.M. (1993) The spectrin-based membrane skeleton and micron-scale organization of the plasma membrane. *Annual Review of Cell Biology*, **9**, 27–66.

Berchtold, M.W., Celio, M.R. and Heizmann, C.W. (1984) Parvalbumin in non-muscle tissues of the rat. Quantitation and immunohistochemical localization. *The Journal of Biological Chemistry*, **259**, 5189–5196.

Berridge, M.J. (2006) Calcium microdomains: organization and function. *Cell Calcium*, **40**, 405–412.

Bi, S. (2007) Role of dorsomedial hypothalamic neuropeptide Y in energy homeostasis. *Peptides*, **28**, 352–356.

Bignami, A., Raju, T. and Dahl, D. (1982) Localization of vimentin, the nonspecific intermediate filament protein, in embryonal glia and in early differentiating neurons. *In vivo* and *in vitro* immunofluorescence study of the rat embryo with vimentin and neurofilament antisera. *Developmental Biology*, **91**, 286–295.

Bogen, I.L., Boulland, J.-L., Mariussen, E., Wright, M.S., Fonnum, F., Kao, H.-T. and Walaas, S.I. (2006) Absence of synapsin I and II is accompanied by decreases in vesicular transport of specific neurotransmitters. *Journal of Neurochemistry*, **96**, 1458–1466.

Boldogh, I.R. and Pon, L.A. (2006) Interactions of mitochondria with the actin cytoskeleton. *Biochimica et Biophysica Acta*, **1763**, 450–462.

Boulland, J.-L., Qureshi, T., Seal, R.P., Rafiki, A., Gundersen, V., Bergersen, L.H., Fremeau, R.T., Edwards, R.H., Storm-Mathisen, J. and Chaudhry, F.A. (2004) Expression of the vesicular glutamate transporters during development indicates the widespread corelease of multiple neurotransmitters. *The Journal of Comparative Neurology*, **480**, 264–280.

Buckmaster, P.S., Otero-Corchón, V., Rubinstein, M. and Low, M.J. (2002) Heightened seizure severity in somatostatin knockout mice. *Epilepsy Research*, **48**, 43–56.

Burgoyne, R.D., Cambray-Deakin, M.A., Lewis, S.A., Sarkar, S. and Cowan, N.J. (1988) Differential distribution of β-tubulin isotypes in cerebellum. *The EMBO Journal*, **7**, 2311–2319.

Cagampang, F.R., Sheward, W.J., Harmar, A.J., Piggins, H.D. and Coen, C.W. (1998) Circadian changes in the expression of vasoactive intestinal peptide 2 receptor mRNA in the rat suprachiasmatic nuclei. *Brain research Molecular Brain Research*, **54**, 108–112.

Caillard, O., Moreno, H., Schwaller, B., Llano, I., Celio, M.R. and Marty, A. (2000) Role of the calcium-binding protein parvalbumin in short-term synaptic plasticity. *Proceedings of the National Academy of Sciences of the United States of America*, **97**, 13372–13377.

Card, J.P., Brecha, N., Karten, H.J. and Moore, R.Y. (1981) Immunocytochemical localization of vasoactive intestinal polypeptide-containing cells and processes in the suprachiasmatic nucleus of the rat: light and electron microscopic analysis. *The Journal of Neuroscience*, **1**, 1289–1303.

Carmo-Fonseca, M. and David-Ferreira, J.F. (1990) Interactions of intermediate filaments with cell structures. *Electron Microscopy Reviews*, **3**, 115–141.

Cauli, B., Porter, J.T., Tsuzuki, K., Lambolez, B., Rossier, J., Quenet, B. and Audinat, E. (2000) Classification of fusiform neocortical interneurons based on unsupervised clustering. *Proceedings of the National Academy of Sciences of the United States of America*, **97**, 6144–6149.

Cauli, B., Audinat, E., Lambolez, B., Angulo, M.C., Ropert, N., Tsuzuki, K., Hestrin, S. and Rossier, J. (1997) Molecular and physiological diversity of cortical nonpyramidal cells. *The Journal of Neuroscience*, **17**, 3894–3906.

Cauli, B., Tong, X.-K., Rancillac, A., Serluca, N., Lambolez, B., Rossier, J. and Hamel, E. (2004) Cortical GABA interneurons in neurovascular coupling: relays for subcortical vasoactive pathways. *The Journal of Neuroscience*, **24**, 8940–8949.

Chen, C.Y. and Balch, W.E. (2006) The Hsp90 chaperone complex regulates GDI-dependent Rab recycling. *Molecular Biology of the Cell*, **17**, 3494–3507.

Chen, G., Racay, P., Bichet, S., Celio, M.R., Eggli, P. and Schwaller, B. (2006) Deficiency in parvalbumin, but not in calbindin D-28k upregulates mitochondrial volume and decreases smooth endoplasmic reticulum surface selectively in a peripheral, subplasmalemmal region in the soma of Purkinje cells. *Neuroscience*, **142**, 97–105.

Ciranna, L. and Cavallaro, S. (2003) Opposing effects by pituitary adenylate cyclase-activating polypeptide and vasoactive intestinal peptide on hippocampal synaptic transmission. *Experimental Neurology*, **184**, 778–784.

Cobos, I., Calcagnotto, M.E., Vilaythong, A.J., Thwin, M.T., Noebels, J.L., Baraban, S.C. and Rubenstein, J.L.R. (2005) Mice lacking Dlx1 show subtype-specific loss of interneurons, reduced inhibition and epilepsy. *Nature Neuroscience*, **8**, 1059–1068.

Collin, T., Chat, M., Lucas, M.G., Moreno, H., Racay, P., Schwaller, B., Marty, A. and Llano, I. (2005) Developmental changes in parvalbumin regulate presynaptic Ca^{2+} signaling. *The Journal of Neuroscience*, **25**, 96–107.

Coyle, J.T. and Enna, S.J. (1976) Neurochemical aspects of the ontogenesis of GABAnergic neurons in the rat brain. *Brain Research*, **111**, 119–133.

Cunha-Reis, D., Ribeiro, J.A. and Sebastião, A.M. (2005) VIP enhances synaptic transmission to hippocampal CA1 pyramidal cells through activation of both VPAC1 and VPAC2 receptors. *Brain Research*, **1049**, 52–60.

D'Adamo, P., Wolfer, D.P., Kopp, C., Tobler, I., Toniolo, D. and Lipp, H.-P. (2004) Mice deficient for the synaptic vesicle protein Rab3a show impaired spatial reversal learning and increased explorative activity but none of the behavioral changes shown by mice deficient for the Rab3a regulator Gdi1. *The European Journal of Neuroscience*, **19**, 1895–1905.

D'Souza, S.M. and Brown, I.R. (1998) Constitutive expression of heat shock proteins Hsp90, Hsc70, Hsp70 and Hsp60 in neural and non-neural tissues of the rat during postnatal development. *Cell Stress Chaperones*, **3**, 188–199.

De Vos, K.J., Allan, V.J., Grierson, A.J. and Sheetz, M.P. (2005) Mitochondrial function and actin regulate dynamin-related protein 1-dependent mitochondrial fission. *Current Biology*, **15**, 678–683.

Deák, F., Shin, O.-H., Tang, J., Hanson, P., Ubach, J., Jahn, R., Rizo, J., Kavalali, E.T. and Südhof, T.C. (2006) Rabphilin regulates SNARE-dependent re-priming of synaptic vesicles for fusion. *The EMBO Journal*, **25**, 2856–2866.

DeFelipe, J., Hendry, S.H. and Jones, E.G. (1989) Visualization of chandelier cell axons by parvalbumin immunoreactivity in monkey cerebral cortex. *Proceedings of the National Academy of Sciences of the United States of America*, **86**, 2093–2097.

DeFelipe, J. and Jones, E.G. (1992) High-resolution light and electron microscopic immunocytochemistry of colocalized GABA and calbindin D-28k in somata and double bouquet cell axons of monkey somatosensory cortex. *The European Journal of Neuroscience*, **4**, 46–60.

Delgado, M., Jonakait, G.M. and Ganea, D. (2002) Vasoactive intestinal peptide and pituitary adenylate cyclase-activating polypeptide inhibit chemokine production in activated microglia. *Glia*, **39**, 148–161.

Dellis, O., Dedos, S.G., Tovey, S.C., Taufiq Ur, R., Dubel, S.J. and Taylor, C.W. (2006) Ca^{2+} entry through plasma membrane IP3 receptors. *Science*, **313**, 229–233.

Dillon, C. and Goda, Y. (2005) The actin cytoskeleton: integrating form and function at the synapse. *Annual Review of Neuroscience*, **28**, 25–55.

Dubé, C. (2007) Neuropeptide Y: potential role in recurrent developmental seizures. *Peptides*, **28**, 441–446.

Dubreuil, R.R. (2006) Functional links between membrane transport and the spectrin cytoskeleton. *The Journal of Membrane Biology*, **211**, 151–161.

Eger, A., Stockinger, A., Wiche, G. and Foisner, R. (1997) Polarisation-dependent association of plectin with desmoplakin and the lateral submembrane skeleton in MDCK cells. *Journal of Cell Science*, **110**(Pt 11), 1307–1316.

Eng, L.F. (1980) The glial fibrillary acidic (GFA) protein, in *Proteins of the Nervous System* (eds R.A. Bradshaw and D.M. Schneider), Raven Press, New York, pp. 85–117.

Földy, C., Neu, A., Jones, M.V. and Soltesz, I. (2006) Presynaptic, activity-dependent modulation of cannabinoid type 1 receptor-mediated inhibition of GABA release. *The Journal of Neuroscience*, **26**, 1465–1469.

Fonseca, M., dél Río, J.A., Martínez, A., Gómez, S. and Soriano, E. (1995) Development of calretinin immunoreactivity in the neocortex of the rat. *The Journal of Comparative Neurology*, **361**, 177–192.

Fournier, A.E. and McKerracher, L. (1997) Expression of specific tubulin isotypes increases during regeneration of injured CNS neurons, but not after the application of brain-derived neurotrophic factor (BDNF). *The Journal of Neuroscience*, **17**, 4623–4632.

Fremeau, R.T., Kam, K., Qureshi, T., Johnson, J., Copenhagen, D.R., Storm-Mathisen, J., Chaudhry, F.A., Nicoll, R.A. and Edwards, R.H. (2004) Vesicular glutamate transporters 1 and 2 target to functionally distinct synaptic release sites. *Science*, **304**, 1815–1819.

Fukuda, T., Kosaka, T., Singer, W. and Galuske, R.A.W. (2006) Gap junctions among dendrites of cortical GABAergic neurons establish a dense and widespread intercolumnar network. *The Journal of Neuroscience*, **26**, 3434–3443.

Gabbott, P.L., Dickie, B.G., Vaid, R.R., Headlam, A.J. and Bacon, S.J. (1997) Local-circuit neurones in the medial prefrontal cortex (areas 25, 32 and 24b) in the rat: morphology and quantitative distribution. *The Journal of Comparative Neurology*, **377**, 465–499.

Gall, D., Roussel, C., Susa, I., D'Angelo, E., Rossi, P., Bearzatto, B., Galas, M.C., Blum, D., Schurmans, S. and Schiffmann, S.N. (2003) Altered neuronal excitability in cerebellar granule cells of mice lacking calretinin. *The Journal of Neuroscience*, **23**, 9320–9327.

Gallopin, T., Geoffroy, H., Rossier, J. and Lambolez, B. (2006) Cortical sources of CRF, NKB, and CCK and their effects on pyramidal cells in the neocortex. *Cerebral Cortex*, **16**, 1440–1452.

Gary, D.S., Sooy, K., Chan, S.L., Christakos, S. and Mattson, M.P. (2000) Concentration- and cell type-specific effects of calbindin D28k on vulnerability of hippocampal neurons to seizure-induced injury. *Brain research Molecular Brain Research*, **75**, 89–95.

Gasnier, B. (2004) The SLC32 transporter, a key protein for the synaptic release of inhibitory amino acids. *Pflugers Archiv: European Journal of Physiology*, **447**, 756–759.

Ghijsen, W.E.J.M. and Leenders, A.G.M. (2005) Differential signaling in presynaptic neurotransmitter release. *Cellular and Molecular Life Sciences*, **62**, 937–954.

Gloster, A., Wu, W., Speelman, A., Weiss, S., Causing, C., Pozniak, C., Reynolds, B., Chang, E., Toma, J.G. and Miller, F.D. (1994) The Talpha1

α-tubulin promoter specifies gene expression as a function of neuronal growth and regeneration in transgenic mice. *The Journal of Neuroscience*, **14**, 7319–7330.

Gloster, A., El-Bizri, H., Bamji, S.X., Rogers, D. and Miller, F.D. (1999) Early induction of Talpha1 α-tubulin transcription in neurons of the developing nervous system. *The Journal of Comparative Neurology*, **405**, 45–60.

Grosse, G., Djalali, S., Deng, D.R., Höltje, M., Hinz, B., Schwartzkopff, K., Cygon, M., Rothe, T., Stroh, T., Hellweg, R., Ahnert-Hilger, G. and Hörtnag, H. (2005) Area-specific effects of brain-derived neurotrophic factor (BDNF) genetic ablation on various neuronal subtypes of the mouse brain. *Brain Research Developmental Brain Research*, **156**, 111–126.

Gurden, H., Schiffmann, S.N., Lemaire, M., Böme, G.A., Parmentier, M. and Schurmans, S. (1998) Calretinin expression as a critical component in the control of dentate gyrus long-term potentiation induction in mice. *The European Journal of Neuroscience*, **10**, 3029–3033.

Gurney, M.E., Heinrich, S.P., Lee, M.R. and Yin, H.S. (1986) Molecular cloning and expression of neuroleukin, a neurotrophic factor for spinal and sensory neurons. *Science*, **234**, 566–574.

Hajós, F., Zilles, K., Schleicher, A. and Kálmán, M. (1988) Types and spatial distribution of vasoactive intestinal polypeptide (VIP)-containing synapses in the rat visual cortex. *Anatomy and Embryology*, **178**, 207–217.

Harmar, A.J., Marston, H.M., Shen, S., Spratt, C., West, K.M., Sheward, W.J., Morrison, C.F., Dorin, J.R., Piggins, H.D., Reubi, J.C., Kelly, J.S., Maywood, E.S. and Hastings, M.H. (2002) The VPAC(2) receptor is essential for circadian function in the mouse suprachiasmatic nuclei. *Cell*, **109**, 497–508.

Hendry, S.H., Jones, E.G., Emson, P.C., Lawson, D.E., Heizmann, C.W. and Streit, P. (1989) Two classes of cortical GABA neurons defined by differential calcium binding protein immunoreactivities. *Experimental Brain Research Experimentelle Hirnforschung Experimentation Cerebrale*, **76**, 467–472.

Hilfiker, S., Pieribone, V.A., Czernik, A.J., Kao, H.T., Augustine, G.J. and Greengard, P. (1999) Synapsins as regulators of neurotransmitter release. *Philosophical Transactions of the Royal Society of London Series B, Biological Sciences*, **354**, 269–279.

Hoffman, P.N. (1989) Expression of GAP-43, a rapidly transported growth-associated protein, and class II β tubulin, a slowly transported cytoskeletal protein, are coordinated in regenerating neurons. *The Journal of Neuroscience*, **9**, 893–897.

Hollenbeck, P.J. and Saxton, W.M. (2005) The axonal transport of mitochondria. *Journal of Cell Science*, **118**, 5411–5419.

Howard, A., Tamas, G. and Soltesz, I. (2005) Lighting the chandelier: new vistas for axo-axonic cells. *Trends in Neuroscience*, **28**, 310–316.

Ikeda, Y., Dick, K.A., Weatherspoon, M.R., Gincel, D., Armbrust, K.R., Dalton, J.C., Stevanin, G., Dür, A, Zühlke, C, Bürk, K., Clark, H.B., Brice, A., Rothstein, J.D., Schut, L.J., Day, J.W. and Ranum, L.P.W. (2006) Spectrin mutations cause spinocerebellar ataxia type 5. *Nature Genetics*, **38**, 184–190.

Ishihama, Y., Sato, T., Tabata, T., Miyamoto, N., Sagane, K., Nagasu, T. and Oda, Y. (2005) Quantitative mouse brain proteomics using culture-derived isotope tags as internal standards. *Nature Biotechnology*, **23**, 617–621.

Jiang, Y.Q. and Oblinger, M.M. (1992) Differential regulation of βIII and other tubulin genes during peripheral and central neuron development. *Journal of Cell Science*, **103**(Pt 3), 643–651.

Johnson, P.R., Dolman, N.J., Pope, M., Vaillant, C., Petersen, O.H., Tepikin, A.V. and Erdemli, G. (2003) Non-uniform distribution of mitochondria in pancreatic acinar cells. *Cell and Tissue Research*, **313**, 37–45.

Joo, K.M., Chung, Y.H., Kim, M.K., Nam, R.H., Lee, B.L., Lee, K.H. and Cha, C.I. (2004) Distribution of vasoactive intestinal peptide and pituitary adenylate cyclase-activating polypeptide

receptors (VPAC1, VPAC2, and PAC1 receptor) in the rat brain. *The Journal of Comparative Neurology*, **476**, 388–413.

Joshi, H.C. and Cleveland, D.W. (1989) Differential utilization of β-tubulin isotypes in differentiating neurites. *The Journal of Cell Biology*, **109**, 663–673.

Julien, J.P. (1999) Neurofilament functions in health and disease. *Current Opinion in Neurobiology*, **9**, 554–560.

Jung, C., Lee, S., Ortiz, D., Zhu, Q., Julien, J.-P. and Shea, T.B. (2005) The high and middle molecular weight neurofilament subunits regulate the association of neurofilaments with kinesin: inhibition by phosphorylation of the high molecular weight subunit. *Brain research Molecular Brain Research*, **141**, 151–155.

Kabir, F. and Nelson, B.D. (1991) Hexokinase bound to rat brain mitochondria uses externally added ATP more efficiently than internally generated ATP. *Biochimica et Biophysica Acta*, **1057**, 147–150.

Kadowaki, K., McGowan, E., Mock, G., Chandler, S. and Emson, P.C. (1993) Distribution of calcium binding protein mRNAs in rat cerebellar cortex. *Neuroscience Letters*, **153**, 80–84.

Kash, S.F., Johnson, R.S., Tecott, L.H., Noebels, J.L., Mayfield, R.D., Hanahan, D. and Baekkeskov, S. (1997) Epilepsy in mice deficient in the 65-kDa isoform of glutamic acid decarboxylase. *Proceedings of the National Academy of Sciences of the United States of America*, **94**, 14060–14065.

Kawaguchi, Y. and Kubota, Y. (1997) GABAergic cell subtypes and their synaptic connections in rat frontal cortex. *Cerebral Cortex*, **7**, 476–486.

Keays, D.A., Tian, G., Poirier, K., Huang, G.-J., Siebold, C., Cleak, J., Oliver, P.L., Fray, M., Harvey, R.J., Molnár, Z., Piñon, M.C., Dear, N., Valdar, W., Brown, S.D.M., Davies, K.E., Rawlins, J.N.P., Cowan, N.J., Nolan, P., Chelly, J. and Flint, J. (2007) Mutations in α-tubulin cause abnormal neuronal migration in mice and lissencephaly in humans. *Cell*, **128**, 45–57.

Kiser, P.J., Cooper, N.G. and Mower, G.D. (1998) Expression of two forms of glutamic acid decarboxylase (GAD67 and GAD65) during postnatal development of rat somatosensory barrel cortex. *The Journal of Comparative Neurology*, **402**, 62–74.

Kislinger, T., Cox, B., Kannan, A., Chung, C., Hu, P., Ignatchenko, A., Scott, M.S., Gramolini, A.O., Morris, Q., Hallett, M.T., Rossant, J., Hughes, T.R., Frey, B. and Emili, A. (2006) Global survey of organ and organelle protein expression in mouse: combined proteomic and transcriptomic profiling. *Cell*, **125**, 173–186.

Kisvárday, Z.F., Beaulieu, C. and Eysel, U.T. (1993) Network of GABAergic large basket cells in cat visual cortex (area 18): implication for lateral disinhibition. *The Journal of Comparative Neurology*, **327**, 398–415.

Kitlinska, J., Abe, K., Kuo, L., Pons, J., Yu, M., Li, L., Tilan, J., Everhart, L., Lee, E.W., Zuknockoutwska, Z. and Toretsky, J.A. (2005) Differential effects of neuropeptide Y on the growth and vascularization of neural crest-derived tumors. *Cancer Research*, **65**, 1719–1728.

Klapstein, G.J., Vietla, S., Lieberman, D.N., Gray, P.A., Airaksinen, M.S., Thoenen, H., Meyer, M. and Mody, I. (1998) Calbindin-D28k fails to protect hippocampal neurons against ischemia in spite of its cytoplasmic calcium buffering properties: evidence from calbindin-D28k knockout mice. *Neuroscience*, **85**, 361–373.

Kodirov, S.A., Takizawa, S., Joseph, J., Kandel, E.R., Shumyatsky, G.P. and Bolshakov, V.Y. (2006) Synaptically released zinc gates long-term potentiation in fear conditioning pathways. *Proceedings of the National Academy of Sciences of the United States of America*, **103**, 15218–15223.

Lazarini, F., Deslys, J.P. and Dormont, D. (1991) Regulation of the glial fibrillary acidic protein, β-actin and prion protein mRNAs during brain development in mouse. *Brain research Molecular Brain Research*, **10**, 343–346.

Lee, M.K., Tuttle, J.B., Rebhun, L.I., Cleveland, D.W. and Frankfurter, A. (1990) The expression and posttranslational modification of a neuron-specific β-tubulin isotype during chick embryogenesis. *Cell Motility and the Cytoskeleton*, **17**, 118–132.

Leenders, A.G., da Silva, F.H.L., Ghijsen, W.E. and Verhage, M. (2001) Rab3a is involved in transport of synaptic vesicles to the active zone in mouse brain nerve terminals. *Molecular Biology of the Cell*, **12**, 3095–3102.

Lencesova, L., O'Neill, A., Resneck, W.G., Bloch, R.J. and Blaustein, M.P. (2004) Plasma membrane-cytoskeleton-endoplasmic reticulum complexes in neurons and astrocytes. *The Journal of Biological Chemistry*, **279**, 2885–2893.

Li, J., Li, Q., Xie, C., Zhou, H., Wang, Y., Zhang, N., Shao, H., Chan, S.C., Peng, X., Lin, S.-C. and Han, J. (2004) β-actin is required for mitochondria clustering and ROS generation in TNF-induced, caspase-independent cell death. *Journal of Cell Science*, **117**, 4673–4680.

Lobsiger, C.S., Garcia, M.L., Ward, C.M. and Cleveland, D.W. (2005) Altered axonal architecture by removal of the heavily phosphorylated neurofilament tail domains strongly slows superoxide dismutase 1 mutant-mediated ALS. *Proceedings of the National Academy of Sciences of the United States of America*, **102**, 10351–10356.

Lonart, G.g. and Simsek-Duran, F. (2006) Deletion of synapsins I and II genes alters the size of vesicular pools and rabphilin phosphorylation. *Brain Research*, **1107**, 42–51.

Loones, M.T., Chang, Y. and Morange, M. (2000) The distribution of heat shock proteins in the nervous system of the unstressed mouse embryo suggests a role in neuronal and non-neuronal differentiation. *Cell Stress Chaperones*, **5**, 291–305.

López-Bendito, G., Sturgess, K., Erdélyi, F., Szabó, G., Molnár, Z. and Paulsen, O. (2004) Preferential origin and layer destination of GAD65-GFP cortical interneurons. *Cerebral Cortex*, **14**, 1122–1133.

Ludueña, R.F. (1993) Are tubulin isotypes functionally significant. *Molecular Biology of the Cell*, **4**, 445–457.

Luo, L. (2002) Actin cytoskeleton regulation in neuronal morphogenesis and structural plasticity. *Annual Review of Cell and Developmental Biology*, **18**, 601–635.

Markram, H., Toledo-Rodriguez, M., Wang, Y., Gupta, A., Silberberg, G. and Wu, C. (2004) Interneurons of the neocortical inhibitory system. *Nature Reviews Neuroscience*, **5**, 793–807.

Mazzola, J.L. and Sirover, M.A. (2002) Alteration of intracellular structure and function of glyceraldehyde-3-phosphate dehydrogenase: a common phenotype of neurodegenerative disorders? *Neurotoxicology*, **23**, 603–609.

McDonald, J.K., Parnavelas, J.G., Karamanlidis, A.N. and Brecha, N. (1982a) The morphology and distribution of peptide-containing neurons in the adult and developing visual cortex of the rat. II. Vasoactive intestinal polypeptide. *Journal of Neurocytology*, **11**, 825–837.

McDonald, J.K., Parnavelas, J.G., Karamanlidis, A.N., Brecha, N. and Koenig, J.I. (1982b) The morphology and distribution of peptide-containing neurons in the adult and developing visual cortex of the rat. I. Somatostatin. *Journal of Neurocytology*, **11**, 809–824.

McGregor, G.P., Woodhams, P.L., O'Shaughnessy, D.J., Ghatei, M.A., Polak, J.M. and Bloom, S.R. (1982) Developmental changes in bombesin, substance P, somatostatin and vasoactive intestinal polypeptide in the rat brain. *Neuroscience Letters*, **28**, 21–27.

Menezes, J.R. and Luskin, M.B. (1994) Expression of neuron-specific tubulin defines a novel population in the proliferative layers of the developing telencephalon. *The Journal of Neuroscience*, **14**, 5399–5416.

Miller, F.D., Naus, C.C., Durand, M., Bloom, F.E. and Milner, R.J. (1987) Isotypes of α-tubulin are differentially regulated during neuronal maturation. *The Journal of Cell Biology*, **105**, 3065–3073.

Minamide, L.S., Striegl, A.M., Boyle, J.A., Meberg, P.J. and Bamburg, J.R. (2000) Neurodegenerative stimuli induce persistent ADF/cofilin-actin rods that disrupt distal neurite function. *Nature Cell Biology*, **2**, 628–636.

Moechars, D., Weston, M.C., Leo, S., Callaerts-Vegh, Z., Goris, I., Daneels, G., Buist, A., Cik, M., van der Spek, P., Kass, S., Meert, T., D'Hooge, R., Rosenmund, C. and Hampson, R.M. (2006) Vesicular glutamate transporter VGLUT2 expression levels control quantal size and neuropathic pain. *The Journal of Neuroscience*, **26**, 12055–12066.

Mogami, H., Nakano, K., Tepikin, A.V. and Petersen, O.H. (1997) Ca^{2+} flow via tunnels in polarized cells: recharging of apical Ca^{2+} stores by focal Ca^{2+} entry through basal membrane patch. *Cell*, **88**, 49–55.

Momiyama, T. and Zaborszky, L. (2006) Somatostatin presynaptically inhibits both GABA and glutamate release onto rat basal forebrain cholinergic neurons. *Journal of Neurophysiology*, **96**, 686–694.

Moore, B.W. (1969) Acidic proteins, in *Handbook of Neurochemistry* (ed. A. Lajtha), Plenum Press, New York, pp. 93–99.

Moore, S.D., Madamba, S.G., Joëls, M. and Siggins, G.R. (1988) Somatostatin augments the M-current in hippocampal neurons. *Science*, **239**, 278–280.

Morales, M., Colicos, M.A. and Goda, Y. (2000) Actin-dependent regulation of neurotransmitter release at central synapses. *Neuron*, **27**, 539–550.

Moran, T.H. and Bi, S. (2006) Hyperphagia and obesity in OLETF rats lacking CCK-1 receptors. *Philosophical Transactions of the Royal Society of London Series B, Biological Sciences*, **361**, 1211–1218.

Morgan, J.R., Prasad, K., Jin, S., Augustine, G.J. and Lafer, E.M. (2001) Uncoating of clathrin-coated vesicles in presynaptic terminals: roles for Hsc70 and auxilin. *Neuron*, **32**, 289–300.

Morrison, J.H., Magistretti, P.J., Benoit, R. and Bloom, F.E. (1984) The distribution and morphological characteristics of the intracortical VIP-positive cell: an immunohistochemical analysis. *Brain Research*, **292**, 269–282.

Moskowitz, P.F. and Oblinger, M.M. (1995) Sensory neurons selectively upregulate synthesis and transport of the β III-tubulin protein during axonal regeneration. *The Journal of Neuroscience*, **15**, 1545–1555.

Motil, J., Chan, W.K.H., Dubey, M., Chaudhury, P., Pimenta, A., Chylinski, T.M., Ortiz, D.T. and Shea, T.B. (2006) Dynein mediates retrograde neurofilament transport within axons and anterograde delivery of NFs from perikarya into axons: regulation by multiple phosphorylation events. *Cell Motility and the Cytoskeleton,* **63**, 266–286.

Müller, A., Kukley, M., Stausberg, P., Beck, H., Müller, W. and Dietrich, D. (2005) Endogenous Ca^{2+} buffer concentration and Ca^{2+} microdomains in hippocampal neurons. *The Journal of Neuroscience,* **25**, 558–565.

Müller, M., Felmy, F., Schwaller, B. and Schneggenburger, R. (2007) Parvalbumin is a mobile presynaptic Ca^{2+} buffer in the calyx of held that accelerates the decay of $Ca2+$ and short-term facilitation. *The Journal of Neuroscience,* **27**, 2261–2271.

Neu, A., Földy, C. and Soltesz, I. (2007) Postsynaptic origin of CB1-dependent tonic inhibition of GABA release at cholecystokinin-positive basket cell to pyramidal cell synapses in the CA1 region of the rat hippocampus. *The Journal of Physiology,* **578**, 233–247.

Olsen, J.V., Nielsen, P.A., Andersen, J.R., Mann, M. and Wišniewski, J.R. (2007) Quantitative proteomic profiling of membrane proteins from the mouse brain cortex, hippocampus, and cerebellum using the HysTag reagent: mapping of neurotransmitter receptors and ion channels. *Brain Research,* **1134**, 95–106.

Ong, S.-E. and Mann, M. (2005) Mass spectrometry-based proteomics turns quantitative. *Nature Chemical Biology,* **1**, 252–262.

Perlson, E., Hanz, S., Ben-Yaakov, K., Segal-Ruder, Y., Seger, R. and Fainzilber, M. (2005) Vimentin-dependent spatial translocation of an activated MAP kinase in injured nerve. *Neuron,* **45**, 715–726.

Peters, A. (1990) The axon terminals of vasoactive intestinal polypeptide (VIP)-containing bipolar cells in rat visual cortex. *Journal of Neurocytology,* **19**, 672–685.

Peters, A., Miller, M. and Kimerer, L.M. (1983) Cholecystokinin-like immunoreactive neurons in rat cerebral cortex. *Neuroscience,* **8**, 431–448.

Pielage, J., Fetter, R.D. and Davis, G.W. (2005) Presynaptic spectrin is essential for synapse stabilization. *Current Biology,* **15**, 918–928.

Poddar, R., Paul, S., Chaudhury, S. and Sarkar, P.K. (1996) Regulation of actin and tubulin gene expression by thyroid hormone during rat brain development. *Brain Research Molecular Brain Research,* **35**, 111–118.

Pollak, D.D., John, J., Hoeger, H. and Lubec, G. (2006) An integrated map of the murine hippocampal proteome based upon five mouse strains. *Electrophoresis,* **27**, 2787–2798.

Porter, J.T., Cauli, B., Staiger, J.F., Lambolez, B., Rossier, J. and Audinat, E. (1998) Properties of bipolar VIPergic interneurons and their excitation by pyramidal neurons in the rat neocortex. *The European Journal of Neuroscience,* **10**, 3617–3628.

Posey, S.C. and Bierer, B.E. (1999) Actin stabilization by jasplakinolide enhances apoptosis induced by cytokine deprivation. *The Journal of Biological Chemistry,* **274**, 4259–4265.

Rogers, J.H. (1987) Calretinin: a gene for a novel calcium-binding protein expressed principally in neurons. *The Journal of Cell Biology,* **105**, 1343–1353.

Romagnoli, A., Oliverio, S., Evangelisti, C., Iannicola, C., Ippolito, G. and Piacentini, M. (2003) Neuroleukin inhibition sensitises neuronal cells to caspase-dependent apoptosis. *Biochemical and Biophysical Research Communications,* **302**, 448–453.

Sáez, D.E. and Slebe, J.C. (2000) Subcellular localization of aldolase B. *Journal of Cellular Biochemistry,* **78**, 62–72.

Said, S.I., Hamidi, S.A., Dickman, K.G., Szema, A.M., Lyubsky, S., Lin, R.Z., Jiang, Y.-P., Chen, J.J., Waschek, J.A. and Kort, S. (2007) Moderate pulmonary arterial hypertension in male mice lacking the vasoactive intestinal peptide gene. *Circulation,* **115**, 1260–1268.

Sánchez, M.P., Frassoni, C., Alvarez-Bolado, G., Spreafico, R. and Fairén, A. (1992) Distribution of calbindin and parvalbumin in the developing somatosensory cortex and its primordium in the rat: an immunocytochemical study. *Journal of Neurocytology*, **21**, 717–736.

Sankaranarayanan, S., Atluri, P.P. and Ryan, T.A. (2003) Actin has a molecular scaffolding, not propulsive, role in presynaptic function. *Nature Neuroscience*, **6**, 127–135.

Sasaki, T., Gotow, T., Shiozaki, M., Sakaue, F., Saito, T., Julien, J.-P., Uchiyama, Y. and Hisanaga, S.-I. (2006) Aggregate formation and phosphorylation of neurofilament-L Pro22 Charcot-Marie-Tooth disease mutants. *Human Molecular Genetics*, **15**, 943–952.

Savel'ev, A.S., Novikova, L.A., Kovaleva, I.E., Luzikov, V.N., Neupert, W. and Langer, T. (1998) ATP-dependent proteolysis in mitochondria. m-AAA protease and PIM1 protease exert overlapping substrate specificities and cooperate with the mtHsp70 system. *The Journal of Biological Chemistry*, **273**, 20596–20602.

Schindler, J., Lewandrowski, U., Sickmann, A., Friauf, E. and Nothwang, H.G. (2006) Proteomic analysis of brain plasma membranes isolated by affinity two-phase partitioning. *Molecular & Cellular Proteomics*, **5**, 390–400.

Schmidt, H., Stiefel, K.M., Racay, P., Schwaller, B. and Eilers, J. (2003) Mutational analysis of dendritic Ca^{2+} kinetics in rodent Purkinje cells: role of parvalbumin and calbindin D28k. *The Journal of Physiology*, **551**, 13–32.

Schurmans, S., Schiffmann, S.N., Gurden, H., Lemaire, M., Lipp, H.P., Schwam, V., Pochet, R., Imperato, A., Böhme, G.A. and Parmentier, M. (1997) Impaired long-term potentiation induction in dentate gyrus of calretinin-deficient mice. *Proceedings of the National Academy of Sciences of the United States of America*, **94**, 10415–10420.

Schwaller, B., Tetko, I.V., Tandon, P., Silveira, D.C., Vreugdenhil, M., Henzi, T., Potier, M.C., Celio, M.R. and Villa, A.E.P. (2004) Parvalbumin deficiency affects network properties resulting in increased susceptibility to epileptic seizures. *Molecular and Cellular Neurosciences*, **25**, 650–663.

Schweitzer, P., Madamba, S.G. and Siggins, G.R. (1998) Somatostatin increases a voltage-insensitive K^+ conductance in rat CA1 hippocampal neurons. *Journal of Neurophysiology*, **79**, 1230–1238.

Selkoe, D.J. (2003) Folding proteins in fatal ways. *Nature*, **426**, 900–904.

Shigeri, Y., Seal, R.P. and Shimamoto, K. (2004) Molecular pharmacology of glutamate transporters, EAATs and VGLUTs. *Brain research Brain Research Reviews*, **45**, 250–265.

Shin, J.-H., Krapfenbauer, K. and Lubec, G. (2005) Column chromatographic prefractionation leads to the detection of 543 different gene products in human fetal brain. *Electrophoresis*, **26**, 2759–2778.

Shinohara, S. and Kawasaki, K. (1997) Electrophysiological changes in rat hippocampal pyramidal neurons produced by cholecystokinin octapeptide. *Neuroscience*, **78**, 1005–1016.

Soghomonian, J.J. and Martin, D.L. (1998) Two isoforms of glutamate decarboxylase: why? *Trends in Pharmacological Sciences*, **19**, 500–505.

Somogyi, J., Baude, A., Omori, Y., Shimizu, H., Mestikawy, S.E., Fukaya, M., Shigemoto, R., Watanabe, M. and Somogyi, P. (2004) GABAergic basket cells expressing cholecystokinin contain vesicular glutamate transporter type 3 (VGLUT3) in their synaptic terminals in hippocampus and isocortex of the rat. *The European Journal of Neuroscience*, **19**, 552–569.

Sorg, O. and Magistretti, P.J. (1992) Vasoactive intestinal peptide and noradrenaline exert long-term control on glycogen levels in astrocytes: blockade by protein synthesis inhibition. *The Journal of Neuroscience*, **12**, 4923–4931.

Staiger, J.F., Freund, T.F. and Zilles, K. (1997) Interneurons immunoreactive for vasoactive intestinal polypeptide (VIP) are extensively innervated by parvalbumin-containing boutons in rat primary somatosensory cortex. *The European Journal of Neuroscience*, **9**, 2259–2268.

Staiger, J.F., Schubert, D., Zuschratter, W., Kötter, R., Luhmann, H.J. and Zilles, K. (2002) Innervation of interneurons immunoreactive for VIP by intrinsically bursting pyramidal cells and fast-spiking interneurons in infragranular layers of juvenile rat neocortex. *The European Journal of Neuroscience*, **16**, 11–20.

Stell, B. and Mody, I. (2003) A tale of timing and transport. *Neuron*, **39**, 729–730.

Sudhof, T.C. (2004) The synaptic vesicle cycle. *Annual Review of Neuroscience*, **27**, 509–547.

Sugino, K., Hempel, C.M., Miller, M.N., Hattox, A.M., Shapiro, P., Wu, C., Huang, Z.J. and Nelson, S.B. (2006) Molecular taxonomy of major neuronal classes in the adult mouse forebrain. *Nature Neuroscience*, **9**, 99–107.

Sullivan, K.F. (1988) Structure and utilization of tubulin isotypes. *Annual Review of Cell Biology*, **4**, 687–716.

Sullivan, K.F., Havercroft, J.C., Machlin, P.S. and Cleveland, D.W. (1986) Sequence and expression of the chicken β5- and β4-tubulin genes define a pair of divergent β-tubulins with complementary patterns of expression. *Molecular and Cellular Biology*, **6**, 4409–4418.

Sun, C., Mtchedlishvili, Z., Bertram, E.H., Erisir, A. and Kapur, J. (2007) Selective loss of dentate hilar interneurons contributes to reduced synaptic inhibition of granule cells in an electrical stimulation-based animal model of temporal lobe epilepsy. *The Journal of Comparative Neurology*, **500**, 876–893.

Sun, X.-Z., Takahashi, S., Cui, C., Inoue, M. and Fukui, Y. (2002) Distribution of calbindin-D28K immunoreactive neurons in rat primary motor cortex. *The Journal of Medical Investigation*, **49**, 35–39.

Suzuki, T., Usuda, N., Murata, S., Nakazawa, A., Ohtsuka, K. and Takagi, H. (1999) Presence of molecular chaperones, heat shock cognate (Hsc) 70 and heat shock proteins (Hsp) 40, in the postsynaptic structures of rat brain. *Brain Research*, **816**, 99–110.

Takamori, S. (2006) VGLUTs: 'exciting' times for glutamatergic research? *Neurosciences Research*, **55**, 343–351.

Tamamaki, N., Yanagawa, Y., Tomioka, R., Miyazaki, J.-I., Obata, K. and Kaneko, T. (2003) Green fluorescent protein expression and colocalization with calretinin, parvalbumin, and somatostatin in the GAD67-GFP knock-in mouse. *The Journal of Comparative Neurology*, **467**, 60–79.

Tarze, A., Deniaud, A., Bras, M.L., Maillier, E., Molle, D., Larochette, N., Zamzami, N., Jan, G., Kroemer, G. and Brenner, C. (2007) GAPDH, a novel regulator of the pro-apoptotic mitochondrial membrane permeabilization. *Oncogene*, **26**, 2606–2620.

Tateno, T., Harsch, A. and Robinson, H.P. (2004) Threshold firing frequency-current relationships of neurons in rat somatosensory cortex: type 1 and type 2 dynamics. *Journal of Neurophysiology*, **92**, 2283–2294.

Tatton, W.G., Chalmers-Redman, R., Brown, D. and Tatton, N. (2003) Apoptosis in Parkinson's disease: signals for neuronal degradation. *Annals of Neurology*, **53**(Suppl 3), S61–S70.

Thorsell, A. (2007) Neuropeptide Y (NPY) in alcohol intake and dependence. *Peptides*, **28**, 480–483.

Toledo-Rodriguez, M., Blumenfeld, B., Wu, C., Luo, J., Attali, B., Goodman, P. and Markram, H. (2004) Correlation maps allow neuronal electrical properties to be predicted from single-cell gene expression profiles in rat neocortex. *Cerebral Cortex*, **14**, 1310–1327.

Toledo-Rodriguez, M., Goodman, P., Illic, M., Wu, C. and Markram, H. (2005) Neuropeptide and calcium-binding protein gene expression profiles predict neuronal anatomical type in the juvenile rat. *The Journal of Physiology*, **567**, 401–413.

Tordera, R.M., Totterdell, S., Wojcik, S.M., Brose, N., Elizalde, N., Lasheras, B. and Rio, J.D. (2007) Enhanced anxiety, depressive-like behaviour and impaired recognition memory in mice with reduced expression of the vesicular glutamate transporter 1 (VGLUT1). *The European Journal of Neuroscience,* **25,** 281–290.

Tsai, M.Y., Morfini, G., Szebenyi, G. and Brady, S.T. (2000) Release of kinesin from vesicles by hsc70 and regulation of fast axonal transport. *Molecular Biology of the Cell,* **11,** 2161–2173.

Tsuboi, T. and Fukuda, M. (2005) The C2B domain of rabphilin directly interacts with SNAP-25 and regulates the docking step of dense core vesicle exocytosis in PC12 cells. *The Journal of Biological Chemistry,* **280,** 39253–39259.

Ungewickell, E. (1985) The 70-kd mammalian heat shock proteins are structurally and functionally related to the uncoating protein that releases clathrin triskelia from coated vesicles. *The EMBO Journal,* **4,** 3385–3391.

Valtorta, F., Pennuto, M., Bonanomi, D. and Benfenati, F. (2004) Synaptophysin: leading actor or walk-on role in synaptic vesicle exocytosis? *Bioessays: News and Reviews in Molecular, Cellular and Developmental Biology,* **26,** 445–453.

Viveros, M.P., Marco, E.M. and File, S.E. (2005) Endocannabinoid system and stress and anxiety responses. *Pharmacology, Biochemistry, and Behavior,* **81,** 331–342.

Voos, W. and Röttgers, K. (2002) Molecular chaperones as essential mediators of mitochondrial biogenesis. *Biochimica et Biophysica Acta,* **1592,** 51–62.

Vos, K.D., Goossens, V., Boone, E., Vercammen, D., Vancompernolle, K., Vandenabeele, P., Haegeman, G., Fiers, W. and Grooten, J. (1998) The 55-kDa tumor necrosis factor receptor induces clustering of mitochondria through its membrane-proximal region. *The Journal of Biological Chemistry,* **273,** 9673–9680.

Wallén-Mackenzie, A., Gezelius, H., Thoby-Brisson, M., Nygård, A., Enjin, A., Fujiyama, F., Fortin, G. and Kullander, K. (2006) Vesicular glutamate transporter 2 is required for central respiratory rhythm generation but not for locomotor central pattern generation. *The Journal of Neuroscience,* **26,** 12294–12307.

Wang, H., Wong, P.T.H., Spiess, J. and Zhu, Y.Z. (2005) Cholecystokinin-2 (CCK2) receptor-mediated anxiety-like behaviors in rats. *Neuroscience and Biobehavioral Reviews,* **29,** 1361–1373.

Wasserman, R.H., Corradino, R.A. and Taylor, A.N. (1968) Vitamin D-dependent calcium-binding protein. Purification and some properties. *The Journal of Biological Chemistry,* **243,** 3978–3986.

Wilson, R.I. and Nicoll, R.A. (2001) Endogenous cannabinoids mediate retrograde signalling at hippocampal synapses. *Nature,* **410,** 588–592.

Winder, S.J. and Ayscough, K.R. (2005) Actin-binding proteins. *Journal of Cell Science,* **118,** 651–654.

Wolff, J.R., Böttcher, H., Zetzsche, T., Oertel, W.H. and Chronwall, B.M. (1984) Development of GABAergic neurons in rat visual cortex as identified by glutamate decarboxylase-like immunoreactivity. *Neuroscience Letters,* **47,** 207–212.

Wood, T.L., Kobayashi, Y., Frantz, G., Varghese, S., Christakos, S. and Tobin, A.J. (1988) Molecular cloning of mammalian 28,000 Mr vitamin D-dependent calcium binding protein (calbindin-D28K): expression of calbindin-D28K RNAs in rodent brain and kidney. *DNA,* **7,** 585–593.

Wu, K., Aoki, C., Elste, A., Rogalski-Wilk, A.A. and Siekevitz, P. (1997) The synthesis of ATP by glycolytic enzymes in the postsynaptic density and the effect of endogenously generated nitric oxide. *Proceedings of the National Academy of Sciences of the United States of America,* **94,** 13273–13278.

Xu, Q., Cobos, I., Cruz, E.D.L., Rubenstein, J.L. and Anderson, S.A. (2004) Origins of cortical interneuron subtypes. *The Journal of Neuroscience,* **24,** 2612–2622.

Xu, X., Roby, K.D. and Callaway, E.M. (2006) Mouse cortical inhibitory neuron type that coexpresses somatostatin and calretinin. *The Journal of Comparative Neurology*, **499**, 144–160.

Xu, Z., Cork, L.C., Griffin, J.W. and Cleveland, D.W. (1993) Increased expression of neurofilament subunit NF-L produces morphological alterations that resemble the pathology of human motor neuron disease. *Cell*, **73**, 23–33.

Yano, K., Subkhankulova, T., Livesey, F.J. and Robinson, H.P.C. (2006) Electrophysiological and gene expression profiling of neuronal cell types in mammalian neocortex. *The Journal of Physiology*, **575**, 361–365.

Yonezawa, N., Nishida, E., Koyasu, S., Maekawa, S., Ohta, Y., Yahara, I. and Sakai, H. (1987) Distribution among tissues and intracellular localization of cofilin, a 21 kDa actin-binding protein. *Cell Structure and Function*, **12**, 443–452.

Yu, L.-R., Conrads, T.P., Uo, T., Kinoshita, Y., Morrison, R.S.,

Lucas, D.A., Chan, K.C., Blonder, J., Issaq, H.J. and Veenstra, T.D. (2004) Global analysis of the cortical neuron proteome. *Molecular & Cellular Proteomics*, **3**, 896–907.

Zomzely-Neurath, C.E. and Walker, W.A. (1980) Nervous system-specific protein 14-3-2 protein, neuron-specific enolase, and S-100 protein In: *Proteins of the Nervous System* (eds R.A. Bradshaw and D.M. Schneider), Raven Press, New York, pp. 1–57.

Zukowska-Grojec, Z., Karwatowska-Prokopczuk, E., Fisher, T.A. and Ji, H. (1998) Mechanisms of vascular growth-promoting effects of neuropeptide Y: role of its inducible receptors. *Regulatory Peptides*, **75–76**, 231–238.

7
Proteome Analysis of Plasma Membranes

Hans Gerd Nothwang

7.1
Introduction

7.1.1
The Dynamic Plasma Membrane Proteome

Plasma membrane proteins are essential to many neural processes, including neurotransmission, the exchange of material and energy between cells and their environment, cell–cell interactions, and signal transduction. To this end, the plasma membrane proteome encompasses a large collection of different proteins such as receptors for neurotransmitters, hormones and growth factors, primary and secondary active transporters, channels, cell adhesion molecules, and molecules that regulate vesicular transport mechanisms. Many of them are involved in human pathologies such as cognitive and affective disorders, rendering them important targets for pharmacological action. Currently, membrane proteins account for ~70% of all known drug targets (Hopkins and Groom, 2002). Many of these therapeutic agents, such as antidepressants and psychostimulants, act on plasma membrane proteins in the brain (Torres *et al.*, 2003).

Highly sensitive mass spectrometry and multidimensional liquid chromatography techniques have paved the way towards efficient identification of plasma membrane proteins. Yet, the comprehensive monitoring of plasma membrane proteins in different physiological and pathophysiological conditions in the nervous system remains an unsettled challenge. First, plasma membrane proteins are in low abundance, amounting to about 2–5% of all cellular proteins (Evans, 1991). Second, there is a large variety in protein species and many of them are specific to certain brain areas or even cell types. The human central nervous system (CNS) alone consists of $10^{10}–10^{11}$ neurons and most likely a 10-fold higher number of glial cells (Temburni and Jacob, 2001). Several thousand cell types can be distinguished, based on function, shape, the extent and complexity of their processes, and their neurochemical and biophysical properties (Masland, 2004). They possess a unique repertoire of

Proteomics of the Nervous System. Edited by H.G. Nothwang and S.E. Pfeiffer
Copyright © 2008 WILEY-VCH Verlag GmbH & Co. KGaA, Weinheim
ISBN: 978-3-527-31716-5

plasma membrane proteins that confer cellular and functional specificity (see Chapter 6). Alternative splicing and posttranslational modification (PTM) add another level of complexity to plasma membrane proteins (see Chapter 11). It is estimated that they increase the number of different protein species by at least one order of magnitude (reviewed in Becker *et al.*, 2006). Interestingly, the transcripts with the highest known degree of alternative splicing, *dscam* (Chen *et al.*, 2006) and the *neurexins*, encode neuronal plasma membrane proteins. The prevalence of PTMs was recently underlined in two studies of postsynaptic density from mouse brain in which a total of 1000 unique phosphorylated peptides (Trinidad *et al.*, 2006) and 65 peptides carrying *O*-linked *N*-acetylglucosamine (Vosseller *et al.*, 2006) were identified in $\sim$1300 different proteins using MS.

Another feature to consider in plasma membrane proteomics is the functional subdivision of the neuronal plasma membrane. The precise location of a protein within the plasma membrane can greatly vary depending on brain area, stimuli, developmental stage, and so on. Important plasma membrane domains include the presynaptic axonal terminal, the postsynaptic dendrite, or the soma. Redistribution of glycinergic receptors from dendrites to the soma of auditory neurons contributes to the refinement of inhibition in the auditory system and most probably reflect an adaptation to improve the encoding of auditory cues with temporal precision and fidelity (Kapfer *et al.*, 2002). Another emerging field is that of plasma membrane microdomains such as detergent-resistant membranes (DRMs). They are increasingly acknowledged as playing essential roles in the proper function of several plasma membrane proteins, such as the serotonin transporter or the excitatory amino acid transporter EAAT2 (Butchbach *et al.*, 2004; Magnani *et al.*, 2004). Similarly, changes in microdomain localization might be associated with disorders. α-Synuclein, a presynaptic protein, is found in DRMs, whereas a mutant form, associated with Parkinson's disease, is localized to non-DRMs (Fortin *et al.*, 2004).

Finally, many proteins are not statically localized in the plasma membrane (Figure 7.1). Depending on the functional state, proteins can move in and out of the plasma membrane in a highly dynamic manner. An instructive example is provided by the ionotropic glutamate receptors of the AMPA and NMDA subtypes. These proteins are delivered to and removed from synapses in response to neuronal activity (Carroll and Zukin, 2002; Esteban, 2003). Furthermore, proteins can move laterally in the plasma membrane. Single-quantum dot tracking demonstrated that receptors switch at unexpected high rates between extrasynaptic and synaptic localizations by lateral diffusion (Triller and Choquet, 2005). This dynamic receptor redistribution within the plasma membrane and between different cellular membranes is important to adjust synaptic strength during development of the nervous system and plays a pivotal role in experience-dependent plasticity such as long-term potentiation and long-term depression. However, most of these changes in plasma membrane localization occur only in specific brain areas at a given time, due to their dependency on activity and varying stimuli provided by the

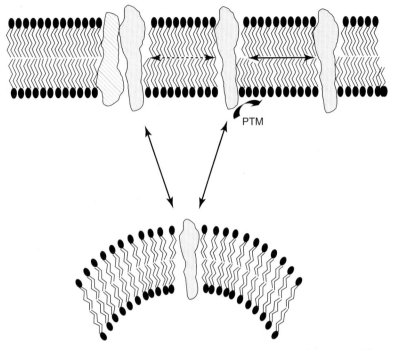

Figure 7.1 Schematic representation of dynamic alterations on the protein level in the plasma membrane. Proteins can be trafficked in and out of the plasma membrane or alter the localization within the plasma membrane by lateral movements. Furthermore, they can be subject to posttranslational modification (PTM). Finally, they can interact to various extents with other plasma membrane proteins. All these changes occur in a region- and activity-dependent way and may reflect pathophysiological conditions.

environment. Furthermore, different areas might use different mechanisms to modulate synaptic transmission.

7.1.2
Protocols for Plasma Membrane Isolation

In light of the above account, it is evident that there is no single protocol for plasma membrane protein analysis in the nervous system. Depending on the focus, a variety of protocols exist. These include protocols for the purification of entire plasma membranes, isolation of postsynaptic densities or presynaptic terminals. Ideally, the protocols should be capable of profiling plasma membrane proteins from functionally or anatomically well-defined areas in the nervous system. In principle, proteins such as PSD-95, which is present at 300 copies/postsynaptic density (Chen *et al.*, 2005), can be detected from 2×10^6 neurons by MS, based on 1000 postsynaptic densities/cells and a sensitivity of 1 pmol in the MS analysis. To keep pace with this progress in the analytical area of proteomics, the commonly used combination of differential centrifugation and density gradient centrifugation has to be replaced by novel, more efficient methods.

Recently, several such approaches have been implemented in proteomic studies. This includes affinity enrichment using immobilized strepta-vidin (Jang and Hanash, 2003; Zhao *et al.*, 2003), colloidal silica parti-cles (Durr *et al.*, 2004), or cell-type specific antibody conjugated to magnetic beads (Watarai *et al.*, 2005). These novel protocols require access to the cell surface for efficient surface protein tagging by an affinity-based agent. As a consequence, they can only be applied to cultured neural cells, but not to bulky brain tissue. Second, protocols relying on antibodies are quite expensive. Finally, most of the protocols are rather time-consuming. These limitations and drawbacks have renewed the interest in aqueous two-phase systems as a rapid, inexpensive, and material-saving isolation procedure. We and oth-ers have recently demonstrated the strength of this method for proteomics when aiming at the entire plasma membrane (Cao *et al.*, 2006; Everberg *et al.*, 2006b; Schindler *et al.*, 2006). The protocol presented below was used to purify plasma membranes from a single rat cerebellum and contained ~40% plasma membrane proteins (Schindler *et al.*, 2006). In the following, the principles un-derlying this protocol are laid down and comments made on some important facts to consider when using aqueous two-phase systems in the lab.

7.1.3
Two-Phase Partitioning

7.1.3.1   Principle of Two-Phase Systems
When solutions of two structurally different polymers are mixed above a certain concentration, they will become immiscible and form two phases. This concentration is called the critical concentration and each phase will be enriched in one of the two polymers. The basis for separation by a two-phase system is the selective enrichment of biomaterial in either of the two phases.

To describe two-phase systems for a given pair of polymers, a phase diagram is used. This summarizes the composition of the two phases for various mixtures of the two polymers (Figure 7.2). A curved line (binodal curve) separates the diagram into two regions. Pairs of polymer concentrations above the binodal curve (open circles in Figure 7.2) give rise to two phases, whereas all compositions represented by points at or below the binodal curve result in a one-phase system. In general, the concentration of polymers required for phase separation increases with decreasing molecular weight of the polymers. Points on the straight lines (tie lines) give polymer concentrations of the entire system. Their intersection with the binodal curve indicates at one end the concentration of each of the two polymers in the top phase (intersection A) and at the opposite end the concentrations in the bottom phase (intersection B). All points on the

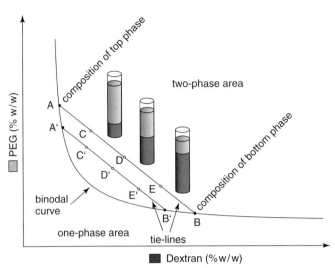

Figure 7.2 Schematic phase diagram for a PEG/dextran system. Two-phase systems are characterized by phase diagrams. The curved line (binodal curve) separates two regions of possible composition of the phase system: polymer compositions above the binodal curve give two phases, all compositions represented by points at or below the binodal curve result in one phase. All points on the binodal curve represent polymer compositions of either top or bottom phase. Each point on the lines connecting the composition of a top phase and a bottom phase in equilibrium (tie lines) represents two-phase systems with the same polymer composition in the top phase and in the bottom phase, respectively. They only differ in the volumes of the two phases. For a detailed explanation of phase diagrams see the text.

same tie line result in two-phase systems with identical polymer concentrations in the top and bottom phase, respectively. They only differ in the volume of each phase. This can be exploited to concentrate biomaterial by simply reducing the amount of the preferred polymer (Figure 7.2). Tie lines become shorter with reduced polymer concentrations. At the critical point, the polymer concentrations in the top and the bottom phase equal each other, resulting in a single phase. Close to the critical point, two-phase systems are very sensitive to alterations such as changes in temperature. Polymer concentrations should therefore be chosen that will lead to a stable two-phase system.

In principle, many different phase-forming polymers can be chosen according to their structure, molecular weight, and ionic group. One of the two polymers can also be substituted by salt. In practice, the most commonly used two-phase systems make use of poly(ethylene glycol) (PEG) and dextran. Both polymers are low priced, require only moderate concentrations (resulting in moderate viscosities), and separate rapidly. Furthermore, they are mild as the material is kept in an aqueous environment. The concentration of water is normally 92–98% in the top phase and 80–90% in the bottom phase. In a PEG/dextran system, PEG is enriched in the top phase and dextran mainly found in the bottom phase. The top phase thereby behaves as if it were more hydrophobic than the bottom phase, since PEG is more hydrophobic than dextran (Albertsson, 1986). The protocol presented below is based on such a PEG/dextran system.

7.1.3.2 Factors Determing Partition Behavior
The distribution of each biomaterial between the two phases is quantitatively described by a partition coefficient, K, which is defined as the ratio between the concentrations of the biomaterial in the two phases. Many factors greatly affect the partition in the PEG/dextran two-phase systems. Important polymer factors are the concentration, type and molecular weight as well as presence of certain chemical groups on the polymers (Table 7.1). Other factors to consider include the size of the biomaterial and the ionic composition and pH of the system (Table 7.1). All of these factors have to be precisely standardized to obtain reproducible results. Increase in polymer concentrations results in larger differences in the composition of the two phases and causes membranes to partition preferentially to the interphase or the bottom phase (Table 7.1). This can be exploited to enrich plasma membranes in the top phase, as they show the

Table 7.1 Influence of different parameters on membrane partitioning.

Increase in	Partition coefficient
Polymer concentration	↓
Molecular weight of prevailing polymer in top phase	↓
Molecular weight of prevailing polymer in bottom phase	↑
Temperature	↓
Interfacial tension	↓
Salt composition	↑↓ [a]
Salt concentration	↑↓ [a]
Affinity ligand coupled to prevailing polymer in top phase	↑
Affinity ligand coupled to prevailing polymer in bottom phase	↓

Increasing the parameters mentioned in the table result in an altered partitioning behavior of membranes of different subcellular origin. An increase in the partitioning coefficient is equivalent with an increased partitioning of the membrane to the top phase. (↓) decrease in the partition coefficient; (↑), increase in the partition coefficient (modified from Schindler and Nothwang, 2006, with permission).
[a] Depending on partition coefficient of the ions and the charge of the biomolecule.

highest affinity for the more hydrophobic top phase, followed by the Golgi, endoplasmic reticulum, and mitochondria. Decreased partition into the top phase can also be obtained by decreasing the molecular weight of PEG. In contrast, increase of the molecular weight of dextran results in an increased partition of membranes to the top phase. Furthermore, phase diagrams are considerably influenced by the temperature. Reduced temperature in the PEG/dextran system requires lower polymer concentrations for phase separation. It is therefore essential to perform two-phase systems at a constant temperature, best at $4\,°C$. Another factor of paramount importance is the composition and concentration of salts present in the system. Ions usually have different affinities for the top phase and for the bottom phase. Cations usually prefer the top phase in the following order: $Li^+ > NH_4^+ > Na^+ > Cs^+ \cong K^+$, whereas anions display a higher affinity for the bottom phase as follows: borate > citrate $\cong$ sulfate $\cong$ hydrogen phosphate > dihydrogen phosphate > halides.

The requirement for electroneutrality in each phase forces one ion to co-partition with its counterion in the absence of additionally charged molecules such as biomembranes. The presence of charged biomaterial will be used by the ions to redistribute between the two phases. This, in turn, will force the charged biomaterial to concomitantly partition in one of the two phases in order to maintain electroneutrality in each of the two phases. Negatively charged membranes can therefore be pushed to the top phase by adding Li_2SO_4, as Li^+ preferentially partitions into the top phase and SO_4^{2-} into the bottom phase. However, one should note that at a pH value that renders the net charge of the membrane patches neutral, partition would occur independent of salts used. Furthermore, already minor changes in salt concentration will affect partition behavior of membranes. This might become a problem when tissue homogenates are used directly as input into the two-phase system. The salt concentration in the total system will differ as a function of the amount of starting material. It is therefore advisable to use a medium-salted buffer to make the final salt concentration independent from the amount and type of tissue added. In the protocol provided below, a microsomal pellet is applied and therefore, salt concentrations are negligible. In theory, the charge of the biomaterial can be altered by adjusting the pH of the buffer. However, most protocols use neutral or only slightly alkaline conditions in order to preserve the native structure of the biomaterial.

7.1.3.3 Increased Selectivity of Partition

So far, conventional two-phase systems have been found to have limited use in fractionation of membranes from animal cells, as the differences between the various membranes are insufficient to obtain a clear-cut separation. To increase selectivity, an affinity ligand can be introduced into one of the phases. Conjugation of a suitable ligand to one of the two polymers will selectively and effectively redirect the target membranes from one phase to the other ligand-containing phase, away from the unwanted material. Affinity partitioning has been applied to isolate membranes enriched in cholinergic receptors (Flanagan *et al.*, 1975) or opiate-binding receptors (Johansson, 1994), as well as to purify plasma membranes from rat liver (Persson *et al.*, 1991), lung (Abedinpour and Jergil, 2003), or brain (Schindler *et al.*, 2006). Recently, the isolation of caveole has been reported (Barinaga-Rementeria *et al.*, 2004). Potential ligands are lectins, antibodies, enzymatic inhibitors, or receptor agonists and antagonists. For plasma membranes, wheat germ agglutinin (WGA) is the ligand of choice, as it is inexpensive. In the PEG/dextran two-phase system, both polymers can be used for conjugation. In the protocol presented below, dextran is used as carrier, as its concentration in the PEG-enriched top phase is lower than the PEG concentration in the dextran-enriched bottom phase. This will cause a higher enrichment of plasma membranes in the dextran-containing bottom phase. Furthermore, the higher molecular weight of dextran is less influenced by the ligand. Major alterations in polymer distribution after conjugation are hence less likely to occur. Finally, dextran has several potential ligand-coupling sites, whereas PEG has only two sites per molecule.

The experimental conditions should be chosen so that all membranes present partition into the top phase in the absence of the polymer–ligand adduct. Under these conditions, the presence of the polymer–ligand adduct in the bottom phase will selectively enrich the plasma membrane in this phase. To favor partition of the ligand–polymer conjugate to the bottom phase, a two-phase system far from the critical point, that is, with higher polymer concentrations, is desirable (Figure 7.2). A drawback of such a system is the partitioning of membranes to the interface. To overcome this problem, first a conventional two-phase system is used with polymer concentrations best suited to enrich plasma membranes in the PEG-enriched phase, and the intracellular membranes in the dextran-enriched phase. In a second step, the so-called affinity partitioning, the PEG-enriched phase is mixed with the affinity ligand conjugated dextran-enriched phase. The plasma membranes will therefore be pulled to the dextran-enriched phase. To counteract partitioning of the residual intracellular membranes from the PEG-enriched top phase to the bottom phase, 2 mM Li_2SO_4 is added. This will increase the partitioning of undesired membranes into the top phase. Alternatively, dextran of higher molecular weight may be used.

7.1.3.4 High pH and High Salt Wash

The protocol is rounded off by a high pH and high salt extraction of the isolated plasma membranes. Under these conditions, plasma membrane vesicles will open and release trapped peripheral proteins (Fujiki *et al.*, 1982). Furthermore, contaminating organelles will be removed. This additional step serves therefore two purposes. First, integral membrane proteins will be twofold enriched. Second, it allows for separate subsequent analysis of integral and peripheral plasma membrane proteins. Many studies aim at a comparative quantitative analysis between two different conditions such as treated versus untreated or between wild-type and disease conditions. Despite recent developments in differential isotope labeling, the work horse for quantification is classic two-dimensional gel electrophoresis with isoelectric focusing in the first dimension and sodium dodecyl sulfate polyacrylamide gel electrophoresis (SDS-PAGE) in the second dimension. The separation of integral from peripheral plasma membrane proteins opens up the possibility of quantifying peripheral proteins by this approach. Comparative quantitative analysis of integral plasma membrane proteins requires techniques such as isotope-coded affinity tagging prior analysis using LC-coupled MS.

7.2
Protocols

Due to the strong influence of ions on membrane partitioning in two-phase systems, double distilled water should be used throughout the experiments.

7.2.1
Preparation of Wheat Germ Agglutinin–Dextran

7.2.1.1   Activation of Dextran

Requirements

Chemicals and materials: DMSO; triethylamine; dichloromethane; Dextran T500, tresyl chloride; dialysis tubes (moleculer weight cut-off 12 000–14 000 Da). DMSO, triethylamine and dichloromethane are dried with molecular sieves prior to use.

1. Dissolve 5 g of freeze-dried Dextran T500 in 25 mL DMSO at room temperature in a glass beaker dried in an oven at 100 °C overnight.
2. Add dropwise 1 mL of triethylamine followed by 5 mL of dichloromethane (~10 min) while stirring on ice to avoid precipitation of dextran.
3. Add slowly 0.35 g (220 µL) of tresyl chloride under vigorous stirring on ice.
4. Stir gently on ice for 1 h, then at room temperature overnight.
5. Add 50 mL of dichloromethane to terminate the reaction and to precipitate dextran. Dextran becomes clear and slimy.
6. Wash four times with 25 mL dichloromethane each time by pressing the slime against the beaker with a glass rod. The product should become white and crystalline.
7. Dissolve the washed precipitate in 30 mL water and dialyze against distilled water until the dialysis tube contains a clear solution. All this is done at room temperature.
8. Freeze-dry tresyl-dextran and store at −20 °C. It is stable for several months under these conditions.

7.2.1.2 Coupling of Wheat Germ Agglutinin

Requirements

Materials: Coupling buffer (500 mM NaCl, 100 mM NaH_2PO_4, pH 7.5); quenching buffer (400 mM Tris-HCl, pH 7.5); dissolve in one glass tube 2 g of tresyl-dextran in 10 mL coupling buffer and in another one 10 mg WGA in 1 mL coupling buffer.

Equipment: Jumbosep centrifugal device (molecular weight cut-off 100 000 Da).

1. Add the WGA solution dropwise with a pipette to the tresyl-dextran solution under vigorous vortexing (approximately 10 min). Incubate the mixture overnight at 4 °C under gentle agitation.
2. Add 10 mL of quenching buffer to terminate the reaction and to inactivate unreacted tresyl groups. Incubate for 2 h at 4 °C with agitation. This step is essential to avoid reactions with amino groups in subsequent procedures.
3. Add the mixture to Jumbosep centrifugal devices, fill with distilled water to a final volume of 60 mL and centrifuge until the volume has decreased to one-third. Repeat the procedure 5 times. This will remove uncoupled ligand and salts.
4. Freeze-dry WGA–dextran. Determine the coupling degree by a Bradford assay (Pierce, Rockford, IL, USA) using WGA as standard.

7.2.2
Preparation of Microsomes

A microsomal membrane preparation is applied to the two-phase system. This crude membrane preparation can be obtained by various differential centrifugation protocols. However, when using other protocols than provided here, keep in mind that altered salt conditions will influence partition behavior.

Requirements

Solutions: Homogenization buffer (250 mM sucrose, 15 mM Tris, complete protease inhibitor (Roche), pH 7.8). Equipment: Glass–Teflon homogenizer.

1. Add 4.5 mL homogenization buffer to 1.5 g of brain tissue and homogenize by 20 strokes at 250 rpm in the glass–Teflon homogenizer.
2. Centrifuge for 10 min at 4 °C with 3000 × g to sediment nuclei and cell debris.
3. Remove the supernatant and store on ice until further use.

4. Re-extract the pellet with a pipette in the same volume of homogenization buffer, as used for initial homogenization. Centrifuge for 10 min at 4 °C with 3000 × g.

5. Repeat steps 3–4.

6. Combine all three supernatants and centrifuge for 12 min at 4 °C with 10 000 × g to sediment mitochondria.

7. Remove the supernatant and store on ice until further use.

8. Re-extract the pellet with a pipette in the same volume of homogenization buffer as removed before. Centrifuge for 12 min at 4 °C with 10 000 × g.

9. Repeat steps 7–8.

10. Combine the three supernatants of the 10 000 × g centrifugation steps and centrifuge for 1 h at 4 °C with 100 000 × g.

11. Discard the supernatant. The resulting pellet represents the microsomes that are further purified by affinity two-phase partitioning. The pellet can be stored at −80 °C.

7.2.3
Affinity Two-Phase Partitioning

All steps of the affinity two-phase partitioning protocol have to be performed at 4 °C, as working at room temperature prevents phase separation.

Requirements

Solutions: Dextran T500 stock solution (20% w/w); PEG 3350 stock solution (40% w/w); 200 mM Tris-H_2SO_4 (pH 7.8, adjusted with H_2SO_4); 200 mM borate buffer (pH 7.8, adjusted with Tris); 200 mM Li_2SO_4 stock solution; WGA–dextran; N-acetyl-D-glucosamine solution (100 mM N-acetyl-D-glucosamine, 250 mM sucrose, 5 mM Tris, pH 7.8).

1. Prepare all two-phase systems with the compositions indicated in Table 7.2 one day prior to use. A two-phase system of 8 g with a final concentration of 6.3% of dextran and 800 µg WGA is required. Mix them by 20 inversions, vortexing for 10 s, and another 20 inversions and store the mixtures at 4 °C overnight. Two-phase systems with the top phase enriched in PEG and the bottom phase enriched in dextran will form overnight.

2. Add 400 µL of microsomes resuspended in homogenization buffer to two-phase system **1**. Mix thoroughly by inversions (2 × 20), interrupted by vortexing for 10 s. Accelerate phase separation by centrifugation for 5 min at 150 × g.

3. Remove the top phase (top phase **A**) without disturbing the interface and store it until further usage. Re-extract the bottom phase by adding a similar volume of fresh top phase from two-phase system **2**. Mix thoroughly as above and accelerate phase separation by centrifugation.

Table 7.2 Composition of two-phase systems.

	Two-phase system				
	1	2	3	4	5
WGA–dextran	–	–	–	X^a	–
Dextran stock solution	1.26 g	1.26 g	1.26 g	X^b	2.52 g
PEG stock solution	0.63 g	0.63 g	0.63 g	1.26 g	1.26 g
Tris-H_2SO_4	0.3 g	0.3 g	0.3 g	–	–
Borate buffer	–	–	–	0.6 g	0.6 g
Li_2SO_4	–	–	–	0.04 g	0.04 g
Water	1.41 g	1.81 g	1.81 g	X^c	3.58 g

[a] $m_{WGA-dextran} = 800\ \mu g/($coupling degree $[\mu g\ mg^{-1}$ dextran$] \times 1000)$.
[b] $m_{dextran} = (0.504\ g - m_{WGA-dextran}) \times 5$.
[c] $m_{water} = 8\ g - (m_{dextran} + m_{WGA-dextran} + m_{PEG} + m_{borate\ buffer} + m_{Li2SO4})$.

4. Remove the top phase (top phase **B**) and combine it with top phase **A**. Layer the combined top phases **A** + **B** onto the bottom phase of two-phase system **2**. Mix as above and accelerate phase separation by centrifugation.
5. Remove the resulting top phase **C** and mix it thoroughly with fresh bottom phase from two-phase system **3**. Accelerate phase separation by centrifugation.
6. Remove the resulting top phase **D** and mix it thoroughly with fresh bottom phase from two-phase system **4**. Accelerate phase separation by centrifugation.
7. Discard the top phase **E** and mix the bottom phase with a similar volume of fresh top phase from two-phase system **5**. Accelerate phase separation by centrifugation. Discard the top phase.
8. Dilute the bottom phase 10-fold in *N*-acetyl-D-glucosamine and centrifuge at $100\,000 \times g$ for 90 min. This will release the plasma membranes from WGA–dextran and will result in the sedimentation of the membranes.

7.2.4
High-Salt and High-pH Washing to Separate Integral and Peripheral Plasma Membrane Proteins

To separate integral and peripheral plasma membrane proteins, high-salt and high-pH washes are recommended. Only peripheral membrane proteins will become solubilized in the washing buffers.

Requirements

Solution: High-salt buffer (1 M KCl, 15 mM Tris, pH 7.4); high-pH buffer (100 mM Na_2CO_3).
1. Resuspend the plasma membrane pellet in ice-cold high-salt buffer with a homogenizer and centrifuge for 1 h at 233 000 × g. Repeat this step twice. Each time, the supernatant, representing peripheral plasma membrane proteins, is collected.
2. Resuspend the final pellet of the high-salt wash in ice-cold high-pH buffer with a homogenizer and centrifuge for 1 h at 233 000 × g. Repeat this step twice. Collect each time the supernatant, which represents peripheral plasma membrane proteins.
3. Combine all six supernatants, enriched in peripheral plasma membrane proteins, and store them as well as the pellet, enriched in integral membrane proteins, at −80 °C.

7.3
Outlook

A major advantage of two-phase systems is the short time required. The above protocol can be performed within 4 h, if microsomes and all reagents are available. To improve the protocol further, two changes can be envisaged. One modification would be the direct use of brain homogenate, omitting the preparation of microsomes. This would further increase the efficiency of the protocol. 90% of the plasma membrane proteins are lost during preparation of microsomes by differential centrifugation, compared to only 50% during affinity partitioning (Schindler *et al.*, 2006). Bypassing microsomes and the concomitant loss of most plasma membrane proteins would likely broaden the application range to CNS areas such as brain nuclei.

Alternatively, the affinity step might be replaced by countercurrent distribution (CCD) experiments. In CCD experiments, multiple extraction steps are carried out in order to separate substances (Figure 7.3). This procedure is based on the fact that the partitioning coefficient K is mainly a function of the properties of the two phases, the nature of the partitioned biomaterial, and the temperature, but independent of the concentration of the biomaterial. The partitioning coefficient hence remains constant during multiple extractions under identical conditions. In CCD experiments, each of the two phases, top and bottom, is re-extracted, respectively, with bottom and top phases. The number of sequential extraction steps required to enrich efficiently plasma membranes depends on the relative solubility of the biomaterial in the two phases (Figure 7.3). Implementation of CCD would further simplify the protocol as no coupling of WGA to dextran has to be performed. This would also make the protocol very inexpensive.

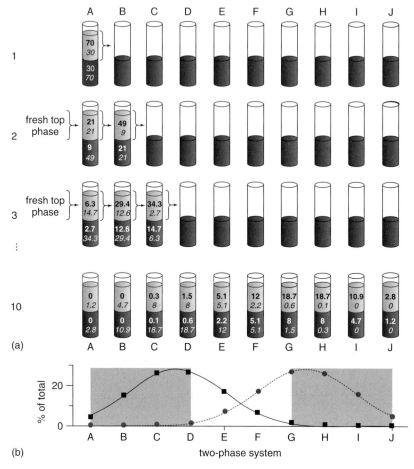

(a)

(b)

Figure 7.3 Schema for countercurrent distribution (CCD). (a) Seventy per cent of a given structure (e.g. plasma membranes) might partition to the top phase and 30% to the bottom phase (bold numbers) in a given two-phase system. Thirty per cent of other structures (e.g. intracellular membranes) might partition to the top phase and 70% to the bottom phase (italic numbers). In CCD experiments, the top phase of the initial two-phase system A is transferred to a fresh bottom phase B and the bottom phase of two-phase system A is re-extracted with a fresh top phase resulting in the distribution indicated. After nine iterations this results in an efficient separation of the biomaterial. (b) The outcome of the CCD procedure is illustrated for each of the resulting two-phase systems. Intracellular membranes (squares) and plasma membrane (circles) are well separated in the gray-shaded two-phase systems. (Modified from Schindler and Nothwang, 2006, with permission.)

A major advantage of two-phase systems is that they are mild and protective of the partitioned biomaterial and display no denaturing effects (Everberg *et al.*, 2006a). Experiences thus far indicate that polymers stabilize, rather than damage the particle structures and the biological activities (Albertsson, 1986). Accordingly, membranes isolated by aqueous two-phase systems preserve their biological functions (Walter and Larsson, 1994). Furthermore, the matrix-free aqueous environment during the separation process minimizes unwanted interactions. Two-phase systems might therefore be the method of choice to enrich plasma membrane protein complexes prior to further purification via affinity columns and so on. Another interesting application might be the analysis of native plasma membrane proteins under defined conditions. This includes studies on the flux rate of plasma membrane transporters by radioactive labeled compounds. In contrast to expression in artificial membranes, the entire native transporter complex could be probed and the effect of modulators such as specific kinases or phosphatases would be possible. As the plasma membrane proteins are already enriched, the sample could rapidly be processed to analyze posttranslational modifications of transporters and other proteins involved in the respective process by mass spectrometry. Finally, efficient isolation of plasma membranes from well-defined brain areas will allow activity-correlated analysis of posttranslational modifications.

References

Abedinpour, P. and Jergil, B. (2003) Isolation of a caveolae-enriched fraction from rat lung by affinity partitioning and sucrose gradient centrifugation. *Analytical Biochemistry*, **313**, 1–8.

Albertsson, P.A. (1986) *Partition of Cell Particles and Macromolecules*, John Wiley & Sons, Inc., New York.

Barinaga-Rementeria, R.I., Abedinpour, P. and Jergil, B. (2004) Purification of caveolae by affinity two-phase partitioning using biotinylated antibodies and NeutrAvidin-dextran. *Analytical Biochemistry*, **331**, 17–26.

Becker, M., Schindler, J. and Nothwang, H.G. (2006) Neuroproteomics—the taks lying ahead. *Electrophoresis*, **27**, 2819–2829.

Butchbach, M.E., Tian, G., Guo, H. and Lin, C.L. (2004) Association of excitatory amino acid transporters, especially EAAT2, with cholesterol-rich lipid raft microdomains: importance for excitatory amino acid transporter localization and function. *The Journal of Biological Chemistry*, **279**, 34388–34396.

Cao, R., Li, X., Liu, Z., Peng, X., Hu, W., Wang, X., Chen, P., Xie, J. and Liang, S. (2006) Integration of a two-phase partition method into proteomics research on rat liver plasma membrane proteins. *Journal of Proteome Research*, **5**, 634–642.

Carroll, R.C. and Zukin, R.S. (2002) NMDA-receptor trafficking and targeting: implications for synaptic transmission and plasticity. *Trends in Neurosciences*, **25**, 571–577.

Chen, B.E., Kondo, M., Garnier, A., Watson, F.L., Puettmann-Holgado, R., Lamar, D.R. and Schmucker, D. (2006) The molecular diversity of Dscam is functionally required for neuronal wiring specificity in Drosophila. *Cell*, **125**, 607–620.

Chen, X., Vinade, L., Leapman, R.D., Petersen, J.D., Nakagawa, T., Phillips, T.M., Sheng, M. and Reese, T.S. (2005) Mass of the postsynaptic density and enumeration of three key molecules. *Proceedings of the National Academy of Sciences of the United States of America*, **102**, 11551–11556.

Durr, E., Yu, J., Krasinska, K.M., Carver, L.A., Yates, J.R., Testa, J.E., Oh, P. and Schnitzer, J.E. (2004) Direct proteomic mapping of the lung microvascular endothelial cell surface *in vivo* and in cell culture. *Nature Biotechnology*, **22**, 985–992.

Esteban, J.A. (2003) AMPA receptor trafficking: a road map for synaptic plasticity. *Molecular Interventions*, **7**, 375–385.

Evans, W.H. (1991) Isolation and characterization of membranes and cell organelles, in *Preparative Centrifugation* (ed. D. Rickwood), IRL Press, Oxford, pp. 233–270.

Everberg, H., Leiding, T., Schioth, A., Tjerneld, F. and Gustavsson, N. (2006a) Efficient and non-denaturing membrane solubilization combined with enrichment of membrane protein complexes by detergent/polymer aqueous two-phase partitioning for proteome analysis. *Journal of Chromatography*, **1122**, 35–46.

Everberg, H., Peterson, R., Rak, S., Tjerneld, F. and Emanuelsson, C. (2006b) Aqueous two-phase partitioning for proteomic monitoring of cell surface biomarkers in human peripheral blood mononuclear cells. *Journal of Proteome Research*, **5**, 1168–1175.

Flanagan, S.D., Taylor, P. and Barondes, S.H. (1975) Affinity partitioning of acetylcholine receptor enriched membranes and their purification. *Nature*, **254**, 441–443.

Fortin, D.L., Troyer, M.D., Nakamura, K., Kubo, S., Anthony, M.D. and Edwards, R.H. (2004) Lipid rafts mediate the synaptic localization of alpha-synuclein. *The Journal of Neuroscience*, **24**, 6715–6723.

Fujiki, Y., Hubbard, A.L., Fowler, S. and Lazarow, P.B. (1982) Isolation of intracellular membranes by means of sodium carbonate treatment: application to endoplasmic reticulum. *The Journal of Cell Biology*, **93**, 97–102.

Hopkins, A.L. and Groom, C.R. (2002) The druggable genome. *Nature Reviews. Drug Discovery*, **1**, 727–730.

Jang, J.H. and Hanash, S. (2003) Profiling of the cell surface proteome. *Proteomics*, **3**, 1947–1954.

Johansson, G. (1994) Synaptic membranes, in *Methods in Enyzmology*, (eds H. Walter

and G. Johansson), Academic Press, San Diego, pp. 496–503.

Kapfer, C., Seidl, A.H., Schweizer, H. and Grothe, B. (2002) Experience-dependent refinement of inhibitory inputs to auditory coincidence-detector neurons. *Nature Neuroscience*, **5**, 247–253.

Magnani, F., Tate, C.G., Wynne, S., Williams, C. and Haase, J. (2004) Partitioning of the serotonin transporter into lipid microdomains modulates transport of serotonin. *The Journal of Biological Chemistry*, **279**, 38770–38778.

Masland, R.H. (2004) Neuronal cell types. *Current Biology*, **14**, R497–R500.

Persson, A., Johansson, B., Olsson, H. and Jergil, B. (1991) Purification of rat liver plasma membranes by wheat-germ-agglutinin affinity partitioning. *The Biochemical Journal*, **273**, 173–177.

Schindler, J., Lewandrowski, U., Sickmann, A., Friauf, E. and Gerd, N.H. (2006) Proteomic analysis of brain plasma membranes isolated by affinity two-phase partitioning. *Molecular & Cellular Proteomics*, **5**, 390–400.

Schindler, J. and Nothwang, H.G. (2006) Aqueous polymer two-phase systems: effective tools for plasma membrane proteomics. *Proteomics*, **20**, 5409–5417.

Temburni, M.K. and Jacob, M.H. (2001) New functions for glia in the brain. [letter; comment]. *Proceedings of the National Academy of Sciences of the United States of America*, **98**, 3631–3632.

Torres, G.E., Gainetdinov, R.R. and Caron, M.G. (2003) Plasma membrane monoamine transporters: structure, regulation and function. *Nature Reviews. Neuroscience*, **4**, 13–25.

Triller, A. and Choquet, D. (2005) Surface trafficking of receptors between synaptic and extrasynaptic membranes: and yet they do move! *Trends in Neurosciences*, **28**, 133–139.

Trinidad, J.C., Specht, C.G., Thalhammer, A., Schoepfer, R. and Burlingame, A.L. (2006) Comprehensive identification of phosphorylation sites in postsynaptic density preparations. *Molecular & Cellular Proteomics*, **5**, 914–922.

Vosseller, K., Trinidad, J.C., Chalkley, R.J., Specht, C.G., Thalhammer, A., Lynn, A.J., Snedecor, J.O., Guan, S., Medzihradszky, K.F., Maltby, D.A., Schoepfer, R. and Burlingame, A.L. (2006) O-Linked N-acetylglucosamine proteomics of postsynaptic density preparations using lectin weak affinity chromatography and mass spectrometry. *Molecular & Cellular Proteomics*, **5**, 923–934.

Walter, H. and Larsson, C. (1994) Partitioning procedures and techniques: cells, organelles, and membranes. *Methods in Enzymology*, **228**, 42–63.

Watarai, H., Hinohara, A., Nagafune, J., Nakayama, T., Taniguchi, M. and Yamaguchi, Y. (2005) Plasma membrane-focused proteomics: dramatic changes in surface expression during the maturation of human dendritic cells. *Proteomics*, **5**, 4001–4011.

Zhao, Y., Zhang, W., White, M.A. and Zhao, Y. (2003) Capillary high-performance liquid chromatography/mass spectrometric analysis of proteins from affinity-purified plasma membrane. *Analytical Chemistry*, **75**, 3751–3757.

8
Proteome Analysis of Synaptic Vesicles

Mads Grønborg, Matthew Holt, Florian Richter, Shigeo Takamori, Dietmar Riedel, Reinhard Jahn and Henning Urlaub

8.1
Introduction

8.1.1
The Synaptic Vesicle

Chemical synapses can be regarded as the elementary structures at which information transfer between neurons occurs. Neurons transmit information through the nervous system by releasing neurotransmitters from the presynaptic terminal. In a resting state, transmitters are stored in small organelles of uniform size and shape called synaptic vesicles. When an action potential (stimulus) arrives in the nerve terminal, the membrane depolarizes and voltage-gated Ca^{2+} channels open. The resulting Ca^{2+} influx triggers fusion (exocytosis) of synaptic vesicles at specialized release sites on the membrane, resulting in the release of neurotransmitter. This transmitter then diffuses to and binds to cognate receptors on the postsynaptic membrane, eliciting a response. At the same, the synaptic vesicle membrane is rapidly retrieved by endocytosis and reutilized for the reformation of synaptic vesicles.

Although a highly specialized process, the synaptic vesicle cycle shares basic properties with other intracellular membrane pathways: these include directed transport to the release site (along cytoskeletal tracks with the aid of a motor protein) (Soldati and Schliwa, 2006), recognition of the target membrane and docking (via rab GTPases) and fusion (executed by the SNARE proteins (Jahn and Scheller, 2006)) followed by several specialized steps including retrieval (interaction of synaptotagmin I with cytosolic proteins) and refilling with neurotransmitter (by specific transporters (Ryan, 2006)). Hence, not only can synaptic vesicles be considered as the basic minimal units of synaptic transmission but they can also be regarded as the basic minimal units of membrane transport, whose integral protein composition serves as the basis for all the functions that a trafficking vesicle

Proteomics of the Nervous System. Edited by H.G. Nothwang and S.E. Pfeiffer
Copyright © 2008 WILEY-VCH Verlag GmbH & Co. KGaA, Weinheim
ISBN: 978-3-527-31716-5

must perform (including the recruitment of protein complexes from the cytoplasm).

The composition of synaptic vesicles is, at present, better understood than any other trafficking organelle (for a detailed characterization of their composition see Takamori *et al.*, 2006) and several proteins first identified in synaptic vesicles have turned out to be members of conserved protein families which operate in all trafficking steps (Jahn *et al.*, 2003; Jahn and Scheller, 2006). This is because synaptic vesicles possess several unique properties that make them amenable to biochemical studies. Synaptic vesicles represent the most abundant class of trafficking organelles known (e.g. the human central nervous system (CNS) alone contains approximately 10^{17} vesicles), and large amounts of nervous tissue can easily be obtained in the laboratory. They are also the most uniform class of organelle in the nervous system, comprising a relatively homogeneous population with diameters between approximately 40 and 50 nm, allowing the application of standard size fractionation techniques. Finally, many of the major integral membrane proteins are already known and provide a further basis for manipulation. In summary, there is no other trafficking organelle of comparable simplicity and abundance that offers biochemical access to the membrane proteins involved in its function. This provides the opportunity of identifying novel trafficking proteins by mass spectrometry, while also providing a platform for the optimization of existing MS protocols, using previously identified membrane proteins.

8.1.2
Purification of Synaptic Vesicles

8.1.2.1   General Remarks

The purity of the sample is one of the most important factors for a successful proteome analysis of any isolated subcellular compartment and/or protein complex. Therefore, much attention is currently devoted to techniques of sample preparation. In particular, purification of synaptic vesicles requires specialized protocols to avoid co-purification of plasma membrane fractions and other trafficking vesicles of similar size, density or composition such as clathrin-coated vesicles (CCVs). Therefore, it is necessary to monitor both the enrichment and the purity of the material at various steps of the purification procedure by the detection of highly specific marker proteins (e.g. synaptobrevin-2, which is an integral synaptic vesicle membrane protein critical for fusion with the plasma membrane; see below).

Synaptic vesicles can be purified in sufficient amounts from rat brain. Purification protocols for synaptic vesicles can be divided into two major groups. The first group involves those that separate exclusively on physical parameters, such as shape and density (Hu *et al.*, 2002). Synaptic vesicles prepared using these methods involve the purification of isolated nerve terminals (synaptosomes) followed by osmotic lysis to release synaptic vesicles (Huttner *et al.*, 1983). Purification of synaptic vesicles from synaptosomes has the advantage that small membrane fragments generated during homogenization are removed before vesicle extraction. Although these purifications are time-consuming and result in comparatively low yields, the vesicles obtained are of exceptionally high purity. The second group involves immunoaffinity purification using known vesicle proteins, for example, synaptophysin (Burger *et al.*, 1989). Using this method, synaptic vesicles can even be isolated directly from rat brain homogenate (without the prior isolation of synaptosomes). The crucial step in this purification method is the homogenization phase, during which relatively harsh conditions have to be used in order to release a sufficient amount of synaptic vesicles from the brain.

An important general point to consider during the sample purification prior to any proteome analysis is whether a particular purification method will select for a biochemically distinct pool of (sub)compartments and/or protein complexes, producing a bias in the final analysis. In neurons, the major sources of variation will arise from (i) differential protein expression within a population of neurons and (ii) the activity status of the cell. This variation may be found in the integral membrane proteins, or in cytosolic factors recruited to the synaptic vesicle at various stages of its life cycle, and is discussed in the following paragraphs in more detail:

(i) Neurons in the brain show differential expression profiles across a range of proteins. Nowhere is this more apparent than in the case of the neurotransmitter transporter proteins carried on the synaptic vesicle. To date, seven transmitter-specific transporters have been identified, namely VMATs 1 and 2 (monoamines), VAChT (acetylcholine), VGLUTs 1, 2, and 3 (l-glutamate), and VGAT (GABA and glycine) (Ahnert-Hilger *et al.*, 2003), and these show non-overlapping but complementary expression profiles in the adult brain. Interestingly, glutamatergic and GABAergic neurons predominate in the CNS and this may reflect why these transporters have been previously identified by mass spectrometry of synaptic vesicles purified from whole brain, while those expressed at low(er) levels (VMAT and VGAT) have remained elusive (Takamori *et al.*, 2006). In addition, other key vesicular proteins, which appear to be present on every vesicle, such as synaptobrevin, synaptotagmin, and synaptophysin, also occur in several isoforms displaying differential localization in the CNS. At present it is impossible to say whether the copy number of these individual vesicle proteins may vary between different neurons, or even between individual vesicles. In addition to the different proteomic expression pattern, some synaptic terminals release neuropeptides from large-dense core vesicles (LDVs), alongside the classical neurotransmitters released by synaptic vesicles (see Chapter 10). Fusion and recycling of these LDVs utilizes many of the same proteins as synaptic vesicles so that differences between these two species are hardly detectable at the proteomic level.

(ii) Synaptic vesicle composition may also be affected by the activity status of the neuron. For instance, some synaptic vesicles seem to be preferentially recycled and released—although it is unclear whether this is related to the molecular composition of the vesicle or a posttranslational modification such as phosphorylation (von Schwarzenfeld, 1979). Recent evidence also suggests that the protein stoichiometry of a vesicle may not be fixed and that synaptic vesicles may exchange proteins with the plasma membrane upon fusion, influencing its composition (Burre *et al.*, 2006a; Wienisch and Klingauf, 2006). Furthermore, recycling of synaptic vesicles in neurons occurs in a clathrin-dependent manner, explaining why the vesicle preparation contains many clathrin-related proteins, in particular the components of the AP-2 adapter complex, responsible for coat recruitment to the vesicle, and why partially decoated vesicles derived from these recycling synaptic vesicles have been shown to cofractionate with synaptic vesicles. It is still unclear whether any, or all, of these recycling synaptic vesicles utilize an early endosomal intermediate that would allow a further opportunity to modify the protein composition of the vesicle. Furthermore, it should also be expected, that there will be some variability in the recovery of soluble proteins that are recruited from the cytosol to the vesicle at various points in the trafficking life cycle, thus resulting in hetereogeneous vesicle populations. Indeed, negatively stained electron micrographs of synaptic vesicles purified from synaptosomes (although perfectly aligning in size and overall shape) show clearly distinct surface staining suggesting different proteins and/or quantities of proteins on the corresponding synaptic vesicles (see Section 8.1.2.5 and Figure 8.3). This individual variation among synaptic vesicles perhaps explains why a differential distribution of synaptic vesicles derived from synaptosomes can be seen in sucrose-density centrifugation (Maycox *et al.*, 1992).

8.1.2.2 Purification of Synaptic Vesicles from Synaptosomes

The standard purification procedure for purification of synaptic vesicles from synaptosomes is based on a modified version of a classical fractionation protocol originally developed by Whittaker and co-workers (Nagy *et al.*, 1976; Huttner *et al.*, 1983). It can be divided into six major steps: (i) homogenization of whole rat brain, (ii) differential centrifugation of the homogenate to obtain a crude synaptosomal pellet, (iii) hypo-osmotic lysis of the syaptosomes to release synaptic vesicles, (iv) differential centrifugation of the crude synaptosomal lysate to obtain a crude synaptic vesicle fraction, (v) purification of the synaptic vesicles by continuous sucrose-density gradient centrifugation and (vi) size-exclusion chromatography on controlled-pore glass. The purification procedure is outlined in Figure 8.1 and in Section 8.2.1.

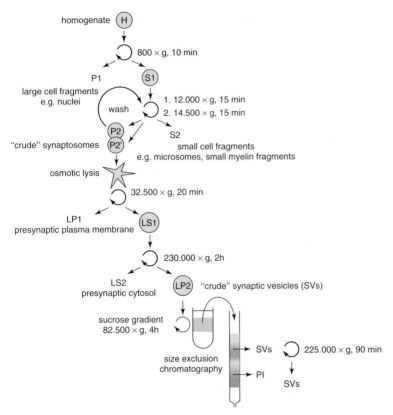

Figure 8.1 Purification of synaptic vesicles from rat brain. Diagram for the purification of synaptic vesicles according to (Huttner et al., 1983). After non-equilibrium sucrose density gradient centrifugation, the zone between approximately 0.04 and 0.4 M sucrose (gray) was collected and separated by chromatography on controlled-pore glass beads (CPG). See text and Section 8.4.1 for further details.

8.1.2.3 Purification of Synaptic Vesicles by Immunoisolation

Analytical amounts of synaptic vesicles may also be obtained by using immunoaffinity purification, which takes advantage of the high binding affinity and specificity of an antibody for its antigen to allow synaptic vesicles to be isolated rapidly. Immunoisolation has been performed both from crude brain homogenate and from isolated synaptosomes. Obviously, using a crude brain homogenate largely avoids the damaging steps associated with purification from synaptosomes (such as osmotic stress), although extra care has to be taken to maintain sample purity. In both cases, the time-consuming size-exclusion chromatography employed in other methods is avoided (Huttner et al., 1983). Moreover, immunoisolation can be used to isolate a distinct synaptic vesicle population, for instance those containing a specific neurotransmitter transporter.

Immunoisolation of synaptic vesicles has recently been carried out using magnetic Dynabeads (Morciano et al., 2005) and the reader is referred to this resource for more detailed protocols. The general requirements for any bead-based system used for immunoisolation however can be summarized as follows: the beads must be small ($1-2$ µm average diameter) to maximize surface-to-volume ratio; they should be non-porous with a hydrophilic surface and a hydrophobic core to restrict the binding of antibody to the bead surface and to allow easy washing; and they should have almost no unspecific binding when assayed with ^{35}S-labeled proteins from cell-homogenates or ^{3}H-labeled glutamate, GABA or acetylcholine. The use of protein A/G sepharose beads coupled with antibodies is not recommended as these beads are porous, resulting in a large amount of "internal" antibody coupling which is not accessible for binding owing to the size of the synaptic vesicles.

In general, any antibody—either affinity-purified polyclonal or mono-clonal—can be successfully used for immunoisolation against proteins on synaptic vesicles. Specific polyclonal antibodies have already been used for the successful isolation of distinct synaptic vesicle populations (Takamori et al., 2000a, 2000b). Antibodies also have the advantage that synaptic vesicles can be eluted under less harsh condition from the beads, that is, by an excess of the antigenic peptide. However, because finding the best antibody/coupling conditions for immunoaffinity purification is an empirical task, and potentially time- and resource-consuming, commercial sources of antibody are rarely an economical option, and, at the least, researchers should consider producing their own polyclonal antibodies.

8.1.2.4 Reducing Contaminating Peripheral Proteins

As mentioned above, the purity of a complex biological sample is an essential prerequisite for a comprehensive analysis of its proteome. In particular, the resolving power and dynamic range of liquid chromatography coupled to mass spectrometry (LC-MS) are drastically decreased by highly abundant protein components that either are naturally present or are contaminants because of their high abundance in the cell. Either such components should be specifically depleted (in case of a highly abundant intrinsic protein component) or the pu-rification protocols should include an additional step to remove contaminating proteins that interact non-specifically with the biological sample.

Synaptic vesicles obtained using either isolation technique contain various amounts of soluble proteins with affinity for membranes such as glyceralde-hydes phosphate dehydrogenase, aldolase, actin, and tubulin. To remove these peripheral proteins from the synaptic vesicles, the purified vesicle fraction can be washed with sodium carbonate (see Figure 8.2 and Section 8.2.2).

8.1.2.5 Assaying the Purity of the Synaptic Vesicle Preparation

Monitoring the purity of the sample during the various steps of purification is another important issue throughout the preparation. The most practical

16 BAC-SDS

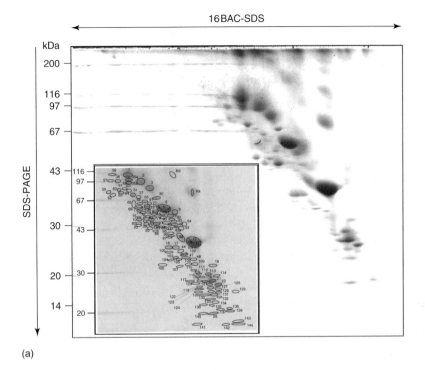

(a)

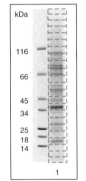
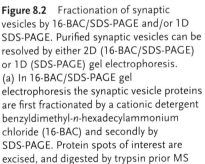

(b)

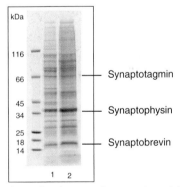

Synaptotagmin

Synaptophysin

Synaptobrevin

Figure 8.2 Fractionation of synaptic vesicles by 16-BAC/SDS-PAGE and/or 1D SDS-PAGE. Purified synaptic vesicles can be resolved by either 2D (16-BAC/SDS-PAGE) or 1D (SDS-PAGE) gel electrophoresis. (a) In 16-BAC/SDS-PAGE gel electrophoresis the synaptic vesicle proteins are first fractionated by a cationic detergent benzyldimethyl-*n*-hexadecylammonium chloride (16-BAC) and secondly by SDS-PAGE. Protein spots of interest are excised, and digested by trypsin prior MS analysis. (b) Alternatively, synaptic vesicle proteins can be resolved by 1D SDS-PAGE. To minimize the number of (contaminating) peripheral proteins, synaptic vesicles can be treated with sodium carbonate prior SDS-PAGE (right panel, lane 1) or left untreated (right panel, lane 2). To maximize the total number of identified proteins in the MS analysis the gel can be divided into 20–25 lanes and subsequently digested by trypsin (left panel).

means of assessing both the degree of enrichment and the purity of the synaptic vesicle preparation is immunoblotting, for which excellent antibodies are available (e.g. Synaptic Systems, Göttingen, Germany, www.sysy.com). During purification, proteins associated with the postsynaptic density (e.g. the NMDA receptor subunit 1 and PSD-95) should be lost, while the integral membrane proteins of synaptic vesicles (e.g. synaptophysin) should be enriched by about 20- to 25-fold in comparison to the homogenate (Jahn *et al.*, 1985). Contamination by other subcellular compartments can also be monitored by assaying for marker enzymes of the plasma membrane, mitochondria or endoplasmic reticulum (Hell *et al.*, 1988). Alternatively, although less sensitive and specific, synaptic vesicles have a well-documented protein profile, as can be observed by sodium dodecyl sulfate polyacrylamide-based gel electrophoresis (SDS-PAGE) followed by staining with Coomassie Brilliant Blue (CBB). Protein bands of the major membrane proteins of synaptobrevin (18 kDa), synaptophysin (38 kDa), and synaptotagmin (65 kDa) are clearly visible (see Figure 8.2b).

Besides the detection of marker proteins, the morphology of synaptic vesicles also adds very valuable information about their purity which can be checked by electron microscopy with negative staining (Takamori *et al.*, 2006). In the final purification step, synaptic vesicles are identified by their small, uniform appearance, with diameters in the range of 40–50 nm (Figure 8.3a). Final confirmation can be obtained by immunogold labeling for the membrane protein synaptophysin (Figure 8.3b). In a highly pure preparation more than 95% of all vesicles must be immunogold stained.

8.1.3
Proteomic Analysis of Synaptic Vesicles

To date, the identification of synaptic vesicle proteins has been limited to biochemical and immunological techniques. The introduction of liquid chromatography coupled to tandem mass spectrometry (LC-MS/MS) and matrix-assisted laser desorption/ionization coupled to tandem time-of-flight mass spectrometry (MALDI-TOF/TOF) either on-line or off-line has provided a very powerful tool for identification of novel synaptic vesicle proteins (Coughenour *et al.*, 2004; Burre *et al.*, 2006a, 2006b; Takamori *et al.*, 2006). Even though synaptic vesicles have been intensively studied as a trafficking organelle, only limited information is available about the overall protein complexity of the synaptic vesicle.

8.1.3.1   Fractionation by 16-BAC/SDS-PAGE or 1D SDS-PAGE
Some issues have to be taken into consideration when a proteomic analysis of synaptic vesicles is to be conducted. First, it has been indicated from previous studies that the synaptic vesicles proteome is rather complex (Takamori *et al.*, 2006). It is therefore recommended that the sample is fractioned prior to MS analysis. Second, synaptic vesicles proteins are mainly membrane-bound proteins or integral membrane proteins and have to be separated by 16-

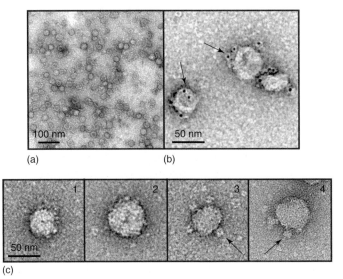

(a) (b)

(c)

Figure 8.3 Electron microscopy of synaptic vesicles. The purity and morphology of synaptic vesicles can be checked by electron microscopy with negative staining. Highly purified synaptic vesicles can be obtained from rat brain homogenate by several differential centrifugation steps combined size-exclusion chromatography.
(a) Negatively stained electron micrographs of purified synaptic vesicles.
(b) Immunogold labeling of synaptic vesicles for the known membrane protein synaptophysin (arrows). (c) Purified synaptic vesicles show distinct surface staining indicating a certain degree of heterogeneity. Panels 1 and 2 show synaptic vesicles with a rough surface while panels 3 and 4 show more smooth synaptic vesicles with ATPases present (arrows). Negative staining: A solution containing synaptic vesicles was applied to glow-discharged carbon-coated grids and stained with 1% uranyl acetate. Images were taken in a Philips CM120 electron microscope (Philips Inc.) at a defocus of 2.3 μm using a TemCam 224A slow scan CCD camera (TVIPS, Gauting, Germany).
Immunogold-labeling: Purified synaptic vesicles were adsorbed to glow-discharged formwar-coated grids and fixed with a mixture of 4% paraformaldehyde and 0.1% glutaraldehyde in 0.1 M potassium–sodium phosphate buffer, pH 7.4. Thereafter unspecific binding sides were blocked with 0.02 M glycin, and 0.5% BSA in phosphate buffer. Labeling with 1 : 500 diluted anti-synaptophysin antibody and 10 nm protein A gold conjugates diluted at 1 : 1000 in 1% BSA in phosphate buffer were performed. The samples were post-fixed for 10 min with 2% glutaraldehyde in phosphate buffer, washed with H_2O, rinsed with three drops of 1% uranyl acetate, and immediately dried with filter paper.

BAC/SDS-PAGE gel electrophoresis (Macfarlane, 1989; Hartinger *et al.*, 1996). This technique has previously been demonstrated to work very well for the fractionation of membrane proteins from synaptic vesicles (Morciano *et al.*, 2005; Burre *et al.*, 2006a, 2006b; Takamori *et al.*, 2006) (Figure 8.2a and Section 8.2.3).

However, when analyzing membrane proteins, one cannot rule out the possibility that some proteins might escape detection when only one fractionation approach is applied so that the proteome is "undersampled". Therefore, it is generally advisable to apply different fractionation approaches in order to increase the total number of proteins identified in the MS analysis (Burre *et al.*, 2006b; Reinders *et al.*, 2006; Takamori *et al.*, 2006). Accordingly, the fractionation of synaptic vesicle proteins can also be performed by traditional one-dimensional SDS-PAGE combined with nanoLC-MS/MS or off-line MALDI-MS/MS (Laemmli, 1970; Takamori *et al.*, 2006). After the electrophoresis, gel lanes can be cut into pieces of equal size instead of cutting single protein bands (Figure 8.2b).

Since gel electrophoresis can be considered the first step in the separation of complex protein samples and because proteins can be differentially stained (or not at all) it is advisable to excise not only bands or single protein spots but rather entire lanes on 1D SDS-PAGEs (Figure 8.2b, left panel). This strategy ensures that proteins that are not detectable by a staining procedure still have a chance of being identified in the subsequent MS analysis. In addition, the total number of proteins identified is usually drastically improved when gel lanes rather than gel spots are analyzed.

Depending on the type and size of the gel, approximately 50–200 µg of purified synaptic vesicles can be loaded as starting material for separation by 1D SDS-PAGE and 16-BAC/SDS-PAGE. The amount of starting material can of course be modified as needed. Figure 8.2 shows the separation of the proteins derived from synaptic vesicles by 16-BAC/SDS-PAGE and 1D SDS-PAGE, respectively.

8.2
Protocols

8.2.1
Purification of Synaptic Vesicles from Synaptosomes

The following method is based on the standard protocol that has been used successfully for many years and is considered to be the "gold-standard" in synaptic vesicle preparation (Hell and Jahn, 1994). Slight variations in centrifugal force and spin time have also been successfully used (Takamori *et al.*, 2006). Note that this method preferentially purifies synaptic vesicles that remain membrane associated after synaptosomal lysis. At present it is unclear whether these synaptic vesicles form a functionally distinct subset in the synaptic terminal.

Requirements

Solutions: Homogenization buffer (320 mM sucrose, 4 mM HEPES (pH 7.40 NaOH)); 1 M HEPES (pH 7.40 NaOH); 40 mM sucrose; 50 mM sucrose; 800 mM sucrose; chromatography buffer (300 mM glycine, 5 mM HEPES (pH 7.4, KOH)), degassed and filtered. Protease inhibitors: 1 mg mL^{-1} pepstatin A in DMSO; 200 mM PMSF in 100% EtOH. Both should be stored at room temperature until use.

Instrumentation: Loose-fitting motor-driven glass–Teflon homogenizer, cooled centrifuge (Sorvall RC5 or comparable with SS34 rotor), ultracentrifuge with fixed-angle and swing-out rotors (Beckman with 50.2Ti and SW28 rotors with corresponding tubes), equipment for column chromatography (peristaltic pump, UV monitor, fraction collector), Corning filter system (0.22 μm polyethersulfone membrane), gradient mixer for forming continuous sucrose gradients.

After collecting the brains, all steps are carried out on ice or at 4 °C.

1. Decapitate 20 rats (180–200 g) and remove the brains into ice-cold homogenization buffer. Wash the brains once with homgenization buffer to remove residual blood. Homogenize the brains in 240 mL homgenization buffer (supplemented with 240 μL PMSF and 240 μL pepstatin A).

2. Centrifuge the homogenate for 10 min at $800 \times g$. Discard the resulting pellet P1 (containing large cell fragments and nuclei) and collect the supernatant (S1).

3. Centrifuge the S1 for 15 min at $12\,000 \times g$. Remove the resulting supernatant (S2), which consists of small cell fragments such as microsomes, small myelin fragments and soluble proteins. The resulting pellet, P2, should be resuspended in homogenization buffer. At this stage care should be taken to avoid the brown bottom part of the pellet that consists of mitochodria. Centrifuge the resuspended pellet at $14\,500 \times g$ for 15 min.

4. The pellet obtained, P2′, represents a crude synaptosomal fraction. To release synaptic vesicles from the synaptosomes, the P2′ is resuspended (again avoiding the brown mitochondrial pellet) to yield a final volume of 24 mL. Transfer 12 mL into a glass–Teflon homogenizer, add 108 mL ice-cold distilled water, and perform three strokes at approximately 2000 rpm. Immediately add 600 μL 1 M HEPES-NaOH and 120 μL PMSF. Repeat for the remaining 12 mL of tissue. Combine both fractions and add 240 μL pepstatin A.

5. Centrifuge the suspension for 20 min at $32\,500 \times g$ to yield a lysate pellet, consisting mainly of presynaptic plama membrane (LP1) and the lysate supernatant LS1. The LS1 should be removed immediately and without disturbing the LP1, which would otherwise significantly reduce the final purity of the synaptic vesicles.

6. The LS1 is centrifuged for 2 h at $230\,000 \times g$ in a 50.2 Ti rotor. The resulting supernatant (presynaptic cytosol; LS2) is discarded and the pellet (LP2; crude synaptic vesicles) is resuspended in 6 mL of 40 mM sucrose, using a small, tight-fitting glass–Teflon homogenizer running at 900 rpm, followed by drawing it through a 20-gauge needle and subsequently out through a 27-gauge needle.

7. During the centrifuge run prepare two linear sucrose gradients from 18 mL of 800 mM sucrose and 18 mL 50 mM sucrose. Layer 3 mL of LP2 onto the top of each gradient and centrifuge for 4 h at $82\,500 \times g$ in

a SW28 rotor. After centrifugation, a turbid (opaque-white) zone is visible in the middle of the gradient (corresponding to 200–400 mM sucrose). This fraction (25–30 mL) is collected with the aid of a peristaltic pump and glass pipette. At this stage synaptic vesicles are enriched approximately 10-fold over the homogenate.

8. The sample is carefully layered onto the top of a controlled-pore glass bead (CPG-3000, see comment below) column pre-equilibrated overnight with glycine buffer. The sample is overlaid and eluted with glycine buffer at a flow rate of 40 mL h^{-1}, with fractions collected every 15 min. The protein content of the eluate is monitored by absorption at 280 nm. Two peaks are obtained from the column. The first contains small amounts of plasma membrane and/or microsomes. The second peak contains the highly purified synaptic vesicles. Fractions comprising the second peak are pooled and centrifuged at 225 000 × g for 90 min. The pellet is resuspended in an appropriate buffer (e.g. PBS). The sample can then be aliquoted and snap-frozen, before storing at −80 °C. Vesicles handled show no obvious deterioration in quality over many months.

The process of size-exclusion chromatography is omitted in many procedures, although this final step has been shown to be important in separating synaptic vesicles from residual amounts of contamination by larger membrane fragments and soluble protein. Unfortunately the controlled-pore glass beads used by our lab are no longer commercially available. An alternative is Sephacryl S-1000 (GE Healthcare) although these columns have a relatively low capacity, do not tolerate overloading and require some experience in their use. In addition, Sephacryl columns have low flow rates, run at low pressure and have a tendency to adsorb proteins and membrane particles, in particular during the first few separation runs in the life of the column. Alternative methods of synaptic vesicle preparation following synaptosomal lysis have also been reported, including the use of flotation on an Optiprep step gradient (Hu *et al.*, 2002).

8.2.2
Reducing Contaminating Peripheral Proteins

Requirements

Solutions: 0.1 M Na$_2$CO$_3$ (pH 11), PBS.

Equipment: Ultracentrifuge with fixed-angle and swing-out rotors (Beckman with 50.2Ti rotor).

1. After purification, the synaptic vesicles are incubated with 0.1 M Na$_2$CO$_3$ (pH 11) on ice for 15 min.
2. The synaptic vesicles are subsequently collected by ultracentrifugation for 20 min at 50 000 rpm.

3. Discard the supernatant after the ultracentrifugation and resuspend the synaptic vesicles in an appropriate buffer (e.g. PBS or SDS/LDS sample buffer).

8.2.3
Fractionation of Synaptic Vesicles by 16-BAC/SDS-PAGE Gel Electrophoresis

Requirements

Chemicals: Benzyldimethyl-*n*-hexadecylammonium chloride (16-BAC), urea, glycerol, β-mercaptoethanol, glycine, phosphoric acid, Tris, acrylamide, bisacryladmide, TEMED, SDS, $FeSO_4$, ascorbic acid, H_2O_2, pyronine Y, EDTA, glycerol, DTT.

Solutions: First dimension:
1. $2 \times$ Sample buffer: 1 g 16-BAC, 4.5 g urea, 1 mL glycerol, 0.5 mL of 1.5 M DTT, 100 µL 5% pyronine Y (w/v) solution (in water), ddH$_2$O to 10 mL. Solubilize detergent and urea in glycerol and 4 mL ddH$_2$O by heating in a microwave, then add DDT and pyronine Y. The solution is finally brought to 10 mL with H_2O.
2. Running buffer (pH 3): 2.5 mM 16-BAC, 150 mM glycine and 50 mM phosphoric acid (a 10× solution can be prepared if needed).
3. Lower gel (7.5%): 10 mL H$_2$O, 10 mL 300 mM potassium phosphate buffer (pH 2.1), 10 mL AMBA (30% acrylamide, 0.8% bisacrylamide), 1.4 mL 1.7% bisacrylamide, 7.2 g urea, 400 µL 10% 16-BAC (heat to 65 °C to solubilize), 64 µL 0.14% FeSO$_4$ (fresh), 2 mL 80 mM ascorbic acid (fresh), start with 1.6 mL H$_2$O$_2$ (1 : 1200, diluted from 30% stock solution, make fresh).
4. Upper gel (4%): 2.5 mL 0.5 M phosphate buffer (pH 4.1), 3.0 mL H$_2$O, 1.33 mL AMBA, 1.38 mL 1.7% bisacrylamide, 1 g urea, 70 µL 250 mM 16-BAC (heat to 65 °C to solubilize), 8.5 µL 5 mM FeSO$_4$ (fresh), 520 µL 80 mM ascorbic acid (fresh), start with 500 µL H$_2$O$_2$ (1 : 750, diluted from 30% stock solution, make fresh).
5. 1 : 750 H$_2$O$_2$ (fresh).
6. Fixing solution: isopropanol:acetic acid:water (3.5 : 1 : 5.5).
7. Staining solution: 0.15% (w/v) Coomassie Brilliant Blue R, 25% (v/v) propanol, 10% (v/v) acetic acid.
8. Re-equilibration solutions: (1) 100 mM Tris-Cl, pH 6.8; (2) 15% (v/v) EtOH, 100 mM Tris-Cl, pH 6.8.

Second dimension:
1. $10 \times$ Running buffer: 150 g Tris, 720 g glycine, 50 g SDS, add ddH$_2$O to 5 L.

2. Upper Tris buffer: 0.5 M Tris, 0.4% (w/v) SDS, pH 6.8.
3. Lower Tris buffer: 1.5 M Tris, 0.4% SDS (w/v), pH 8.8.
4. AMBA (acrylamide stock): 300 g acrylamide, 8 g bisacrylamide, fill up to 1 L with ddH$_2$O.
5. 3× Sample buffer: 45 g SDS, 124.8 mL upper Tris (pH 6.8), 15.0 mL 0.1 M EDTA, 150 g sucrose or 150 mL glycerol, ddH$_2$O to 450 mL. Remember to add β-mercaptoethanol (10% final concentration).
6. TEMED and 10% APS.
7. Coomassie stain: 0.15% Coomassie Brilliant Blue R, 25% isopropanol, 10% acetic acid.
8. Destain: 25% isopropanol, 10% acetic acid.

16-BAC discontinuous gel (first dimension):
1. The glass plates used for the gel apparatus are first washed with ethanol and assembled according to the manufactures instructions. The 16-BAC gel is prepared as a slab gel using a stacking gel casted on top of a resolving gel.
2. The 7.5% resolving gel (40 mL final volume) is made accordingly to the above method (lower gel). The polymerization is initiated by adding the H$_2$O$_2$ and should be completed in approximately 30 min at room temperature. For optimal results the gel should be allowed to polymerize over night.
3. The 4% stacking gel prepared accordingly to the above method (upper gel) and is poured on top on the resolving gel. The polymerization is initiated by adding H$_2$O$_2$ and should be completed in approx 20–30 min. Appropriate gel combs are inserted into the stacking gel before it polymerizes.

First-dimension electrophoresis:
1. After the comb has been removed from the gel, the wells are washed with 1× running buffer.
2. The samples are diluted in the prepared 2× sample buffer (to 1×) and heated for 5 min at 65 °C. Do not boil the samples. The samples are then loaded on the gel.
3. Remember that the electrophoresis is carried out such that the proteins move towards the cathode (opposite of SDS gels!).
4. For mini-gels (0.75 mm) run the gel at 10 mA/gel until the dye front enters the separation gel, then 20 mA/gel until the dye front has completely run out of the gel (approx 1.5 h). For larger gels (14 × 16 cm) the current is initially 25 mA/gel and subsequent at 80 mA/gel (approx 7.5 h).

Note: Never store samples in sample buffer. Due to unfolding of the proteins in the presence of urea they are more susceptible to proteases and can degrade overnight. If dealing with membrane proteins which are hard to dissolve one may tip-sonicate samples before adding sample buffer and centrifuge them before loading.

Staining, destaining, and re-equilibration:
1. After first-dimension electrophoresis the gel is fixed in fixing solution for at least 1 h. Several changes should be made during fixation.
2. Stain the gel with Coomassie Blue (15–30 min).
3. Destain the gel with fixing solution (several changes).
4. For re-equilibration, the gel is first incubated for 3 × 10 min with re-equilibration solution 1 and subsequently for 5–10 min with re-equilibration solution 2.
5. The strip of interest is carefully excised by cutting with the edge of a glass plate (0.3 and 0.6 cm for mini-gels and larger gels, respectively) and stored at 4 °C.

Second-dimension electrophoresis:
1. The SDS-PAGE is done under standard conditions using the lower Tris buffer for the separations gel and the upper Tris buffer for the stacking gel. Either a gradient (9–15%) or a 10% gel can be used depending on the complexity of the sample to be analyzed. Remember to prepare the stacking gel with a large well that can accommodate the strip generated from the first dimension. There should also be an extra lane for molecular mass markers.
2. After polymerization, the gel is placed in the appropriate gel apparatus and the well is filled with 1× running buffer.
3. Place the strip at the bottom of the well (stacking gel) with the aid of a spatula.
4. Fill the well with 100–300 μL 3× sample buffer and incubate for 5 min.
5. The gel is first run at 5 mA for mini-gels and 12 mA for larger gels (16 × 16 cm, 1 mm thick) until the dye front enters the separation gel. Separation is carried out at 20 mA for mini-gels and 80 mA for larger gels. The electrophoresis will run for approx 1 h for mini-gels and 3–3.5 h for larger gels (10%).
6. The gel apparatus is dismantled carefully and the gel stained with colloidal Coomassie Blue stain.

8.2.4
Fractionation by 1D SDS-PAGE

This protocol is based on the use of pre-cast gels which can be bought from several vendors. This paragraph is based on the NuPAGE system (Invitrogen).

Requirements

Equipment: Novex Bis-Tris pre-cast gels (10% or 4–12% gradient gels), gel chamber, running buffer (MES or MOPS), molecular weight markers, LDS sample buffer, reducing agent and power supply. The Novex Bis-Tris gels come in thickness of 1 mm (approx 30 μL loading capacity) and 1.5 mm (approx 40 μL loading capacity).

Sample preparation:
1. The sample is dissolved in LDS sample buffer (1×) containing reducing agent.
2. Heat (do not boil) the samples for 5–10 min at 70 °C.
3. Prepare 1 L of running buffer (MES for low molecular weight proteins or MOPS for mid-size molecular weight proteins).
4. After heating, the sample is loaded in the gel (10% or 4–12% gradient gel).
5. 200 mL 1× running buffer containing 500 μL antioxidant is placed in the inner gel chamber.
6. 600 mL 1× running buffer is placed in the outer gel chamber.

Gel electrophoresis:

Buffer type	Voltage	Expected current	Run time
Novex Bis-Tris gels with MES running buffer	200 V constant	Start: 110–125 mA/Gel	35 min
		End: 70–80 mA/Gel	
Novex Bis-Tris gels with MOPS running buffer	200 V constant	Start: 100–115 mA/Gel	50 min
		End: 60–70 mA/Gel	

After end gel electrophoresis the gel is stained with colloidal Coomassie Blue or other staining procedure compatible with MS.

8.2.5
In-Gel Digestion

Requirements

Equipment: Clean scalpel, spatula, 0.5 mL safe-lock reaction tubes.

8.2.5.1 Excision of Protein Spots/Lanes from 16-BAC/SDS-PAGE and 1D SDS-PAGE gel
Protein spots/bands of interest are excised from either the 16-BAC-SDS-PAGE or the 1D SDS-PAGE gels. A clean scalpel is used for this purpose. Cut as

close as possible to the edge of the spot/lane to avoid extra gel material. The excised spot/lane is further cut into smaller pieces of approx 1×1 mm. The gel particles are transferred into a 0.5-mL reaction test tube.

8.2.5.2 In-Gel Reduction, Alkylation, and Digestion

Chemicals: H_2O, acetonitrile, NH_4HCO_3, dithiothreitol, iodoacetamide, $CaCl_2$, formic acid, trypsin.

Solutions: 100 mM NH_4HCO_3 (pH 8.0), 10 mM DTT in 100 mM NH_4HCO_3, 55 mM iodoacetamide in 100 mM NH_4HCO_3, 5% (v/v) formic acid, trypsin $(0.1\ \mu g\ \mu L^{-1})$, 100 mM $CaCl_2$.

Digestion buffer (prepared fresh):

	1	2
Trypsin (0.1 μg μL^{-1})	15 μL	–
NH_4HCO_3 (100 mM)	50 μL	50 μL
CaCl$_2$ (100 mM)	5 μL	5 μL
H_2O	50 μL	50 μL
Total	120 μL	120 μL

The amount of buffer is sufficient for approximately 10–15 digestions.

1. Wash the gel pieces with 150 μL ddH$_2$O. Incubate for 5 min at 25 °C (1.050 rpm) in a thermomixer.
2. Spin gel pieces down and remove all liquid with thin pipette tips.
3. Add 150 μL acetonitrile and incubate for 15 min at 25 °C (1.050 rpm) in a thermomixer to shrink (dehydrate) the gel pieces (they become white and stick together).
4. Spin the gel pieces down and remove all liquid.
5. Dry the gel pieces for approx 5 min in a SpeedVac.
6. Swell the gel pieces in 100 μL 10 mM DTT (the gel pieces must be covered completely). Incubate at 56 °C for 50 min to reduce the cysteine residues within the protein.
7. Spin the gel pieces down and remove all liquid.
8. Add 150 μL acetonitrile and incubate for 15 min at 25 °C (1050 rpm) in a thermomixer (until the gel pieces have shrunk).
9. Spin the gel pieces down and remove all liquid with a thin tip.
10. Incubate the gel pieces with 55 mM iodoacetamide for 20 min at room temperature in the dark to modify (alkylate) the cysteines.

11. Spin the gel pieces down and remove all liquid with a thin tip.
12. Add 150 μL of 100 mM NH_4HCO_3, incubate for 15 min at 25 °C (1050 rpm) in a thermomixer.
13. Spin the gel pieces down and add 150 μL of acetonitrile. Incubate for 15 min at 25 °C (1050 rpm) in a thermomixer.
14. Spin the gel pieces down and remove all liquid with a thin tip.
15. Shrink the gel pieces in 150 μL acetonitrile by incubating for 15 min at 25 °C (1050 rpm) in a thermomixer.
16. Spin the gel pieces down and remove all liquid with a thin tip.
17. Dry the gel pieces for 5–10 min in a SpeedVac.
18. Rehydrate the gel pieces at 4 °C in digestion buffer **1** (see above) containing trypsin for 30–45 min. Use only small amounts of digestion buffer. Check the samples after 15–20 min and add more buffer if all liquid is absorbed by the gel pieces. Add 10–20 μL of digestion buffer **2** (without trypsin) to cover the gel pieces completely and to keep them wet during enzymatic cleavage.
19. Incubate samples in incubator at 37 °C overnight.

8.2.5.3   Extraction of Peptides from In-Gel Digests

1. Prepare fresh 0.5 mL reaction tubes to collect the supernatant.
2. Spin the gel pieces down.
3. Add 10–15 μL water to the digest, so that the gel pieces are completely covered with liquid.
4. Spin the gel pieces down and incubate for 15 min at 37 °C and 1050 rpm in a thermomixer.
5. Spin the gel pieces down.
6. Add at least 50 μL of acetonitrile (a volume twice as large as the volume of the gel pieces should be added) and incubate for 15 min at 37 °C (1050 rpm) in a thermomixer.
7. Spin the gel pieces down and collect the supernatant in the new reaction tubes.
8. Add 50 μL of 5% formic acid to the gel pieces and incubate for 15 min at 37 °C (1050 rpm) in a thermomixer.
9. Spin the gel pieces down and add 50 μL of acetonitrile, then incubate for 15 min at 37 °C (1050 rpm) in a thermomixer.
10. Spin the gel pieces down and collect the supernatant and pool the extracts in the new reaction tubes.
11. Add 100 μL acetonitrile and incubate for 15 min at 37 °C (1050 rpm) in a thermomixer.
12. Spin the gel pieces down and transfer the supernatant to the pooled extracts in the new reaction tubes.
13. Evaporate the samples to dryness in the SpeedVac.

8.2.6
On-Line and Off-Line Nano Liquid Chromatography (NanoLC)

8.2.6.1 Pre- and Analytical Columns from Vendors

Requirements

C18-analytical columns: C18 PepMap 100, 75 μm ID, 3 μm 100 Å (LC Packings). PreproSil-Pur 120 C18-AQ, 3 μm and/or 5 μm (Dr Maisch GmbH). Onyx Monolithic C18, 100 μm ID (Phenomenex).

C18-pre columns: μ-Precolumn Cartridge; C18 PepMap 100, 300 μm ID (5 mm length), 5 μm 100 Å (LC Packings).

8.2.6.2 Preparation of Pre- and Analytical Nano-Flow Reverse-Phase Columns

Requirements

Chemicals and materials: Formamide, methanol, 0.1% (v/v) trifluoroacetic acid (TFA) in water (solvent A), 80% (v/v) acetonitrile, 0.1% (v/v) TFA in water (solvent B), Kvasil1 (PQ Europe), fused silica capillaries (375 μm outer diameter and 75 μm inner diameter for analytical columns, 375 μm OD and 150 μm ID for pre-columns (Polymicro Technologies), MicroTight Fittings with 5 μM PEEK filter end fitting (UpChurch Scientific Inc.), MicroTight Sleeve Green (0.0155 × 0.025, UpChurch Scientific Inc.), polymer tubing PEEK Gray 1/16 × 0.015 (400 μm ID, Up-Church Scientific Inc.), reverse-phase material (e.g. Vydac MS218, 5 μm 300 Å beads (Vydac) or Reprosil-Pur 120 C18-AQ, 3 μm (Dr Maisch GmbH).

Instrumentation: Pressure vessel (for packing the columns; Bruchbuehler) connected to a high-pressure helium cylinder. Pressure valve should allow up to 200 bar (e.g. Messer Griesheim).

8.2.6.2.1 Generation of a "frit" restrictor in the fused silica capillary for analytical columns

1. Mix 88 μL Kvasil1 and 16 μL formamide in a 1.5-mL test tube.
2. Vortex rigorously for 2–3 min (the solution becomes viscous).
3. Dip one end of a 30–40-cm-long fused silica capillary (375 μm OD 75 μm ID) in the solution for 1–2 s (the solution will move upward into the fused silica by capillary action).
4. Wipe off excess solution. Polymerization is achieved by leaving the capillary at room temperature overnight or by heating at 50 °C for 2–3 h.
5. Check the frit under the microscope/binocular. It should be 2–5 mm in length. Cut the frit if it is too long.

8.2.6.2.2 Packing reverse-phase analytical columns

1. The fused silica capillary (with the frit) is inserted into the pressure vessel and the open end is placed in a reaction tube (within the pressure vessel) containing 100% methanol. The vessel is closed properly and the helium pressure is raised until the methanol flows through the capillary. This step assures that the capillary is clean before column-packing and that the frit stays intact under higher pressure.
2. Resuspend approx 5–10 mg of reverse-phase material with 500 µL methanol in a reaction tube. Place the reaction tube in the pressure vessel and the capillary in methanol slurry as above. Pack the column with the slurry according to the cleaning procedure above, but with higher pressure (up to 70 bar). In order to keep the reverse-phase material in suspension during the packing procedure, a very small magnetic stirrer should be put into the reaction tube and the entire vessel should be placed on a magnetic stirring device. Column packing can be observed under the microscope/binocular. The column should be packed for 25–20 cm. After the helium pressure has been turned off, the column should remain in the vessel to slowly minimize the pressure and thus avoiding any back-flushing of sample material.
3. The open end (without the frit) is covered with a peek sleeve (400 µm ID) and is tightly fixed with a stainless nut and ferule compatible with the valve port of the nanoLC system.
4. The packed column is mounted in a capillary/nanoLC system and equilibrated first with solvent B and then with solvent A for the 30 min each, with a flow rate of 400–800 nL min^{-1} (depending on the back pressure, which should not exceed 160 bar).
5. The performance of the column is tested in several test runs with a tryptic digest of a standard protein (e.g. 10–100 fmol BSA).

Pre-columns are made in the same way as described above for analytical columns using a fused silica with an OD of 375 µm and ID of 75 µm (for LC-MS/MS) or 150 µm (for LC-MALDI). When pre-columns for LC-MALDI are generated, a column (after end packing) with an approximate length of 2 cm is cut out from the fused silica and subsequently closed by MicroTight fittings on both sides.

8.2.6.3 On-Line NanoLC-ESI MS/MS

Requirements

Chemicals: Water, acetonitrile, formic acid.

Solutions: Solvent A, 0.1% formic acid (v/v) in water; solvent B, 100% acetonitrile (v/v), 0.1% formic acid (v/v) in water; solvent C, 0.1% formic acid (v/v) in water; Solvent D: 10% acetonitrile (v/v), 0.15% formic acid (v/v) in water.

Instrumentation: Waters Q-TOF Ultima ESI mass spectrometer equipped with a capillary LC system and autosampler. Columns from vendors and/or self-packed pre- and analytical columns are described above.

1. Extracted peptides derived from in-gel digested synaptic vesicle proteins are dissolved in an appropriate volume of solvent D (e.g. 10–30 µL).
2. Samples (max. 6 µL) are loaded onto the pre-column with solvent C at a flow rate of 10 µL min^{-1} for 10 min.
3. Peptides are eluted onto the analytic column by backflush and subsequently separated with the following gradient with a flow rate of 180 nL min^{-1}: 7% (v/v) solvent B to 40% (v/v) solvent B for 50 min, 40% B to 80% B for 1 min, isocratic elution at 80% B for 10 min, 80% B to 7% for 1 min, isocratic equilibration at 7% B for 10 min.
4. Peptides are chosen for MS/MS analysis by performing a survey scan of the ionized species that elute from the column into the instrument (automated MS and MS/MS analysis). The settings for the survey scan have to be optimized according to the corresponding ESI instrument.
5. MS/MS spectra of the peptides are processed (smoothing, centroiding) and searched against databases using Mascot as search engine according to the above mentioned settings (see Section 8.3.4).

8.2.6.4 Off-Line NanoLC

Requirements

Chemicals: α-Cyano-cinnamic acid, water, acetonitrile, TFA (Sigma-Aldrich), o-phosphoric acid (H_3PO_4, Merck).

Solutions: Solvent A, 0.1% TFA (v/v) in water; solvent B, 80% ACN (v/v), 0.1% TFA (v/v) in water; solvent C, 3.5% ACN (v/v), 0.1% TFA (v/v) in water; MALDI matrix, 10 mg mL^{-1} HCCA in 70% ACN (v/v), 0.1% TFA (v/v) in water.

Instrumentation: Dual Gradient System (Dionex) equipped with an autosampler; LC-MALDI Spotter Probot (Dionex) with a 300-nL mixing chamber (UpChurch Scientific Inc.); MALDI-TOF/TOF 4800 analyzer (Applied Biosystems/Sciex MDS).

- Samples (complex peptide mixtures derived from in-gel digestion of synaptic vesicles) are dissolved in 10–30 µL of 10% (v/v) acetonitrile, 0.1% (v/v) TFA and injected via the autosampler onto the pre-column with solvent C at a flow rate of 5 µL min^{-1} for 25 min.
- The desalted peptides are eluted from the pre-column and subsequently separated on the analytical column by the following gradient: 15 min 10%

(v/v) solvent B, 10–60% (v/v) solvent B for 60 min, 60–100% (v/v) solvent B for 3 min, 100% (v/v) solvent B for 9 min, 100% (v/v) solvent B—10% solvent B for 1 min. The gradient can be adjusted according to the complexity of the sample.

- Fractions are spotted every 15 s onto stainless steel LC-MALDI plates (Applied Biosystems) with α-cyanocinnamic acid as matrix. Matrix is delivered with a flow rate of 0.9 µL min⁻¹ and is mixed with the eluate using a T-piece mounted in before the spotter needle.
- Fully automated MALDI-MS and MS/MS analysis of the spotted fraction is performed according to the manufacturer's instructions for the MALDI instrument.
- Settings for data analysis are according to the analysis of data acquired by LC-ESI-MS/MS, except that the number of missed cleavages (see above) for the database search is higher (2–3 missed cleavages) than in the ESI analysis.

8.3
Summary and Outlook

A comprehensive proteomic analysis of highly purified synaptic vesicles has provided a detailed map of the protein constituents involved in the synaptic vesicle life cycle in addition to vesicle-associated proteins (Takamori *et al.*, 2006). These proteins include already known players in addition to novel proteins. Since the synaptic vesicle proteome is rather complex, with more than 400 identified proteins, the sample has to be fractionated before MS analysis. A combination of 1D SDS-PAGE and 16-BAC/SDS-PAGE is recommended to ensure maximum recovery of both soluble and (integral) membrane proteins. In a new study, synaptic vesicles were fractionated by a combination of 1D SDS-PAGE and 16-BAC/SDS-PAGE and subsequently analyzed by nanoLC-MS/MS; this resulted in the identification of 321 and 262 proteins, respectively (Table 8.1). Of these, 149 proteins were uniquely identified by 1D SDS-PAGE, and a further 90 proteins were uniquely identified by 16-BAC/SDS-PAGE. Even though 172 proteins were found to be common between the two analyses the relatively high number of unique proteins identified in each method emphasizes that the two fractionation strategies are complementary. As seen in Table 8.1, the proteins identified include a variety of protein classes including trafficking proteins, small endocytosis-related GTPases, transporters/channels, cytoskeleton proteins, cell surface protein, signaling molecules, metabolic enzymes, chaperones, proteasome proteins, RNA-processing proteins, and novel proteins (for a detailed description of the individual proteins see Takamori *et al.*, 2006). Interestingly, even though proteomics approaches have failed to identify all known synaptic vesicle proteins (in particular integral membrane proteins such as the low abundant transporters and the chloride channels), the total number of identified proteins

Table 8.1 *Comparison of SV proteins identified by LC-MS after fractionation by either 16-BAC-SDS PAGE or 1D SDS PAGE.

	Total	Overlap	16-BAC-SDS	1D SDS
Trafficking proteins	18	11	12	17
Endocytosis-related proteins	19	8	12	15
Small GTPases + related proteins	50	32	45	37
Other trafficking proteins	39	22	29	32
Transporter/ channel	45	27	33	39
Cytoskeleton	29	12	14	27
Cell surface	24	7	14	17
Signaling molecules	38	13	25	26
Metabolic enzymes	42	15	25	32
Others	43	9	16	37
Chaperones	12	4	6	10
Proteasome	11	5	6	10
RNA processing	22	4	15	11
Novel	18	3	11	11

* Table 8.1 lists the number of proteins identified from purified SV when separated by either 16-BAC-SDS PAGE or 1D-SDS PAGE followed by LC-MS/MS analysis. The total numbers of proteins identified by both fractionation methods combined are indicated (Total) in addition to the overlap between the two methods (Overlap). The identified proteins are grouped according to protein function.

is still considered surprisingly high. The large number of proteins identified can be explained to some extent by proteins that are thought to associate only transiently with synaptic vesicles. Another explanation might be that heterogeneous populations of synaptic vesicles exist where not all proteins reside on the same vesicle. This phenomenon is already observed for the transporters (i.e. VGLUT and GABA) which represent a specific pool of synaptic vesicles (Takamori et al., 2000a, 2000b). A proteomic analysis of different subpopulations of synaptic vesicles will therefore be helpful to elucidate such differences. Finally it might be the case that many novel synaptic vesicle proteins are still to be identified. These proteins include known proteins which have not been assigned as synaptic vesicle proteins before and proteins which have only been identified by automated genome annotation. A functional characterization of these proteins as novel synaptic vesicle proteins will play an important role in understanding the detailed mechanism of the synaptic vesicle life cycle.

Acknowledgments

Mads Grønborg is supported by the Danish Agency for Science, Technology and Innovation (DASTI).

References

Ahnert-Hilger, G., Holtje, M., Pahner, I., Winter, S. and Brunk, I. (2003) Regulation of vesicular neurotransmitter transporters. *Reviews of Physiology, Biochemistry and Pharmacology*, **150**, 140–160.

Burger, P.M., Mehl, E., Cameron, P.L., Maycox, P.R., Baumert, M., Lottspeich, F., De Camilli, P. and Jahn, R. (1989) Synaptic vesicles immunoisolated from rat cerebral cortex contain high levels of glutamate. *Neuron*, **3**, 715–720.

Burre, J., Beckhaus, T., Corvey, C., Karas, M., Zimmermann, H. and Volknandt, W. (2006a) Synaptic vesicle proteins under conditions of rest and activation: analysis by 2-D difference gel electrophoresis. *Electrophoresis*, **27**, 3488–3496.

Burre, J., Beckhaus, T., Schagger, H., Corvey, C., Hofmann, S., Karas, M., Zimmermann, H. and Volknandt, W. (2006b) Analysis of the synaptic vesicle proteome using three gel-based protein separation techniques. *Proteomics*, **6**, 6250–6262.

Coughenour, H.D., Spaulding, R.S. and Thompson, C.M. (2004) The synaptic vesicle proteome: a comparative study in membrane protein identification. *Proteomics*, **4**, 3141–3155.

Hartinger, J., Stenius, K., Hogemann, D. and Jahn, R. (1996) 16-BAC/SDS-PAGE: a two-dimensional gel electrophoresis system suitable for the separation of integral membrane proteins. *Analytical Biochemistry*, **240**, 126–133.

Hell, J.W. and Jahn, R. (1994) *Cell Biology: A Laboratory Handbook*, 1st edn, Academic, New York.

Hell, J.W., Maycox, P.R., Stadler, H. and Jahn, R. (1988) Uptake of GABA by rat brain synaptic vesicles isolated by a new procedure. *EMBO Journal*, **7**, 3023–3029.

Hu, K., Carroll, J., Fedorovich, S., Rickman, C., Sukhodub, A. and Davletov, B. (2002) Vesicular restriction of synaptobrevin suggests a role for calcium in membrane fusion. *Nature*, **415**, 646–650.

Huttner, W.B., Schiebler, W., Greengard, P. and De Camilli, P. (1983) Synapsin I (protein I), a nerve terminal-specific phosphoprotein. III. Its association with synaptic vesicles studied in a highly purified synaptic vesicle preparation. *The Journal of Cell Biology*, **96**, 1374–1388.

Jahn, R. and Scheller, R.H. (2006) SNAREs—engines for membrane fusion. *Nature Reviews. Molecular Cell Biology*, **7**, 631–643.

Jahn, R., Schiebler, W., Ouimet, C. and Greengard, P. (1985) A 38,000-dalton membrane protein (p38) present in synaptic vesicles. *Proceedings of the National Academy of Sciences of the United States of America*, **82**, 4137–4141.

Jahn, R., Lang, T. and Sudhof, T.C. (2003) Membrane fusion. *Cell*, **112**, 519–533.

Laemmli, U.K. (1970) Cleavage of structural proteins during the assembly of the head of bacteriophage T4. *Nature*, **227**, 680–685.

Macfarlane, D.E. (1989) Two dimensional benzyldimethyl-n-hexadecylammonium chloride–sodium dodecyl sulfate preparative polyacrylamide gel electrophoresis: a high capacity high resolution technique for the purification of proteins from complex mixtures. *Analytical Biochemistry*, **176**, 457–463.

Maycox, P.R., Link, E., Reetz, A., Morris, S.A. and Jahn, R. (1992) Clathrin-coated vesicles in nervous tissue are involved primarily in synaptic vesicle recycling. *The Journal of Cell Biology*, **118**, 1379–1388.

Morciano, M., Burre, J., Corvey, C., Karas, M., Zimmermann, H. and Volknandt, W. (2005) Immunoisolation of two synaptic vesicle pools from synaptosomes: a proteomics analysis. *Journal of Neurochemistry*, **95**, 1732–1745.

Nagy, A., Baker, R.R., Morris, S.J. and Whittaker, V.P. (1976) The preparation and characterization of synaptic vesicles of high purity. *Brain Research*, **109**, 285–309.

Reinders, J., Zahedi, R.P., Pfanner, N., Meisinger, C. and Sickmann, A. (2006) Toward the complete yeast mitochondrial proteome: multidimensional separation techniques for mitochondrial proteomics. *Journal of Proteome Research*, **5**, 1543–1554.

Ryan, T.A. (2006) A pre-synaptic to-do list for coupling exocytosis to endocytosis. *Current Opinion in Cell Biology*, **18**, 416–421.

Soldati, T. and Schliwa, M. (2006) Powering membrane traffic in endocytosis and recycling. *Nature Reviews. Molecular Cell Biology*, **7**, 897–908.

Takamori, S., Riedel, D. and Jahn, R. (2000a) Immunoisolation of GABA-specific synaptic vesicles defines a functionally distinct subset of synaptic vesicles. *The Journal of Neuroscience*, **20**, 4904–4911.

Takamori, S., Rhee, J.S., Rosenmund, C. and Jahn, R. (2000b) Identification of a vesicular glutamate transporter that defines a glutamatergic phenotype in neurons. *Nature*, **407**, 189–194.

Takamori, S., Holt, M., Stenius, K., Lemke, E.A., Gronborg, M., Riedel, D., Urlaub, H., Schenck, S., Brugger, B., Ringler, P., Muller, S.A., Rammner, B., Grater, F., Hub, J.S., De Groot, B.L., Mieskes, G., Moriyama, Y., Klingauf, J., Grubmuller, H., Heuser, J., Wieland, F. and Jahn, R. (2006) Molecular anatomy of a trafficking organelle. *Cell*, **127**, 831–846.

von Schwarzenfeld, I. (1979) Origin of transmitters released by electrical stimulation from a small metabolically very active vesicular pool of cholinergic synapses in guinea-pig cerebral cortex. *Neuroscience*, **4**, 477–493.

Wienisch, M. and Klingauf, J. (2006) Vesicular proteins exocytosed and subsequently retrieved by compensatory endocytosis are nonidentical. *Nature Neuroscience*, **9**, 1019–1027.

9
Proteomics Analysis of the Synapse

A.B. Smit and K.W. Li

9.1
Introduction

9.1.1
The Synapse

The brain is a most complex and dynamic organ. Its high degree of computational ability enables an animal to perceive and integrate information and to respond to environmental and physiological inputs. Central to the neuronal circuitry of the brain is the extensive connectivity, in particular the 100 billion central neurons and their 10^{15} synaptic connections.

A typical synapse consists of a presynaptic bouton and a postsynaptic spine. In the bouton, a number of synaptic vesicles are docked around the active zone. A depolarizing potential from the axon causes the influx of extracellular calcium ions into the bouton, leading to the priming of synaptic vesicles and their subsequent fusion with the plasma membrane of the active zone (see Chapter 8). The released transmitter diffuses through the synaptic cleft, binds and activates the corresponding receptors and/or ion channels located in the postsynaptic density (PSD) of the spine.

Synaptic transmission is not a static process; depending on the history of neuronal activity, synaptic efficacy can be strengthened or weakened. This phenomenon is called synaptic plasticity (Malenka and Bear, 2004). These plastic changes of synaptic efficacy have been correlated to morphological changes in the PSD and the spines (Connor *et al.*, 2006). Recent studies indicate that PSDs contain a high protein complexity (Li *et al.*, 2004), and the residing proteins are believed to be clustered differentially to form distinct transient molecular machineries that regulate different forms of plasticity of the synapse, such as long-term potentiation or depression (Merrill *et al.*, 2005). In particular, neuronal activity elicits signal transduction cascades that regulate posttranslational modifications, especially protein phosphorylation (Miyamoto, 2006) (see Chapter 11). These processes drive downstream events, notably alteration of protein–protein interactions as

Proteomics of the Nervous System. Edited by H.G. Nothwang and S.E. Pfeiffer
Copyright © 2008 WILEY-VCH Verlag GmbH & Co. KGaA, Weinheim
ISBN: 978-3-527-31716-5

well as protein trafficking, resulting in a change of protein constituents in distinct synaptic subdomains leading to an alteration of synapse physiology.

Classical approaches focusing on single or a few synaptic proteins have advanced our understanding of the components of neurotransmission. However, in view of the fact that synaptic transmission involves coordinated molecular events with intricate networks of proteins, it becomes clear that a global spatio-temporal analysis of synapse (sub)proteomes will be required to reveal the dynamics of synapses in order to describe the molecular mechanisms of neurotransmission and synaptic plasticity.

With the advancement of mass spectrometry technology, it became possible to characterize large numbers of proteins at high sensitivity. Recently, studies have been reported on the proteomes of several synaptic subdomains (Li *et al.*, 2005; Morciano *et al.*, 2005; Phillips *et al.*, 2005), and the posttranslational modifications of synaptic proteins including protein phosphorylation (Collins *et al.*, 2005; Trinidad *et al.*, 2006) and glycosylation (Vosseller *et al.*, 2006). In all cases focus was on glutamatergic synapses because they are the major excitatory neurotransmission pathway of the brain. Furthermore, glutamatergic synapses form stable structures during isolation, which facilitates subsequent analysis of their protein constituents.

9.1.2
Protocols for the Isolation of Synapse and Subdomains

The methodology for the preparation and isolation of synapses and distinct synaptic subdomains is well established (Carlin *et al.*, 1980). In most studies, detached synapses from brain regions are enriched by means of ultracentrifugation in sucrose density gradients to yield a synaptosome preparation. Synaptosomes are sealed membraneous particles that contain small clear transmitter vesicles (presynaptic boutons), and are often conjugated to the electron-dense postsynaptic membranes. Synaptosomes can also be isolated using Percoll density gradients (Dunkley *et al.*, 1988). This bears several advantages; Percoll gradients require shorter centrifugation time, and provide iso-osmotic conditions throughout the gradient, which might be vital to maintain synapse physiology for functional studies. On the other hand, the boundaries of the step Percoll gradient will gradually merge during centrifugation. The shape of the self-forming Percoll gradient is critically dependent on the centrifugation force and the time of centrifugation. We routinely use a sucrose density gradient because of its ease of preparation and stability.

Synaptosomes are often used as the starting material to prepare synapse subdomains such as the PSD (Li *et al.*, 2005), presynaptic particles (Phillips *et al.*, 2005), and dendritic rafts (Suzuki *et al.*, 2001). To prepare the PSD or dendritic rafts, most studies make use of the advantage that these two structures are insoluble in mild detergent and treat synaptosomes in 0.5–1%

Triton X-100 at low temperature. An additional sucrose density gradient ultracentrifugation step will separate the cholesterol-rich, low-density dendritic raft from the protein-rich, high-density PSD. Several hundreds of proteins and their phosphorylation sites have been identified from PSD preparations. It should be realized that these preparations still contain some contaminants (Li et al., 2005). A high-purity PSD preparation can be obtained with affinity isolation, but the yield of PSD will be lower, and the cost of antibodies is substantial.

The isolation of presynaptic compartments is more challenging than that of the PSD and dendritic rafts. In one study, monoclonal antibodies were used to purify two synaptic vesicle-containing fractions from a synaptosome preparation (Morciano et al., 2005). In another study, a presynaptic particle fraction and PSD was obtained by sequential extraction of synaptosomes in Triton X-100 first at pH 6 and then at pH 8 (Phillips et al., 2005).

9.1.3
Proteomics Analysis of the Synapse

The classic approach for proteomics analysis is based on two-dimensional gel electrophoresis to separate proteins that are solubilized from a cellular extract. We have used this approach to separate PSD proteins (Li et al., 2004), detected 250 protein spots, and characterized many synaptic proteins including scaffolding proteins and signaling proteins. Unfortunately, many membrane proteins that are known to be major PSD constituents, such as glutamate receptors and ion channels, were not detected. This result is in agreement with the limitations of 2D gel electrophoresis, that is, it is not effective in resolving hydrophobic proteins, proteins larger than 100 kDa, and very basic and acidic proteins (see Chapter 2).

To circumvent the problems associated with 2D gel electrophoresis, we pursued a gel-free two-step liquid chromatography–mass spectrometry (LC-MS) approach (Li et al., 2004, 2005). PSD proteins are first digested with trypsin, and subsequently separated by means of cation-exchange chromatography followed by nano reversed-phase LC. Small peptide fragments are often easy to separate using this system thereby bypassing the previously mentioned limitations of 2D gel electrophoresis. This approach detects all protein classes, including the ionotropic and metabotropic glutamate receptors, ion channels, high molecular weight proteins (>500 kDa), and basic proteins (pH > 10).

9.1.4
Quantitative Analysis of Synaptic Proteins

There are only a few reports on the quantitative proteomics analysis of synaptic proteins (Li, 2007). Currently, we are using isobaric tags for

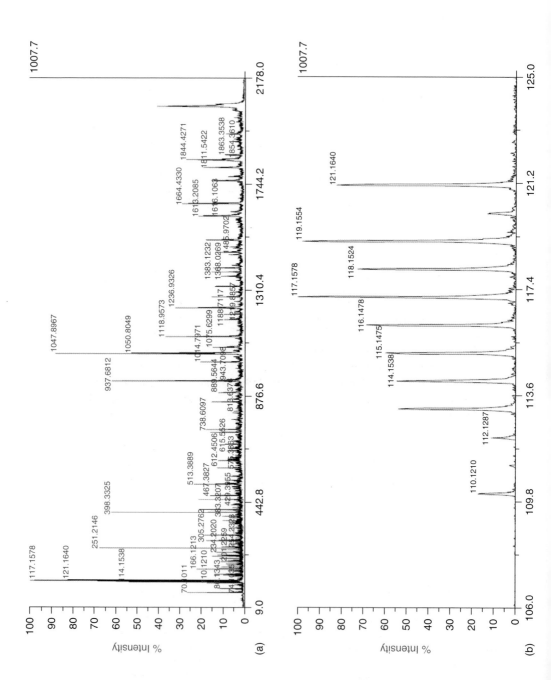

relative and absolute quantitation (iTRAQ) in conjunction with tandem mass spectrometry (MS/MS) to examine the difference in expression pattern of synaptic membrane proteins in different brain regions and under different experimental conditions. The iTRAQ reagents are a multiplexed set of four isobaric reagents that are identical in total mass and covalently bind to lysine side-chains and the N-terminal group of a peptide (Ross *et al.*, 2004). Hence, the mass of the tagged peptides from sample and control remain identical. The abundance ratio of a given peptide from sample and control is revealed in the product ion spectrum (MS/MS). Recently, 8-plex iTRAQ reagents became available. Tryptic peptides from up to eight samples can be tagged each with one of the eight isobaric reagents and then pooled into a single sample. Upon collision-induced dissociation of a tagged peptide, signature ions of each iTRAQ reagent will be produced. The peak ratios of the iTRAQ signature ions represent the relative quantities of this peptide contained in the original eight samples (Figure 9.1). We routinely quantify 400–500 synaptic proteins per experiment with standard deviation in the technical replicates being smaller than 20%.

We use a matrix-assisted laser desorption/ionization coupled to tandem time-of-flight (MALDI-TOF/TOF) mass spectrometer for this analysis. This off-line approach decouples MS analysis from the chromatography separations allowing comprehensive MS and MS/MS analysis without the time constraints of an LC run. In a typical experiment the mass spectrometer performs a scan of all the fractions collected on a metal MALDI plate from a single LC run. Precursor ions are then selected at the maximum point of the peak's elution profile, allowing optimum MS/MS sensitivity. Electrospray quadrupole/TOF-type mass spectrometers have also been successfully applied for iTRAQ experiments (Chong *et al.*, 2006). Usually a survey MS scan is followed by 2–5 MS/MS analyses of the most intense molecular ions. The total cycle time ranges from 1 to 5 s. Electrospray ion trap mass spectrometers have a very high sensitivity and the fastest scan time currently available. However, the upper limit on the ratio between precursor m/z and the lowest trapped fragment ion in an ion trap is ~0.3. Therefore, the iTRAQ reporter ions with the masses of 113.1 to 121.1 could not be detected.

◄ **Figure 9.1** Representative example of an 8-plex iTRAQ reagents-based quantitative analysis of a sample with control and experimental treated groups. Upper panel shows an MS/MS spectrum of iTRAQ reagent-labeled peptide with good ion series for peptide sequencing. Lower panel focuses on the mass range encompassing the reporter ions used for quantitation. The reporter ions of 113.1–116.1 represent four independent biological replicates of the control group; the reporter ions of 117.1–119.1 and 121.1 the experimental treated group. Comparison of the reporter ions reveals upregulation of this protein in the treated group. The x-axis is mass-to-charge ratio; y-axis is in arbitrary units with the most intense peak set to 100%. (Please find a color version of this figure in the color plates.)

9.2
Protocols

9.2.1
Preparation of Synaptosomes and Postsynaptic Densities

Requirements

Chemicals: Complete protease inhibitor (Roche).

Solutions: HEPES stock solution (500 mM, pH 7.4); sucrose stock solution (2 M); 10% Triton X-100.

Instrumentation: Glass–Teflon Potter homogenizer; bench-top temperature-controlled centrifuge (e.g. Centrifuge 5417R from Eppendorf); ultracentrifuge with swing-out rotor (e.g. Optima LE-80K, with SW 32.1 Ti from Beckman Coulter).

1. Prepare the sucrose gradient solution from stock solution with composition indicated in Table 9.1.
2. Dissolve 1 tablet of Roche complete protease inhibitor in 50 mL 0.32 M sucrose solution.
3. Pipette 15 mL of this sucrose solution into the glass Potter, and keep it on ice.
4. Pipette 10 mL 1.2 M sucrose into a 37-mL polycarbonate ultracentrifuge tube, and layer on top 10 mL 0.85 M sucrose solution while keeping the tubes on ice.
5. Drop frozen brain tissue (1–2 g) directly into the glass Potter.
6. Place the Teflon pestle into the glass Potter with your sample, switch on the rotation at 900 rpm and homogenize the sample with 12 strokes.
7. Remove the homogenate to a tube and centrifuge for 10 min at $1000 \times g$, $4\,^{\circ}$C.
8. Using a Pasteur pipette, carefully layer the supernatant onto the ultracentrifuge tube containing the 0.85/1.2 M sucrose step gradient.

Table 9.1 Composition of 50 mL of sucrose density gradient buffers prepared from the stock solutions.

Buffer	500 mM HEPES	2 M sucrose	Distilled water
0.32 M sucrose	0.5 mL	8 mL	41.5 mL
0.85 M sucrose	0.5 mL	21.25 mL	28.25 mL
1.2 M sucrose	0.5 mL	30 mL	19.5 mL
1.5 M sucrose	0.5 mL	37.5 mL	12 mL

9. Balance ultracentrifuge buckets with tubes on a balance. The difference between two opposite tubes should not exceed 0.02 g.
10. Centrifuge the gradients for 2 h at 100 000 × g in a swing-out rotor (SW 32.1 Ti from Beckman Coulter) at 4 °C.
11. Collect the synaptosome fraction from the 0.85/1.2 M interface, and dilute 4–5 times with 5 mM HEPES buffer.
12. Centrifuge the sample at 25 000 × g for 30 min at 4 °C.
13. Remove the supernatant until about 0.5 mL solution above the pellet.
14. Resuspend the pellet with 5 mL 5 mM HEPES buffer containing complete protease inhibitor, and transfer to a pre-cooled glass vial with a small magnetic stirrer inside, and stir on a stirring platform at 250 rpm for 15 min over ice.
15. Layer the hypotonic shocked sample on a 17-mL ultracentrifuge tube containing a sucrose density gradient of 0.85/1.2 M, 5 mL each.
16. Centrifuge for 2 h at 100 000 × g in a swing-out rotor at 4 °C.
17. Collect the synaptic membrane fraction from the 0.85/1.2 M interface. This fraction can be used for (quantitative) proteomics analysis, or proceed further to prepare PSD (steps 18–22).
18. Dilute the synaptic membrane fraction to 7 mL with 5 mM HEPES buffer containing complete protease inhibitor.
19. Add 7 mL 2% Triton X-100 solution to the synaptic membrane, and stir with a magnetic bar at 250 rpm for 30 min over ice.
20. Layer 7 mL sample on a 17-mL ultracentrifuge tube containing a sucrose step density gradient of 1.5/2 M, 4.5 mL each.
21. Centrifuge for 2 h at 100 000 × g in a swing-out rotor at 4 °C.
22. Collect the PSD fraction from the 1.5/2 M interface, and proceed with (quantitative) proteomics analysis.

9.2.2
iTRAQ Labeling of Synaptic Membrane

The same procedure can be applied for the analysis of other synaptic structures.

Requirement

Chemicals: iTRAQ reagents from Applied Biosystems; Rapigest from Waters.

Solutions: 1% Trifluoroacetic acid (TFA).

Instrumentation: Table centrifuge; SpeedVac.
1. Dilute the synaptic membrane fraction 4 times with distilled water, centrifuge the sample at 25 000 × g for 30 min at 4 °C.
2. Remove the supernatant until about 0.5 mL solution above the pellet.

3. Add 0.5 mL distilled water and resuspend the pellet.
4. Determine protein concentration, transfer 100 μg protein for each sample to a 1.5-mL reaction tube, and centrifuge in a table centrifuge at maximum speed for 20 min.
5. Remove the supernatant, and dry the pellet with a SpeedVac for about 20 min.
6. Dissolve one vial of Rapigest in 125 μL dissolution buffer (from the iTRAQ reagent kit, Applied Biosystems), and add 28 μL to each dried synaptic membrane preparation.
7. Add 2 μL reducing buffer (from the iTRAQ reagent kit) to each sample, and vortex for 1 h at room temperature.
8. Add 1 μL blocking buffer (from the iTRAQ reagent kit), vortex briefly and let it stand for 10 min at room temperature.
9. Add 25 μL distilled water to a vial of trypsin (from Applied Biosystems), and vortex.
10. Transfer 10 μL trypsin solution to each sample, vortex and incubate overnight at 37 °C.
11. Add 80 μL ethanol to each iTRAQ reagents, and vortex for 1 min.
12. Transfer each iTRAQ reagents to one of maximum 8 samples and vortex gently for 2 h. As there are 8 iTRAQ reagents, up to 8 different samples can be labeled individually.
13. Pool the iTRAQ reagents labeled samples, add 400 μL 1% TFA to lower the pH to about 3, and vortex gently for 1 h.
14. Centrifuge the pooled samples on a table centrifuge for 5 min at maximum speed.
15. Transfer the supernatant to a new 1.5-mL reaction tube, and dry in a SpeedVac.
16. The sample may be stored at −20 °C or proceed for LC separation.

9.2.3
Liquid Chromatography Separation of iTRAQ-Labeled Peptides

Requirements

Solutions: Running solvent A (10 mM KH_2PO_4 in 20% acetonitrile, pH 2.9); running solvent B (500 mM KCl in 10 mM KH_2PO_4, 20% acetonitrile, pH 2.9); running solvent C (0.1% TFA); running solvent D (0.1% TFA and 80% acetonitrile).

Instrumentation: High-performance liquid chromatography (HPLC) system for cation-exchange chromatography; a 100 × 2.1-mm cation-exchange column, packed with 3 μm polysulfoethyl A (from polyLC); a nano-HPLC system (from LC packings) for reversed-phase chromatography, the column is packed with 3 µm C18 beads in a fused-silica capillary of 100 µm internal diameter.

1. Redissolve the dried synaptic membrane fraction in 250 µL running solvent A.
2. Centrifuge the sample 10 min on a table centrifuge at maximum speed.
3. Remove supernatant and load it into a cation-exchange column. The protein amount is high and will exceed the binding capability of microbore/capillary column. We therefore use a conventional 2.1 × 100 mm column at a flow rate of 200 µL min^{-1} for peptide separation. The 3-µm particle size results in better resolution, but the column is more susceptible to deterioration in performance due to sudden change of pressure and so on. The column should be used with care and/or needs more frequent replacement.
4. Wash the sample with 5 column volumes of running solvent A.
5. Elute the peptides from the column with a linear salt gradient from 100% running solvent A to 100% running solvent B in 20 min. It is possible to use a shallower salt gradient to get a better separation of the peptides. The disadvantage is that the number of fractions to be analyzed will be higher. Furthermore, due to the moderate resolution of the ion-exchange column a shallow salt gradient will elute individual peptides in multiple fractions.
6. Collect 1-min fractions, and dry the fractions in a SpeedVac. Generally 15 peptide-containing fractions will be obtained for further reversed-phase LC separation.
7. Redissolve each fraction in 50 µL running solvent C.
8. Inject the fractions into a nano reversed-phase column. Generally, a column diameter of 75 µm is used for electrospray ionization (ESI)-MS. Elute the peptides from the column with a linear gradient from 100% running solvent C to 40% running solvent C/60% running solvent D in 30 min, and to 100% solvent D in 5 min. If the fractions are collected off-line for MALDI-MS analysis, the internal diameter of the column may be bigger, that is, around 100–150 µm. This will increase the loading capability of the column and facilitate the mass spectrometric detection of minor peptides.
9. The peptides are either directly infused to ESI-MS/MS or collected off-line on a metal plate and subjected to MALDI-MS/MS (see Chapters 2 and 10 for specific requirements of ESI- and MALDI-MS/MS, respectively).

9.3
Outlook

A major advantage of using iTRAQ reagents is the possibility to analyze multiple samples simultaneously, allowing samples to be compared directly and/or to include replicates offering statistical analysis. This new technology, therefore, opens up new avenues for brain research. For example, it allows one to follow the temporal global changes of the synapse proteome induced by neuronal activity, developmental changes of synaptic protein constituents, and the comparison of the synapse proteome from different brain regions. The recent development of >4 isobaric iTRAQ reagents, such as the 8-plex reagents, will certainly facilitate the quantitative synapse proteome analysis and advance its use in biology.

While MALDI TOF/TOF mass spectrometry provides high-quality iTRAQ-based data for the quantitative analysis of synapse proteome, it has a relatively low throughput. New-generation mass spectrometry such as the electrospray LTQ-Orbitrap may provide substantial higher throughput while maintaining the high confidence of protein identification with accurate mass measurements at <5 ppm level. Due to the MS^n capability, the LTQ-Orbitrap will be extremely useful for the analysis of posttranslational modifications.

References

Carlin, R.K., Grab, D.J., Cohen, R.S. and Siekevitz, P. (1980) Isolation and characterization of postsynaptic densities from various brain regions: enrichment of different types of postsynaptic densities. *The Journal of Cell Biology*, **86**, 831–845.

Chong, P.K., Gan, C.S., Pham, T.K. and Wright, P.C. (2006) Isobaric tags for relative and absolute quantitation (iTRAQ) reproducibility: implication of multiple injections. *Journal of Proteome Research*, **5**, 1232–1240.

Collins, M.O., Yu, L., Coba, M.P., Husi, H., Campuzano, I., Blackstock, W.P., Choudhary, J.S. and Grant, S.G. (2005) Proteomic analysis of *in vivo* phosphorylated synaptic proteins. *The Journal of Biological Chemistry*, **280**, 5972–5982.

Connor, S., Williams, P.T., Armstrong, B., Petit, T.L., Ivanco, T.L. and Weeks, A.C. (2006) Long-term potentiation is associated with changes in synaptic ultrastructure in the rat neocortex. *Synapse*, **59**, 378–382.

Dunkley, P.R., Heath, J.W., Harrison, S.M., Jarvie, P.E., Glenfield, P.J. and Rostas, J.A. (1988) A rapid Percoll gradient procedure for isolation of synaptosomes directly from an S1 fraction: homogeneity and morphology of subcellular fractions. *Brain Research*, **441**, 59–71.

Li, K.W. (2007) Proteomics of synapse. *Analytical and Bioanalytical Chemistry*, **387**, 25–28.

Li, K.W., Hornshaw, M.P., Van Der Schors, R.C., Watson, R., Tate, S., Casetta, B., Jimenez, C.R., Gouwenberg, Y., Gundelfinger, E.D., Smalla, K.H. and Smit, A.B. (2004) Proteomics analysis of rat brain postsynaptic density. Implications of the diverse protein functional groups for the integration of synaptic physiology. *The Journal of Biological Chemistry*, **279**, 987–1002.

Li, K.W., Hornshaw, M.P., van Minnen, J., Smalla, K.H., Gundelfinger, E.D. and Smit, A.B. (2005) Organelle proteomics of rat synaptic proteins: correlation-profiling by isotope-coded affinity tagging in conjunction with liquid chromatography-tandem mass spectrometry to reveal post-synaptic density specific proteins. *Journal of Proteome Research*, **4**, 725–733.

Malenka, R.C. and Bear, M.F. (2004) LTP and LTD: an embarrassment of riches. *Neuron*, **44**, 5–21.

Merrill, M.A., Chen, Y., Strack, S. and Hell, J.W. (2005) Activity-driven postsynaptic translocation of CaMKII. *Trends in Pharmacological Sciences*, **12**, 645–653.

Miyamoto, E. (2006) Molecular mechanism of neuronal plasticity: induction and maintenance of long-term potentiation in the hippocampus. *Journal of Pharmacological Sciences*, **100**, 433–442.

Morciano, M., Burre, J., Corvey, C., Karas, M., Zimmermann, H. and Volknandt, W. (2005) Immunoisolation of two synaptic vesicle pools from synaptosomes: a proteomics analysis. *Journal of Neurochemistry*, **95**, 1732–1745.

Phillips, G.R., Florens, L., Tanaka, H., Khaing, Z.Z., Fidler, L., Yates, J.R., 3rd, Colman, D.R. (2005) Proteomic comparison of two fractions derived from the transsynaptic scaffold. *Journal of Neuroscience Research*, **81**, 762–775.

Ross, P.L., Huang, Y.N., Marchese, J.N., Williamson, B., Parker, K., Hattan, S., Khainovski, N., Pillai, S., Dey, S., Daniels, S., Purkayastha, S., Juhasz, P., Martin, S., Bartlet-Jones, M., He, F., Jacobson, A. and Pappin, D.J. (2004) Multiplexed protein quantitation in Saccharomyces cerevisiae using amine-reactive isobaric tagging reagents. *Molecular & Cellular Proteomics*, **3**, 1154–1169.

Suzuki, T., Ito, J., Takagi, H., Saitoh, F., Nawa, H. and Shimizu, H. (2001) Biochemical evidence for localization of AMPA-type glutamate receptor subunits in the dendritic raft. *Brain research Molecular Brain Research*, **89**, 20–28.

Trinidad, J.C., Specht, C.G., Thalhammer, A., Schoepfer, R. and Burlingame, A.L. (2006) Comprehensive identification of phosphorylation sites in postsynaptic density preparations. *Molecular & Cellular Proteomics*, **5**, 914–922.

Vosseller, K., Trinidad, J.C., Chalkley, R.J., Specht, C.G., Thalhammer, A., Lynn, A.J., Snedecor, J.O., Guan, S., Medzihradszky, K.F., Maltby, D.A., Schoepfer, R. and Burlingame, A.L. (2006) O-linked N-acetylglucosamine proteomics of postsynaptic density preparations using lectin weak affinity chromatography and mass spectrometry. *Molecular & Cellular Proteomics*, **5**, 923–934.

10
Peptidomics of the Nervous System

K.W. Li and A.B. Smit

10.1
Introduction

10.1.1
Neuropeptides

Peptide messengers occur in the nervous systems of all animals. Peptides may function as a hormone, neuromodulator, or neurotransmitter, and they are involved in the regulation of a large number of processes including reproduction, feeding, growth, pain, and various behaviors, such as anxiety, stress, and reward response (Hokfelt *et al.*, 2000).

The structural diversity of neuropeptides is large and amounts to hundreds, as compared to a few classical neurotransmitters (Fricker *et al.*, 2006; Hummon *et al.*, 2006). Neuropeptides are synthesized in the form of precursor proteins, and packaged in dense core vesicles. In most cases the precursor proteins contain multiple peptide domains, and they are cleaved by peptide-processing endopeptidases (e.g. prohormone convertases 1 and 2) at sites containing multiple basic amino acids Lys and Arg. The C-terminal basic amino acids generated through this processing step are further trimmed off by the action of carboxypeptidase E. In addition, some precursor protein processing may occur at single basic amino acids, especially at Arg and to a lesser extend at Lys. Processing at non-basic residues has also been reported (Jensen *et al.*, 2005). Not all the potential processing sites are used; the precursor proteins may be cleaved in a tissue-specific or stimulation-dependent manner. Finally, the processed peptides may be posttranslationally modified by acetylation, phosphorylation, glycosylation, C-terminal amidation, sulfation, and hydroxylation. These modifications change the bio-activity of the peptides (e.g. Jimenez *et al.*, 2006b).

Peptide precursor proteins are often coexpressed in single neurons (Jimenez *et al.*, 2006b), but their expression patterns may be differentially regulated, depending on the physiological states of the animals, or more precisely, as part of the cellular response to external stimuli. As a result, different ratios of distinct

Proteomics of the Nervous System. Edited by H.G. Nothwang and S.E. Pfeiffer
Copyright © 2008 WILEY-VCH Verlag GmbH & Co. KGaA, Weinheim
ISBN: 978-3-527-31716-5

peptides are generated and released under different conditions conveying different messages to the target cells (Brezina *et al.*, 1996; Jimenez *et al.*, 2006a). This process can be considered as a means to increase information-handling capacity of the nervous system.

In order to better understand the interactive effects of the distinct peptides and peptide mixtures on neuronal physiology and circuitry, there is an urgent need to perform global quantitative analysis of peptides in the nervous system. Classical antibody-based assays have been used successfully to detect and quantify single peptides. However, this method is not suitable for global analysis. Also, it cannot be used to detect novel peptides, or their various posttranslational modifications.

With the development of nano-liquid chromatography (nanoLC) and mass spectrometry methods, it is becoming routine to carry out peptidomics analysis to reveal peptide messengers contained in neuronal tissues (Baggerman *et al.*, 2002; El Filali *et al.*, 2006). In principle, MS can detect all the peptides contained in the sample, including novel peptides and peptides with posttranslational modifications. In practice, sample complexity and peptide concentration set constraints on the analysis.

Several peptidomics approaches have been developed for the analysis of neuronal samples. For instance, single cell analysis has been carried out on a number of invertebrate and vertebrate species (Li *et al.*, 2000; Hummon *et al.*, 2006). An important issue here is to positively identify, isolate, and transfer the neurons of interest to the mass spectrometer. As the peptide content from single cells is generally low, the use of a mass spectrometer with high sensitivity is desirable.

Studies of peptidomics from brain regions are often confounded by a large number of molecular ion species in the sample, many of which represent protein degradation products. Furthermore, it is fairly common to find various oxidized forms of single peptides formed by chemical modifications during the extraction and separation steps. In face of the complexity of the samples, all peptidomics studies of neuronal tissue employ single to multiple LC steps to fractionate the molecular ion species. As structurally unrelated molecular ion species in a complex sample may have similar masses, a simple single-stage MS analysis does not have enough discriminative power to identify the peptides. Therefore, tandem MS (MS/MS) with good mass accuracy is the method of choice, and is used in most peptidomics studies of nervous tissues.

10.1.2
Instruments for Peptidomics Analysis

10.1.2.1 **Mass Spectrometer**
Peptide mass measurement and quantitation are at the core of every modern peptidomics experiment. Currently, for the analysis of peptides, there are two

main types of desorption and ionization techniques: electrospray ionization (ESI) and matrix-assisted laser desorption/ionization (MALDI).

The ESI source can be coupled to different types of mass analyzers including quadrupole and ion trap, and at the high end to the hybrid mass analyzers, such as quadrupole-TOF, ion trap-TOF, ion trap-orbitrap, and ion trap-fourier transform ion cyclotron resonance mass spectrometry. In particular, the fourier transform ion cyclotron resonance mass spectrometry and orbitrap mass analyzers give high mass accuracy routinely at 1–5 ppm level. In conjunction with the ion trap they allow MS^n analysis, which facilitates the identification of posttranslational modifications.

Peptides are usually electrosprayed on-line from an LC system directly into the mass spectrometer. ESI often generates multiple-charged peptide species. The charge state is roughly correlated to the number of basic residues of the peptides, and more than one charge state per peptide species may be formed. There are many small neuropeptides with masses <1000 Da, and the doubly charged species would be measured in the mass spectrometer at less than 500 m/z (mass-to-charge ratio). Unfortunately, at this low mass range many abundant contaminants, for example from the collection vial, are present and may in part mask the signals of the peptides.

The most popular mass analyzer for MALDI source has a TOF or TOF/TOF configuration. Peptides are always analyzed off-line (Li et al., 2005). MALDI generates singly charged peptide species and therefore the peptide ion species do not overlap with the masses of the major background peaks at <600 Da. It is also more tolerant to salt and other impurities from the sample. Therefore, MALDI-MS is the method of choice for direct single cell analysis that does not require prior sample handling. Furthermore, MALDI-TOF/TOF MS is very effective for structural identification of peptides up to 3000 Da. Higher molecular weight peptides are less amenable for structural characterization because they tend to be fragmented poorly. In these cases an ESI-based method should be used.

10.1.2.2 Nano-Liquid Chromatography

The purposes of a nanoLC step are: (i) reduction of sample complexity to a level that can be handled by the MS; (ii) concentration of peptides into a smaller volume/fraction to increase signal-to-noise level in the MS and to facilitate detection of (low abundant) peptides; (iii) removal of undesirable constituents in the sample such as salts that may interfere with mass spectrometric measurements.

The current trend of nanoLC for peptide separation is to use a capillary column of ≈100 μM internal diameter at a flow rate of 100–400 nL min^{-1}, using a high-resolution resin such as the 3 μm reversed-phase C18 silica. The capillary C18 column can be purchased from a number of vendors, such as LC-Packings. The column can also be easily packed in-house at low cost. The preferable running solvents contain 0.1% trifluoroacetic acid (TFA) that serves to improve LC resolution, and an increasing concentration of acetonitrile to sequentially elute peptides from the column. A typical peak width of an eluting peptide is 20–30 s. The peptides can then be analyzed off-line with MALDI-MS, or on-line coupled to an ESI-MS. If the nanoLC column is connected on-line to an ESI mass spectrometer, TFA should be avoided because it reduces the mass spectrometry sensitivity. Other acidic additives such as acetic acid and formic acid that do not affect MS performance should be used. The LC resolution in this case is only slightly compromised.

It is possible to obtain ultra-high LC resolution with peak width in the range of seconds using monolithic resin or reversed-phased silica particles of less than 2 µm. This will increase sensitivity and peak capacity, and it has found application in experiments that aimed at measuring exact masses of the peptides with mass accuracy at sub-ppm levels. For experiments that require MS/MS analysis, such as structural characterization of peptides, ultra-high LC resolution may not be desirable because the elution time window of the peptides may be too narrow for MS/MS experiments.

10.2
Protocols

10.2.1
Single Cell Peptidomics Analysis

A number of studies have demonstrated the separation of peptides from a single cell by nanoLC (Hsieh *et al.*, 1998) or capillary electrophoresis (Stuart and Sweedler, 2003), followed by MS or laser-induced fluorescence detection. As a peptidergic neuron contains only several to tens of different peptides, it is also possible to carry out direct analysis of peptides by MALDI-MS without prior sample preparation and fractionation. Direct peptide profiling from a single neuron is simple, robust, and sensitive. A major concern of single neuron analysis is to identify the neuron of interest. Immunocytochemistry has been applied to color-mark the cells of interest. The cells are then isolated and analyzed by MALDI-TOF-MS (Redeker *et al.*, 1998). Alternatively, neurons can be identified on the basis of their electrical properties. We exploited the fact that functionally connected neurons often share a common nerve innervating the same or overlapping targets, and therefore, they can be retrograde-labeled from the nerve. These back-filled cells can then be isolated for subsequent analysis (El Filali *et al.*, 2003).

10.2.1.1 Retrograde Labeling of Neurons of Interest
We have used the brain of the freshwater snail, *Lymnaea stagnalis*, as a model. The protocol described, however, can be applied to other invertebrate animal species with a well-formed brain and nerve trunks. For vertebrates, *in vivo*

injection of dye into the target field of the neurons of interest should be carried out to assist dissection.

Requirements

Chemicals and material: Sylgard dish (Dow Corning); Vaseline.

Solutions: Saline buffer (4 mM $CaCl_2$, 1.7 mM KCl, 1.5 mM $MgCl_2$, 30 mM NaCl, 5 mM $NaHCO_3$, 10 mM $NaCH_3SO_4$, and 10 mM N-2-hydroxyethylpiperazine-N-2-ethanesulfonic acid); saturated rubeanic acid (dithiooxamide); nickel-lysine solution (1.7 g $NiCl_2 \times 6\ H_2O$ and 3.5 g of L-lysine-free base in 20 mL H_2O).

1. Dissect the brain and pin it down in a Sylgard dish containing saline buffer.
2. Cut off all the nerves that are connected to the brain, except the nerve of interest.
3. Cut the nerve of interest several tens of centimeters away from the brain.
4. Transfer the brain to a dry Sylgard dish.
5. Construct a dam with Vaseline around the cut nerve. Immerse the cut edge of the nerve of interest within the dam in a drop of nickel-lysine solution.
6. Apply a thick mass of Vaseline to completely cover the nickel-lysine solution to avoid diffusion of the nickel-lysine into the rest of the preparation. This procedure should be completed within 1–2 min, otherwise the nerve may partially dry out.
7. Immerse the preparation completely in saline buffer, and leave it at room temperature overnight.
8. Transfer the brain to another Sylgard dish containing saline buffer.
9. Wash the brain once in fresh saline buffer.
10. Add rubeanic acid to ethanol until it is saturated. Add this saturated rubeanic acid solution to the Sylgard dish containing the brain. Use 1 drop of rubeanic acid solution per 1 mL of saline buffer. After 15–20 min, the retrograde labeled neurons appear brownish black in color.
11. Desheath the brain to expose the cells.
12. Remove individual neurons for MALDI-MS/MS analysis.

10.2.1.2 **MALDI Single Cell Analysis**

Requirements

Solutions: MALDI matrix (7 mg α-cyano-4-hydroxycinnamic acid/mL in 50% acetonitrile/50% water containing 0.1% TFA).

Instrumentation: Dissection microscope; MALDI mass spectrometer (e.g. 4800 proteomic analyzer from Applied Biosystems).

1. Place the preparation under a dissection microscope at 40× magnification and carefully suck up the neuron of interest into a glass pipette, and transfer it onto a stainless steel MALDI sample plate.
2. Add 0.3–0.5 μL of matrix to the neuron. It is important to use high-quality matrix. To obtain the desirable quality we always use the recrystallized α-cyano-4-hydroxycinnamic acid matrix, see Section 10.2.1.3 for preparation of the matrix.
3. Rupture the neuron with a glass pipette in the matrix.
4. Dry the sample at room temperature; this may take about 3 to 5 min.
5. Redissolve the sample in 50% acetonitrile/50% water containing 5 mM diammonium citrate. This will reduce the generation of matrix polymer.
6. Dry the sample again at room temperature for several minutes.
7. Insert the sample plate into the mass spectrometer for MALDI-MS analysis.

10.2.1.3 Recrystallization of MALDI Matrix

Requirements

Chemicals and material: Ethanol; α-cyano-4-hydroxycinnamic acid; Whatman paper.

Solutions: Solvent of 50% acetonitrile/50% water containing 0.1% TFA; solvent of 50% acetonitrile/5% water and 10 mM ammonium monobasic phosphate.

Instrumentation: Water bath; Buchner funnel.

1. Heat 100 mL ethanol in a boiling water bath, and then add α-cyano-4-hydroxycinnamic acid to the ethanol until it is saturated.
2. Pour the saturated matrix into a vial, and store it at −20 °C for several days.
3. Pour off the solution and collect the pale yellow precipitate of the matrix.
4. Put the matrix on a Whatman paper, break it up and transfer it to a Buchner funnel.
5. Wash the matrix with a few volumes of ice cold ethanol onto the Whatman paper to wash off the ethanol still on the dried matrix.
6. Transfer the matrix to a fresh filter paper and air dry.
7. Weigh about 7 mg of matrix and put it in a 1.5-mL Eppendorf tube.
8. Store the matrix at −20 °C.
9. Redissolve the matrix in 1 mL solvent of 50% acetonitrile/50% water containing 0.1% TFA. The matrix can now be used for direct single cell

analysis. If the matrix is used for off-line mixing with LC eluents and MALDI-TOF/TOF MS analysis, the matrix should be redissolved in 50% acetonitrile/50% water and 10 mM ammonium monobasic phosphate (Smirnov *et al.*, 2004).

10.2.2
Peptidomics Analysis of Nervous Tissue

The first step in peptidomics analysis of nervous tissue is to set up an appropriate method to extract neuropeptides. The brain and nerves of an invertebrate can be extracted by homogenization and brief sonication in 10 volumes of 1 M acetic acid or solvent consisting of acetone/HCl/water (40 : 1 : 6). For vertebrate brain tissue, the extraction is confounded by the high fat content of the tissue, and the rapid degradation of proteins into peptide fragments. Postmortem protein degradation is prevented by sacrificing mice/rats using a standard decapitation procedure and then immediately irradiating the head in a conventional microwave oven (Che *et al.*, 2005) (1.6-kW oven at power level 5 for 5–8 s). Peptides are then extracted with acidic solvent and sonication.

The extracted peptides are fractionated by LC and then analyzed by MS either on-line with ESI-MS/MS or off-line with MALDI-MS/MS. MALDI-MS detects singly charged peptides, which is advantageous because most contaminants are <600 Da and are smaller than the majority of neuropeptides. ESI-MS often detects peptides as doubly charged species. Unfortunately, most of the contaminants remain singly charged, and therefore may overlap with the doubly charged small neuropeptides of $m/z < 600$ Da. Figure 10.1 indicates three clusters of singly charged polymer which may come from the collection tube during extraction of the nervous tissue. It is useful to run a blank extraction experiment and measure the masses of the contaminants, and place these molecular ion species into the exclusion list for MS analysis of the subsequent samples.

It should be realized that tandem MS must be performed. The sample contains a large population of low mass molecular ion species; some of the structural distinct peptides will have similar masses and can only be distinguished by MS/MS analysis.

In the following section we use the brain of the snail *Lymnaea stagnalis* as an example for global peptide analysis.

10.2.2.1   Protocol

Requirements

Chemicals: Methanol, acetonitrile.

Solutions: 1 M acetic acid; 0.1% TFA; 60% acetonitrile in 0.1% TFA.

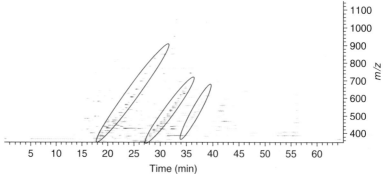

Figure 10.1 Electrospray ionization mass spectrometric analysis of a peptide extract from an invertebrate nerve. Peptides were extracted from the nerve by homogenization in a 1.5-mL reaction tube with acidic solvent. After centrifugation, the supernatant was injected into a nano-C18 column and eluted with an increasing gradient of acetonitrile. The eluents were electrosprayed on-line into a LTQ-Orbitrap mass spectrometer. There were many endogenous peptides scattered across the whole elution time and m/z value. Three well-defined clusters of singly charged polymers were also prominently present (enclosed in elliptical circles), and they may interfere with the analysis of the peptides. The x-axis is elution time from the column; y-axis is mass-to-charge ratio. (Please find a color version of this figure in the color plates.)

Instrumentation: Glass Potter, sonicater; bench-top temperature-controlled centrifuge (e.g. Centrifuges 5417R from Eppendorf); solid-phase C18 extraction column (e.g. Supeclean from Supelco); a high-performance nanoLC system with 3 μm nano-C18 LC column (e.g. Ultimate system from LC Packings); SpeedVac.

1. Pipette 10 mL of 1 M acetic acid into a glass Potter, and keep it on ice.
2. Drop the brains directly into the homogenizer.
3. Place the Teflon pestle into the glass Potter with your sample, switch on the rotation at 900 rpm and homogenize the sample with 12 strokes.
4. Remove the homogenate to a 1.5-mL reaction tube, and centrifuge in a pre-cooled table centrifuge at 4 °C for 10 min at maximum speed.
5. Pipette the supernatant to a new 1.5-mL reaction tube.
6. Resuspend the pellet in 1 mL 1 M acetic acid and sonicate 5 × 5 s over ice.
7. Centrifuge the sample in a pre-cooled table centrifuge for 10 min at maximum speed.
8. Pipette the supernatant and pool it together with the previously collected supernatant.
9. Activate a solid-phase C18 extraction column with 5 mL methanol, and wash the extraction with 10 mL 0.1% TFA.
10. Load the supernatant into the extraction column, and wash the column with 10 mL 0.1% TFA.

11. Elute the peptides in 2 column volumes of 60% acetonitrile in 0.1% TFA. This solid-phase extraction chromatography step cleans up the sample, thereby protecting the nanoLC column.
12. Dry the eluent in a SpeedVac.
13. Redissolve the peptides in 40 μL 0.1% TFA.
14. Inject the peptides into a 3 μm nano-C18 LC column, and fractionate the peptides with increasing concentrations of acetonitrile.
15. Most neuropeptides elute from the column between 10 and 40% acetonitrile, therefore, the gradient should be optimized around 10–40% acetonitrile.
16. Analyze the peptides with MS/MS.

10.3
Outlook

Two recent developments in proteomics studies may be highly relevant for neuropeptide analysis. First, the analysis of peptides is facilitated by the use of a mass spectrometer that has high mass accuracy, high sensitivity, and MS^n capability, for example the ion trap-fourier transform ion cyclotron resonance mass spectrometer and the ion trap-orbitrap mass spectrometer. These mass spectrometers are particularly useful for *de novo* peptide sequencing, which is indispensable for the characterization of peptides with posttranslational modifications, and peptides from species of which the genome sequences have not yet been completely determined. Second, due to technical difficulty only a few quantitative peptidomics studies have been reported so far. Recently, a label-free LC-MS-based quantitative approach has been developed for shotgun proteomics (Old *et al.*, 2005). This approach could be implemented for (large-scale) quantitative peptidomics analysis. In conclusion, using peptidomics technology we may be able to map the neuropeptide constituents in distinct brain regions, and start deciphering the interactive effects of these peptides on neuronal physiology and properties of neuronal circuitry.

References

Baggerman, G., Cerstiaens, A., De Loof, A. and Schoofs, L. (2002) Peptidomics of the larval Drosophila melanogaster central nervous system. *The Journal of Biological Chemistry*, **277**, 40368–40374.

Brezina, V., Orekhova, I.V. and Weiss, K.R. (1996) Functional uncoupling of linked neurotransmitter effects by combinatorial convergence. *Science*, **273**, 806–810.

Che, F.Y., Lim, J., Pan, H., Biswas, R. and Fricker, L.D. (2005) Quantitative neuropeptidomics of microwave-irradiated mouse brain and pituitary. *Molecular & Cellular Proteomics*, **4**, 1391–1405.

El Filali, Z., Hornshaw, M., Smit, A.B. and Li, K.W. (2003) Retrograde labeling of single neurons in conjunction with MALDI high-energy collision-induced dissociation MS/MS analysis for peptide profiling and structural characterization. *Analytical Chemistry*, **75**, 2996–3000.

El Filali, Z., Van Minnen, J., Liu, W.K., Smit, A.B. and Li, K.W. (2006) Peptidomics analysis of neuropeptides involved in copulatory behavior of the mollusk Lymnaea stagnalis. *Journal of Proteome Research*, **5**, 1611–1617.

Fricker, L.D., Lim, J., Pan, H. and Che, F.Y. (2006) Peptidomics: identification and quantification of endogenous peptides in neuroendocrine tissues. *Mass Spectrometry Reviews*, **25**, 327–344.

Hokfelt, T., Broberger, C., Xu, Z.Q., Sergeyev, V., Ubink, R. and Diez, M. (2000) Neuropeptides—an overview. *Neuropharmacology*, **39**, 1337–1356.

Hsieh, S., Dreisewerd, K., van der Schors, R.C., Jimenez, C.R., Stahl-Zeng, J., Hillenkamp, F., Jorgenson, J.W., Geraerts, W.P. and Li, K.W. (1998) Separation and identification of peptides in single neurons by microcolumn liquid chromatography-matrix-assisted laser desorption/ionization time-of-flight mass spectrometry and postsource decay analysis. *Analytical Chemistry*, **70**, 1847–1852.

Hummon, A.B., Amare, A. and Sweedler, J.V. (2006) Discovering new invertebrate neuropeptides using mass spectrometry. *Mass Spectrometry Reviews*, **25**, 77–98.

Jensen, H., Yamamoto, K., Bundgaard, J.R., Rehfeld, J.F. and Johnsen, A.H. (2005) Processing of chicken progastrin at post-Phe bonds by an aspartyl protease. *Biochimica et Biophysica Acta*, **1748**, 43–49.

Jimenez, C.R., Li, K.W., Smit, A.B. and Janse, C. (2006a) Auto-inhibitory control of peptidergic molluscan neurons and reproductive senescence. *Neurobiology of Aging*, **27**, 763–769.

Jimenez, C.R., Spijker, S., de Schipper, S., Lodder, J.C., Janse, C.K., Geraerts, W.P., van Minnen, J., Syed, N.I., Burlingame, A.L., Smit, A.B. and Li, K.W. (2006b) Peptidomics of a single

identified neuron reveals diversity of multiple neuropeptides with convergent actions on cellular excitability. *Journal of Neuroscience*, **26**, 518–529.

Li, K.W., Hornshaw, M.P., van Minnen, J., Smalla, K.H., Gundelfinger, E.D. and Smit, A.B. (2005) Organelle proteomics of rat synaptic proteins: correlation-profiling by isotope-coded affinity tagging in conjunction with liquid chromatography-tandem mass spectrometry to reveal post-synaptic density specific proteins. *Journal of Proteome Research*, **4**, 725–733.

Li, L., Garden, R.W. and Sweedler, J.V. (2000) Single-cell MALDI: a new tool for direct peptide profiling. *Trends in Biotechnology*, **18**, 151–160.

Old, W.M., Meyer-Arendt, K., Aveline-Wolf, L., Pierce, K.G., Mendoza, A., Sevinsky, J.R., Resing, K.A. and Ahn, N.G. (2005) Comparison of label-free methods for quantifying human proteins by shotgun proteomics. *Molecular & Cellular Proteomics*, **4**, 1487–1502.

Redeker, V., Toullec, J.Y., Vinh, J., Rossier, J. and Soyez, D. (1998) Combination of peptide profiling by matrix-assisted laser desorption/ionization time-of-flight mass spectrometry and immunodetection on single glands or cells. *Analytical Chemistry*, **70**, 1805–1811.

Smirnov, I.P., Zhu, X., Taylor, T., Huang, Y., Ross, P., Papayanopoulos, I.A., Martin, S.A. and Pappin, D.J. (2004) Suppression of alpha-cyano-4-hydroxycinnamic acid matrix clusters and reduction of chemical noise in MALDI-TOF mass spectrometry. *Analytical Chemistry*, **76**, 2958–2965.

Stuart, J.N. and Sweedler, J.V. (2003) Single-cell analysis by capillary electrophoresis. *Analytical and Bioanalytical Chemistry*, **375**, 28–29.

11
Analysis of Posttranslational Modifications

Daniel S. Spellman and Thomas A. Neubert

11.1
Introduction

11.1.1
Posttranslational Modification of Proteins

The primary structure of virtually all eukaryotic proteins is modified posttranslationally through addition or removal of biochemically functional species such as phosphate, sulfate, carbohydrates, and lipids, as well as through the cleavage of peptide backbones and side-chain bonds. These alterations extend the range of functions that a given amino acid sequence can perform. Many of these modifications are transient in nature, providing cells with elaborate on/off switches and attenuation devices to control and modulate biological processes. The importance of posttranslational modification (PTM) has come into particular focus over the past decade as sequencing of the human and other genomes revealed what many never predicted. The genomes of organisms such as human, mouse, yeast, nematode, fruitfly, and arabidopsis do not differ on a scale that one would predict given the observed differences in complexity of organization and function (Gregory, 2001; Gregory *et al.*, 2007). This is exaggerated in the neurosciences where perhaps the most dramatic differences between humans and other organisms are observed. From where does this great complexity and diversity in function arise? How can dramatic leaps in complexity between organisms such as worms and humans be achieved with just one third more genes?

Many mechanisms for generating phenotypic complexity have emerged, including regulatory functions of intergenic material, alternative splicing of pre-mRNA, posttranscriptional regulation of mRNA, and new functional roles for mature RNA. But perhaps the greatest contributor, adding an enormous potential for combinatorial diversity on top of the above mentioned diversifying phenomena are PTMs. For example, addition of only two independent amino acid-specific modifications on a protein of 100 amino acids, with each amino acid occurring at a rate of 1 in 20, would provide the potential for

Proteomics of the Nervous System. Edited by H.G. Nothwang and S.E. Pfeiffer
Copyright © 2008 WILEY-VCH Verlag GmbH & Co. KGaA, Weinheim
ISBN: 978-3-527-31716-5

approximately 1000 additional amino acid combinations (i.e. a 50% probability of modification times 2 modifications, times 5 occurrences of the amino acid in the protein $= (1/2^{(2\times5)}) = 1/1024$ probability for each modification state). A more realistic combination of several potential PTMs, with varied amino acid occurrences and PTM occupancies at sub-stoichiometric levels, could provide truly enormous potential for molecular diversity.

11.1.2
PTMs and the Nervous System

A large body of literature relates PTMs to the control of numerous processes in the nervous system including cytoskeletal regulation, neuronal morphogenesis and neurite outgrowth, and protein distribution, recycling and trafficking. Roles for PTMs are best characterized in cytoskeletal systems such as tubulin (Kobayashi and Mundel, 1998; Saragoni *et al.*, 2000), neurofilaments (Grant and Pant, 2000; Pant *et al.*, 2000), microtubule-associated proteins (Avila *et al.*, 1994; Mandell and Banker, 1996; Sanchez *et al.*, 2000), kinesins and dynein motors (Shea, 2000), and actin and actin-binding proteins (reviewed in Sarmiere and Bamburg, 2004). Beyond these basic functions, one of the more fascinating roles of PTMs is their participation in the process of memory formation. In most accepted models of memory, changes occur at specific synapses in response to particular stimuli, modifying both the structure and content of the synapse and allowing for the persistence of a given memory trace (McGaugh, 2000). The immediate changes at the synapse are widely attributed to activity-dependent PTM of proteins (Routtenberg, 1979; Sweatt, 2001) with longer term stabilization of the synapse being attributed to activity-dependent protein turnover and synthesis (Kandel, 2001). It has been argued as of late that PTM of synaptic proteins may be the only mechanism required for long-term memory (Routtenberg and Rekart, 2005). Given the importance of PTMs in such essential functions, it is no surprise that many diseases of the nervous system, including neurodegenerative disorders such as multiple sclerosis (Kim *et al.*, 2003) and Alzheimer's disease (Maccioni *et al.*, 2001), involve PTM-specific misregulation of the above mentioned processes. In addition to neurodegenerative diseases, several psychological disorders such as schizophrenia (Klushnik *et al.*, 1991; Hans *et al.*, 2004), bipolarism (Grimes and Jope, 2001), and depression (Dwivedi *et al.*, 2004) have hypothesized links to misregulation of enzymatic processes and aberrant PTMs.

Numerous PTMs have important roles in brain function and pathology. In this chapter, we focus on three PTMs: phosphorylation, ubiquitination, and glycosylation. These have demonstrated roles in the nervous system and their analysis benefits from established enrichment and/or mass spectrometry-based detection protocols. For the analysis of oxidation, the reader is referred to Chapter 14. A more thorough list of common PTMs is presented in Table 11.1.

Table 11.1 Common posttranslational modifications.

Modification	Sites affected	Δm MS (Da)	Enrichment methods
Acetylation	N-terminus, K	42.011	Immunoaffinity
Citrullination	R	0.984	Immunoaffinity
Disulfide bond	C	2.0 intact, −2.0 reduced	Chemical labeling and chemical affinity
Formylation	N-terminus	27.995	Specific method N/A
Glycosyl phosphatidylinosiol (GPI)	C-terminus	Various, dependent upon type and number of carbohydrate and lipid groups	Specific method N/A, but present in membrane fraction after cellular fractionation
Glycosylation	N, S, T	Various, dependent upon type and number of carbohydrate groups	Lectin affinity (N-linked), chemical affinity
Methylation	R, K	14.016($\times$N)	Immunoaffinity
Myristoylation	N-terminus	210.198	Specific method N/A, but present in membrane fraction after cellular fractionation
Palmitoylation	C	238.230	Specific method N/A, but present in membrane fraction after cellular fractionation
Phosphorylation	S, T, Y	79.966	Strong cation exchange, immobilized metal affinity chromatography, isoelectric focusing, immunoaffinity
Polyglutamylation	E	128.131($\times$N)	Specific method N/A
Proteolytic Cleavage	General	Various, enzyme-dependent	Specific method N/A
Sulfation	Y	79.957	Strong cation exchange, immobilized metal affinity chromatography, isoelectric focusing
SUMOylation	K	Various, dependent upon genetic incorporation of tryptic cleavage site	Genetic affinity tag incorporation
Transglutamination	Q	Various, dependent upon available amine substrate	Chemical labeling, immunoaffinity, affinity chromatography
Ubiquitination	K	114.043 (after tryptic cleavage)	Genetic affinity tag incorporation, Unbiquitin-binding proteins

($\times$N), modification can be added at one residue multiple times,
N/A, not available.

Protein phosphorylation, the addition of phosphate (PO_4) to serine, threonine, or tyrosine, serves as one of the most common, important, and well-studied PTMs. This is demonstrated by the fact that kinases constitute the largest enzyme family in the human genome and it is estimated that up to 50% of predicted proteins are phosphorylated at some time (Hubbard and Cohen, 1993; Kalume *et al.*, 2003). Phosphorylation plays a prominent role in the regulation of many critical neuronal functions such as those discussed above.

Ubiquitination is another important PTM with an established role in signal transduction, endocytosis, and the recycling and degradation of proteins (Ciechanover *et al.*, 1980; Hershko *et al.*, 1980; Hershko and Ciechanover, 1998; Pickart, 2001; Finley *et al.*, 2004). During ubiquitination, a linkage between its C-terminal glycine and a lysine side-chain of the target protein is established through an isopeptide bond. Differential outcomes in this process are often dependent upon the presence and degree of protein ubiquitination (Pickart and Fushman, 2004). The awarding of the 2004 Nobel Prize in chemistry for work that brought to light the role of ubiquitin in regulating protein degradation has led to a rapid development of strategies for the detection and characterization of ubiquitin-modified proteins. In the brain, much recent evidence has pointed to a prominent role for ubiquitin-dependent regulation of the structure and function of the synapse (reviewed in DiAntonio and Hicke, 2004).

Glycosylation plays a vital role in complex tissues such as the brain through defining and modulating cell–cell contact. This is exemplified by its participation in the effective labeling of subsets of neuronal populations. Different glycol epitopes are presented by cell adhesion molecules (CAM), primarily the neuronal-specific NCAM, and these are in turn recognized by lectins on opposing cell surfaces (Dodd and Jessell, 1985; Key and Akeson, 1991; Pays and Schwarting, 2000). To this end, differences in carbohydrate signaling have been hypothesized to control sequential steps in synaptic growth (Tai and Zipser, 2002). There are two classes of glycosylation, *N*-linked glycosylation to the amide nitrogen of asparagine side-chains, and *O*-linked glycosylation to the hydroxy oxygen of serine and threonine side-chains. It has been demonstrated that the brain contains an unusually high amount of neutral *N*-linked glycans compared to other organs (Chen *et al.*, 1998), and *O*-linked glycosylations such as *O*-acetylglucosamine have also been shown to have important roles in the brain. This is evidenced by the high expression levels of enzymes responsible for addition and removal of this modification in the nervous system (Gao *et al.*, 2001).

11.1.3
Strategies for Characterization of Posttranslational Modifications

The simplest and most general strategy for characterization of PTM of a protein of interest is to purify the protein, measure the mass of the intact protein and/or its proteolytic peptides, and compare these masses with the predicted masses (Neubert and Johnson, 1995). The advantage of this strategy is that all PTMs of a given protein can in theory be characterized in this way, even those that have not previously been described. The disadvantage is that (often) large amounts of relatively pure protein are required. Today, methods for analysis of PTMs typically consist of one or more steps of modification-specific enrichment as well as targeted MS detection schemes. At times enrichment or targeted detection is sufficient for characterization, and in these cases such an approach is preferred for gains made in throughput. However, given the inherent complexity of biological matrices such as cell and tissue homogenates, a combined approach is typically the most effective. Below we will discuss such methodological approaches, most of which are amenable to combinatorial use. MS detection schemes will be specific to the type of instrumentation available whereas enrichment approaches should be applicable to most samples. The general strategy for PTM characterization is presented in Figure 11.1.

11.1.3.1 Enrichment of Posttranslationally Modified Proteins and Peptides

Biological matrices such as tissue and plasma can contain up to 12 orders of magnitude in dynamic range of protein concentrations (Anderson and Anderson, 2002). At best, mass spectrometers are only capable of observing 3 or 4 orders of magnitude in concentration at any given time. The inherent complexity of the proteome usually necessitates targeted enrichment of specific posttranslationally modified proteins or peptides in order to work within the dynamic range of available instrumentation. Enrichment strategies will be dependent upon the type of question being asked. These typically fall into one of two general categories: (i) Complete PTM characterization of a specific protein or a small group of proteins or, (ii) characterization of specific PTM sub-proteomes, for example, the phosphotyrosine proteome.

The first approach requires targeted enrichment of a hypothesized post-translationally modified protein. This is most often accomplished through immunopurification when good antibodies are available, or more often, the genetic incorporation of affinity or epitope tags such as the FLAG hydrophilic octapeptide (FLAG), glutathione-*S*-transferase (GST) fusion protein, polyhistidine-tag (His), green fluorescing protein (GFP), or biotinylation sites into the amino acid sequence of the target protein. Affinity tags allow for isolation of a target protein and often those proteins associated with it. After targeted isolation one can rely on PTM-specific MS detection methods such as those discussed below in Section 11.1.3.2 or could use a secondary enrichment of modified peptides like the ones discussed in this section.

A large proportion of the work done in the area of PTM-specific enrichment has focused on phosphorylation. Consequently, numerous methods

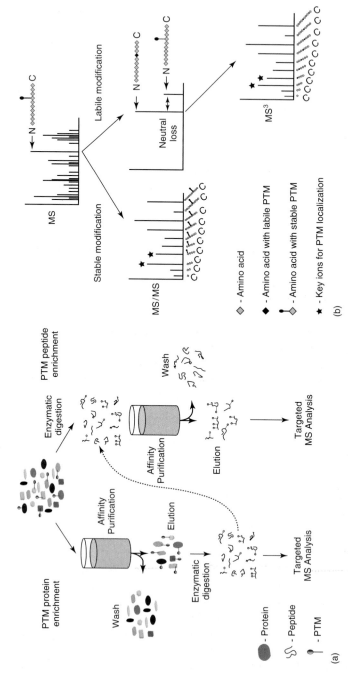

Figure 11.1 Posttranslational modification (PTM)-specific enrichment and mass spectrometric analysis. (a) A general strategy for PTM-specific enrichment of modified proteins before enzymatic digestion, and enrichment of modified peptides after enzymatic digestion using PTM-targeted affinity chromatography is depicted. (b) Mass spectrometric analysis of a hypothetical PTM is shown. In the case of a stable modification, fragment ions (idealized y ion series) observed in MS/MS reveal the position and identity of the PTM. In the case of a labile modification, the major process observed in MS/MS is neutral loss of the modification. Selection of the neutral loss species for further fragmentation and MS^3 analysis, allows for fragmentation of peptide bonds, and identification of the position and identity of the PTM.

have been developed for phospho-specific enrichment. These include immunoprecipitation using phosphotyrosine (Blagoev *et al.*, 2003; Amanchy *et al.*, 2005; Rush *et al.*, 2005; Zhang and Neubert, 2006) or phosphoserine/threonine (Gronborg *et al.*, 2002) antibodies, affinity chromatography such as immobilized metal-ion affinity chromatography (IMAC) (Stensballe *et al.*, 2001; Ficarro *et al.*, 2002) and TiO_2 (Pinkse *et al.*, 2004; Larsen *et al.*, 2005), strong cation exchange (SCX) (Beausoleil *et al.*, 2004), and chemical modification strategies centered around β-elimination of phosphate groups and Michael-type addition of nucleophiles that can be further modified to incorporate affinity tags such as biotin (Oda *et al.*, 2001; Goshe *et al.*, 2002). Here, we have provided three methods that have proven particularly useful in our lab as well as others (Section 11.2.1). One protocol enriches phosphotyrosine-proteins by immunoprecipitation, and two protocols enrich on the peptide level: TiO_2 pipette tip chromatography and immunoprecipitation of phosphotyrosine-containing peptides (Oda *et al.*, 2001; Goshe *et al.*, 2002).

The limited availability and usefulness of ubiquitin-specific antibodies as well as a lack of chemical affinity strategies has made it difficult to apply approaches similar to those used for other PTMs to the ubiquitin modification. Several alternative approaches such as epitope-tagged ubiquitin have shown promise, but these studies are primarily limited to simple eukaryotes such as yeast in which all genes encoding ubiquitin can be genetically inactivated (Peng *et al.*, 2003). Enrichment using ubiquitin-binding proteins is another recently developed method that allows for the analysis of other types of samples such as cultured mammalian cells and tissue samples (Mayor *et al.*, 2005). The usefulness of this approach is also limited given the minimal knowledge of the identities and specificities of ubiquitin-binding proteins. Given the novelty of this area of proteomic research and lack of effective tools, particularly in its application to complex mammalian systems such as neuronal tissue, detailed protocols for the enrichment of ubiquitin-modified proteins and peptides are not yet available.

The development of general strategies for the enrichment of glycosylated proteins and peptides are complicated by the complexity and diversity of these modifications. Instead, more common is the targeting of a specific class or subtype of glycosylation. A popular example of such an approach is targeted lectin affinity purification. Lectins are a class of cell surface proteins that bind specifically to certain oligosaccharide structures on glycoconjugates, and they display a variety of binding specificities. Lectins have been extensively used to purify glycoproteins, glycopeptides, and oligosaccharides from a host of biological sources (Ghosh *et al.*, 2004; Manning *et al.*, 2004; Nawarak *et al.*, 2004; Vosseller *et al.*, 2006). We have provided methods for lectin affinity approaches at both the protein and peptide level (Section 11.2.3). Other strategies, such as the purification of N-linked carbohydrates based on the conjugation of glycoproteins to a solid support using hydrazide chemistry (Zhang *et al.*, 2003; Zhang *et al.*, 2005), and varied chemical derivation and affinity tagging approaches (Khidekel *et al.*, 2003; Brittain *et al.*, 2005; Sprung *et al.*, 2005) show great promise.

11.1.3.2 Detection of Posttranslationally Modified Peptides and Localization of Sites of Modification by Mass Spectrometry

To gain yet another level of sensitivity and specificity, it is often useful or even necessary to use a PTM-specific mass spectrometric detection method when small amounts of protein or low stoichiometry modifications are studied. One approach developed in our lab for phospho-specific MS detection takes advantage of the fact that the high acidity of phosphopeptides gives them increased signal intensities in negative ion mode when compared to positive ion mode in matrix-assisted laser desorption/ionization time-of-flight (MALDI-TOF) MS (Ma *et al.*, 2001). An additional step of methyl esterification of peptide mixtures before analysis can reduce the signal of non-phosphopeptides in negative ion mode, greatly enhancing the specificity of positive/negative ion mode scanning (Xu *et al.*, 2005). Other methods such as detection of loss of the modification from the peptide precursor (neutral loss scanning), and detection of product and marker ions are effective for identifying phosphopeptides in complex mixtures (Annan *et al.*, 2001; Bateman *et al.*, 2002; Steen and Mann, 2002; Schroeder *et al.*, 2004). We have provided detailed descriptions of how to detect phosphopeptides using both MALDI and electrospray ionization (ESI) approaches (Section 11.2.1).

Direct detection of ubiquitinylated peptides is also a quickly developing area. After tryptic digestion, ubiquitin-modified peptides contain a signature diglycine-modified lysine residue that is the result of a tryptic cleavage between the C-terminal Arg and Gly of ubiquitin. Diglycine-modified lysine can be identified by database search engines using this signature as a variable modification. This approach has proven to be effective and both large-scale and targeted studies have been performed (Marotti *et al.*, 2002; Hitchcock *et al.*, 2003; Coulombe *et al.*, 2004; Starita *et al.*, 2004). The corresponding protocol is presented below (Section 11.2.2). Similarly, ubiquitin–ubiquitin linkages can be detected providing a means to characterize the degree and linkage sites of polyubiquitination (Wu-Baer *et al.*, 2003; Nishikawa *et al.*, 2004; Saeki *et al.*, 2004). It has also been demonstrated that the N-terminal sulfonation of peptides can generate unique fragmentation patterns for ubiquitin-modified peptides, facilitating their identification (Wang and Cotter, 2005; Wang *et al.*, 2006) and offering a promising approach that has yet to be applied on a proteomic scale.

Detection of glycosylated peptides is another area of intense research. As discussed in the context of enrichment, tremendous difficulty results from the heterogeneous nature of glycosylations and the likely presence of several glycoforms of a given glycopeptide, each present at relatively low concentration in the total peptide pool. More difficulty arises from the fact that glycans are labile and easily lost during ionization, making neutral loss and glycan fragmentation the primary dissociation processes during tandem mass spectrometry (MS/MS). Several specialized MS^n and fragmentation methods have been used to characterize the nature of glycosylation on purified proteins, but the interpretation of spectra from large branched molecules like glycans with numerous degrees of freedom is difficult (Jebanathirajah *et al.*, 2003; Budnik *et al.*, 2006; Wuhrer *et al.*, 2006). To date, the most effective method for identification of glycosylation sites is to enrich glycosylated proteins by affinity chromatography, then deglycosylate the enriched proteins before analysis by MS. This is recommended if one simply wishes to determine the site of glycosylation, whereas characterization of the glycans is a much more difficult process and beyond the scope of this chapter. The use of enzymes such as peptide-*N*-glycosidase F (PNGase F) in the case of *N*-linked glycans will convert the modified Asn to Asp (Xie *et al.*, 2006). In high-resolution mass spectrometers this mass difference of 1 Da is enough for detection of the site of glycosylation. Furthermore, this difference can be highlighted by performing digestion in 50% heavy water ($H_2^{18}O$), creating an easily observed mass increase of 2 Da in addition to the $H_2^{16}O$ version (Kuster and Mann, 1999; Zhou *et al.*, 2001). A protocol for this procedure has been provided (Section 11.2.3).

11.2
Protocols

11.2.1
Phosphorylation

11.2.1.1 Enrichment by Protein–Phosphotyrosine Immunoprecipitation

It is recommended that the best antibody or mix of antibodies, as well as the appropriate ratio of sample to antibody for a particular experimental system, are determined empirically with small-scale (usually Western blot) analyses before proceeding with proteome-scale experiments.

Requirements

Chemicals: Complete protease inhibitors (Roche); agarose/sepharose-immobilized anti-phosphotyrosine antibodies such as pY99 (Santa Cruz Biotechnology, Inc.), 4G10 (Upstate), pY100 (Invitrogen).

Solutions: Phosphatase inhibitors (2 mM Na_3VO_4 and 2 mM NaF); 100 mM phenyl phosphate; 25 mM NH_4HCO_3.
1. Prepare desired protein isolate such as cell or tissue homogenate. Include fresh protease inhibitors (such as commercially available tablets) and phosphatase inhibitors.
2. Combine protein isolate with a 50% suspension in homogenate buffer of agarose/sepharose-immobilized anti-phosphotyrosine antibodies at a

ratio of 20 μL bead suspension to 500 μL protein isolate (may vary based on sample type).

3. Incubate the mixture for 5 h to overnight at 4 °C with gentle mixing on an apparatus such as an end-over-end rocker.

4. Elute proteins by incubating beads in 100 mM phenyl phosphate (30 min at 4 °C with gentle shaking), or reducing Laemmli buffer (mix and boil 5 min) if IgG contamination is not a concern.

5. After phenyl phosphate elution, dialyze proteins against 25 mM NH_4HCO_3 for a minimum of 1 h in a volume 50× or greater than the volume of the sample and repeat at least three times. Digest the sample in-solution with trypsin, or concentrate eluate by preferred method (TCA precipitation, centrifugal concentration, etc.), and separate sample on sodium dodecyl sulfate polyacrylamide-based gel electrophoresis (SDS-PAGE) for subsequent in-gel digestion.

6. For reducing Laemmli elution, separate sample directly on to SDS-PAGE for subsequent in-gel digestion.

11.2.1.2 Enrichment by Peptide-Pipette Tip TiO_2 Chromatography

Requirements

Material: TiO_2 tips (NuTip, 1–10 μL, Glygen Corp.)

Solutions: Loading buffer (1.0% trifluoroacetic acid (TFA) in 80% acetonitrile); 0.1% TFA in 80% acetonitrile; 500 mM NH_4OH.

1. Prepare in-solution or in-gel tryptic digest and dry peptide mixture under vacuum.

2. Condition TiO_2 tips (NuTip, 1–10 μL, Glygen Corp.) by pipetting 10 μL of 1.0% TFA in 80% acetonitrile loading buffer through the tip 5 times.

3. Dissolve peptides in 10 μL of loading buffer and load on to tip by pipetting peptide solution through the tip at least 10 times.

4. Wash the tip with an additional 10 μL of loading buffer, pipetting the solution through the tip at least 10 times.

5. Wash the tip again with 10 μL of 0.1% TFA in 80% acetonitrile by pipetting the solution through the tip at least 10 times.

6. Elute bound peptides by pipetting 3.5–10 μL of 500 mM NH_4OH through the tip 10 times.

7. Remove solvent by lyophilization and redissolve sample in matrix or LC loading buffer for MS analysis.

11.2.1.3 Enrichment by Peptide Phosphotyrosine Immunoprecipitation

Take note that the use of a non-ionic detergent such as *n*-octyl glucoside, above its critical micelle concentration, in the immunoprecipitation buffer is crucial for attaining high selectivity and sensitivity with this protocol for peptide phosphotyrosine immunoprecipitation.

Requirements

Chemicals and material: High-performance liquid chromatography (HPLC)-grade water; agarose/sepharose-immobilized anti-phosphotyrosine antibody (see Section 11.2.1.1).

Solutions: Immunoprecipitation buffer (150 mM NaCl, 20 mM Tris pH 8), 1% *n*-octyl glucoside; 1.0% formic acid in 50% acetonitrile.
1. Prepare in-solution or in-gel tryptic digest and dry peptide mixture under vacuum.
2. Wash 5 µL of agarose/sepharose-immobilized anti-phosphotyrosine antibody such as pY99 (Santa Cruz Biotechnology, Inc.), 4G10 (Upstate), pY100 (Invitrogen) with 50 µL immunoprecipitation buffer (150 mM NaCl, 20 mM Tris pH 8, 1% *n*-octyl glucoside).
3. Redissolve peptide mixture in 50 µL immunoprecipitation buffer, mix with anti-phosphotyrosine beads, and incubate for 2 h at 4 °C with gentle mixing.
4. Spin the beads down in a bench top centrifuge (refer to bead manufacturer's instructions for recommended speed of centrifugation) and remove the supernatant.
5. Wash the beads once with 50 µL of immunoprecipitation buffer and 3 times with HPLC-grade water.
6. Add 10 µL of elution buffer (1% formic acid in 50% acetonitrile) to the washed beads and mix for 15 min.
7. Spin the beads down once again and remove the peptide-containing supernatant.
8. Dry the eluate under vacuum and redissolve the sample in matrix or LC loading buffer for MS analysis.

11.2.1.4 Analysis of Methyl Esterified Peptides

Requirements

Chemicals: Dry methanol; acetyl chloride

Solutions: 0.2% TFA in 30% acetonitrile.
1. Prepare methanolic HCl solution by dropwise addition of 160 µL of acetyl chloride to 1 mL of dry methanol (Ficarro *et al.*, 2002).
2. Lyophilize protein tryptic digests and redissolve peptides in 50 µL of 2 M methanolic HCl reagent (for up to 250 pmol of protein, larger amounts will require a larger volume of methanolic HCl).

3. Allow methyl esterification to proceed for 2–3 h at room temperature.
4. Remove solvent by lyophilization, and redissolve peptide mixture in 0.2% TFA, 30% acetonitrile.
5. Prepare matrix (depending on laser energy used) for MALDI analysis and mix with sample at a ratio of 1 : 1 (v/v), and spot 1.2 µL of this mixture onto MALDI sample stage.
6. Acquire positive and negative ion MALDI mass spectra.
7. Carboxyl methylation can be observed as +14 atomic mass units and asparagine/glutamine methylation side-products as +15 atomic mass units.
8. Phosphopeptides can be observed as those peptides that have large relative increases in signal intensity in negative ion mode as compared to positive ion mode and whose masses correspond to candidate peptides + phosphorylation + methylation.

11.2.1.5 ESI-MS Positive Ion Mode Neutral Loss Scanning

Most instrumentation capable of MS/MS or MS^n experiments such as triple quadrupoles and ion traps are capable of neutral loss scanning. Most modern instrumentation and software allow this analysis to be done in an automated, data-dependent fashion.

1. Instrument operation methods should be programmed to select the top 3–10 most intense ions (depending upon instrument type and scan speeds) from each MS survey scan for MS/MS analysis.
2. The instrument operation method should also be programmed to search MS/MS spectra for a neutral loss ion of 98, 49 or 32.7 m/z (corresponding to +1, +2, +3 charge states of the loss of phosphate), and if this loss is observed as one of the top 3 most intense fragment ions, an MS^3 event should be triggered on this ion.
3. MS^3 spectra should yield readily interpretable b and y ion series.

11.2.2
Ubiquitination

11.2.2.1 Characterization of Diglycine-Modified Lysine Residues

1. Digest the protein or protein mixture of interest either in-solution or in-gel with trypsin.
2. After tryptic digestion ubiquitin-modified peptides will contain a signature diglycine-modified lysine residue that is the result of a tryptic cleavage between the C-terminal Arg and Gly of ubiquitin.
3. If a ubiquitin diglycine is not a PTM option for the database search engine you are using, create a custom modification of lysine of 114 atomic mass units.
4. Diglycine-modified lysine should be detected by search engines with treatment of this signature as a variable modification.

11.2.3
Glycosylation

11.2.3.1 Enrichment by Protein–Lectin Affinity

Several lectins such as concanavalin A (ConA) or wheat germ agglutinin (WGA) immobilized on agarose or sepharose resins are commercially available. The lectin and eluting sugar used should be chosen only after careful consideration of the lectin selectivity. The following protocol can be performed in a self-packed column for bead volumes larger than 200 µL or in a 1.5 mL conical sample tube or 1.5 mL spin cup for smaller volumes.

Requirements

Material: Immobilized lectins.

Solutions: Buffer A (10 mM Tris-HCl, 150 mM NaCl, 1 mM $CaCl_2$ and 1 mM $MnCl_2$); wash buffer (10 mM Tris-HCl, 1 M NaCl, 1 mM $CaCl_2$, and 1 mM $MnCl_2$); 1 M methyl α-mannopyranoside for ConA or 1 M N, N'-diacetylchitobiose for WGA; 25 mM NH_4HCO_3.

1. Wash and equilibrate selected immobilized lectin with at least fivefold resin volume excess of buffer A.
2. Mix prepared protein isolate (preferably in buffer A or a 1:1 mix with buffer A) with lectin resin at a ratio of 100 µL bead volume to 1 mg protein at a maximum concentration of 0.1 mg mL^{-1}, and incubate at room temperature for 30 min with gentle mixing using a device such as an end-over-end rocker.
3. Decant unbound protein and wash resin with at least 10 resin volumes of wash buffer.
4. Elute bound proteins by incubating resin with 1 M methyl α-mannopyranoside (for ConA) or 1 M N, N'-diacetylchitobiose (for WGA) in wash buffer for 30 min at room temperature.
5. Dialyze proteins against 25 mM NH_4HCO_3 for a minimum of 1 h in a volume $50\times$ or greater the sample and repeat at least three times, and digest in-solution with trypsin, or separate eluate by SDS-PAGE for in-gel digestion.

Glycopeptide affinity purification can be performed in a similar way using a lyophilized in-solution tryptic digest reconstituted in Tris-buffered saline as sample.

11.2.3.2 Deglycosylation and Stable Isotope Tagging of Glycopeptides

This protocol is specific to N-linked glycopeptides. It should be performed on a simplified mixture such as an in-solution tryptic digest of a purified glycoprotein or affinity captured glycopeptides.

Requirements

Chemicals and material: $H_2^{18}O$ and $H_2^{16}O$ water; lyophilized PNGase F.

Solution: 0.1 M Tris base, adjust to pH 9 using acetic acid.

1. To minimize the dilution of $H_2^{18}O$ before the tagging reaction, dry sample completely under vacuum to remove any $H_2^{16}O$ water.
2. Redissolve peptides in 0.1 M Tris base, pH 9 in 50% $H_2^{18}O$/50% $H_2^{16}O$.
3. Dissolve lyophilized PNGase F in 50% $H_2^{18}O$/50% $H_2^{16}O$, add 1 mU/10 μg peptide to the peptide solution and incubate overnight at 37 °C.
4. Remove solvent by lyophilization and redissolve sample in matrix or LC loading buffer for MS analysis.
5. Formerly N-glycosylated peptides should be readily observable as peptides that were not observable in tryptic digests before deglycosylation. Isotopic distribution of formerly glycosylated peptides is unique and appears as a pair of isotopic clusters, one distributed as usual and a second similar cluster adjacent to the first, but shifted by +2 Da.

11.3
Outlook

Interest and progress in the analysis of PTMs of proteins in the nervous system is rapidly increasing. The growing popularity of this field is due to many factors, including increased awareness of the importance of PTMs in the proper functioning as well as diseases of the nervous system, novel and innovative application of biochemistry to the enrichment and analysis of PTMs, and improvement and increased availability of MS technology for the analysis of PTMs. More rigorous assessment of PTMs in the context of brain function and pathology will include identification of what modifications are present, where, and how they change in time in correlation with specific functions such as memory formation and disease. Most likely, the future of PTM proteomics will focus on developing better ways of obtaining PTM-specific, quantitative measurements with temporal resolution. Improvements in chromatography, MS instrumentation, protein identification strategies, data processing, quantitative techniques, and PTM-specific isolation and detection techniques will be of great help.

Acknowledgments

We acknowledge Dr Vivekananda Shetty for assistance with glycosylation protocols, Drs Chong-Feng Xu and Guoan Zhang for assistance in phosphorylation protocols, and the rest of our colleagues at the New York University

Protein Analysis Facility for their ideas and discussions which contributed to the strategies presented in this manuscript. Our work on proteomics of the nervous system was supported by NIH Grants R21 NS44184 and P30 NS050276 to T.A.N.

References

Amanchy, R., Kalume, D.E., Iwahori, A., Zhong, J. and Pandey, A. (2005) Phosphoproteome analysis of HeLa cells using stable isotope labeling with amino acids in cell culture (SILAC). *Journal of Proteome Research*, **4**, 1661–1671.

Anderson, N.L. and Anderson, N.G. (2002) The human plasma proteome: history, character, and diagnostic prospects. *Molecular & Cellular Proteomics*, **1**, 845–867.

Annan, R.S., Huddleston, M.J., Verma, R., Deshaies, R.J. and Carr, S.A. (2001) A multidimensional electrospray MS-based approach to phosphopeptide mapping. *Analytical Chemistry*, **73**, 393–404.

Avila, J., Dominguez, J. and Diaz-Nido, J. (1994) Regulation of microtubule dynamics by microtubule-associated protein expression and phosphorylation during neuronal development. *The International Journal of Developmental Biology*, **38**, 13–25.

Bateman, R.H., Carruthers, R., Hoyes, J.B., Jones, C., Langridge, J.I., Millar, A. and Vissers, J.P. (2002) A novel precursor ion discovery method on a hybrid quadrupole orthogonal acceleration time-of-flight (Q-TOF) mass spectrometer for studying protein phosphorylation. *Journal of the American Society for Mass Spectrometry*, **13**, 792–803.

Beausoleil, S.A., Jedrychowski, M., Schwartz, D., Elias, J.E., Villen, J., Li, J., Cohn, M.A., Cantley, L.C. and Gygi, S.P. (2004) Large-scale characterization of HeLa cell nuclear phosphoproteins. *Proceedings of the National Academy of Sciences of the United States of America* **101**, 12130–12135.

Blagoev, B., Kratchmarova, I., Ong, S.E., Nielsen, M., Foster, L.J. and Mann, M. (2003) A proteomics strategy to elucidate functional protein-protein interactions applied to EGF signaling. *Nature Biotechnology*, **21**, 315–318.

Brittain, S.M., Ficarro, S.B., Brock, A. and Peters, E.C. (2005) Enrichment and analysis of peptide subsets using fluorous affinity tags and mass spectrometry. *Nature Biotechnology*, **23**, 463–468.

Budnik, B.A., Lee, R.S. and Steen, J.A. (2006) Global methods for protein glycosylation analysis by mass spectrometry. *Biochimica et Biophysica Acta*, **1764**, 1870–1880.

Chen, Y.J., Wing, D.R., Guile, G.R., Dwek, R.A., Harvey, D.J. and Zamze, S. (1998) Neutral N-glycans in adult rat brain tissue—complete characterisation reveals fucosylated hybrid and complex structures. *European Journal of Biochemistry*, **251**, 691–703.

Ciechanover, A., Heller, H., Elias, S., Haas, A.L. and Hershko, A. (1980) ATP-dependent conjugation of reticulocyte proteins with the polypeptide required for protein degradation. *Proceedings of the National Academy of Sciences of the United States of America* **77**, 1365–1368.

Coulombe, P., Rodier, G., Bonneil, E., Thibault, P. and Meloche, S. (2004) N-Terminal ubiquitination of extracellular signal-regulated kinase 3 and p21 directs their degradation by the proteasome. *Molecular and Cellular Biology*, **24**, 6140–6150.

DiAntonio, A. and Hicke, L. (2004) Ubiquitin-dependent regulation of the synapse. *Annual Review of Neuroscience*, **27**, 223–246.

Dodd, J. and Jessell, T.M. (1985) Lactoseries carbohydrates specify subsets of dorsal root ganglion neurons projecting to the superficial dorsal horn of rat spinal cord. *Journal of Neuroscience,* 5, 3278–3294.

Dwivedi, Y., Rizavi, H.S., Shukla, P.K., Lyons, J., Faludi, G., Palkovits, M., Sarosi, A., Conley, R.R., Roberts, R.C., Tamminga, C.A. and Pandey, G.N. (2004) Protein kinase A in postmortem brain of depressed suicide victims: altered expression of specific regulatory and catalytic subunits. *Biological Psychiatry,* 55, 234–243.

Ficarro, S.B., McCleland, M.L., Stukenberg, P.T., Burke, D.J., Ross, M.M., Shabanowitz, J., Hunt, D.F. and White, F.M. (2002) Phosphoproteome analysis by mass spectrometry and its application to Saccharomyces cerevisiae. *Nature Biotechnology,* 20, 301–305.

Finley, D., Ciechanover, A. and Varshavsky, A. (2004) Ubiquitin as a central cellular regulator. *Cell,* 116, S29–S32.

Gao, Y., Wells, L., Comer, F.I., Parker, G.J. and Hart, G.W. (2001) Dynamic O-glycosylation of nuclear and cytosolic proteins: cloning and characterization of a neutral, cytosolic beta-N-acetylglucosaminidase from human brain. *Journal of Biological Chemistry,* 276, 9838–9845.

Ghosh, D., Krokhin, O., Antonovici, M., Ens, W., Standing, K.G., Beavis, R.C. and Wilkins, J.A. (2004) Lectin affinity as an approach to the proteomic analysis of membrane glycoproteins. *Journal of Proteome Research,* 3, 841–850.

Goshe, M.B., Veenstra, T.D., Panisko, E.A., Conrads, T.P., Angell, N.H. and Smith, R.D. (2002) Phosphoprotein isotope-coded affinity tags: application to the enrichment and identification of low-abundance phosphoproteins. *Analytical Chemistry,* 74, 607–616.

Grant, P. and Pant, H.C. (2000) Neurofilament protein synthesis and phosphorylation. *Journal of Neurocytology,* 29, 843–872.

Gregory, T.R. (2001) Coincidence, coevolution, or causation? DNA content, cell size, and the C-value enigma. *Biological Reviews of the Cambridge Philosophical Society,* 76, 65–101.

Gregory, T.R., Nicol, J.A., Tamm, H., Kullman, B., Kullman, K., Leitch, I.J., Murray, B.G., Kapraun, D.F., Greilhuber, J. and Bennett, M.D. (2007) Eukaryotic genome size databases. *Nucleic Acids Research,* 35, D332–D338.

Grimes, C.A. and Jope, R.S. (2001) The multifaceted roles of glycogen synthase kinase 3beta in cellular signaling. *Progress in Neurobiology,* 65, 391–426.

Gronborg, M., Kristiansen, T.Z., Stensballe, A., Andersen, J.S., Ohara, O., Mann, M., Jensen, O.N. and Pandey, A. (2002) A mass spectrometry-based proteomic approach for identification of serine/threonine-phosphorylated proteins by enrichment with phospho-specific antibodies: identification of a novel protein, Frigg, as a protein kinase A substrate. *Molecular & Cellular Proteomics,* 1, 517–527.

Hans, A., Bajramovic, J.J., Syan, S., Perret, E., Dunia, I., Brahic, M. and Gonzalez-Dunia, D. (2004) Persistent, noncytolytic infection of neurons by Borna disease virus interferes with ERK 1/2 signaling and abrogates BDNF-induced synaptogenesis. *The FASEB Journal,* 18, 863–865.

Hershko, A. and Ciechanover, A. (1998) The ubiquitin system. *Annual Review of Biochemistry,* 67, 425–479.

Hershko, A., Ciechanover, A., Heller, H., Haas, A.L. and Rose, I.A. (1980) Proposed role of ATP in protein breakdown: conjugation of protein with multiple chains of the polypeptide of ATP-dependent proteolysis. *Proceedings of the National Academy of Sciences of the United States of America* 77, 1783–1786.

Hitchcock, A.L., Auld, K., Gygi, S.P. and Silver, P.A. (2003) A subset of membrane-associated proteins is ubiquitinated in response to mutations in the endoplasmic reticulum degradation machinery. *Proceedings of the National Academy of Sciences of the United States of America* 100, 12735–12740.

Hubbard, M.J. and Cohen, P. (1993) On target with a new mechanism for the regulation of protein phosphorylation. *Trends in Biochemical Sciences,* 18, 172–177.

Jebanathirajah, J., Steen, H. and Roepstorff, P. (2003) Using optimized collision energies and high resolution, high accuracy fragment ion selection to improve glycopeptide detection by precursor ion scanning. *Journal of the American Society for Mass Spectrometry*, **14**, 777–784.

Kalume, D.E., Molina, H. and Pandey, A. (2003) Tackling the phosphoproteome: tools and strategies. *Current Opinion in Chemical Biology*, **7**, 64–69.

Kandel, E.R. (2001) The molecular biology of memory storage: a dialogue between genes and synapses. *Science*, **294**, 1030–1038.

Key, B. and Akeson, R.A. (1991) Delineation of olfactory pathways in the frog nervous system by unique glycoconjugates and N-CAM glycoforms. *Neuron*, **6**, 381–396.

Khidekel, N., Arndt, S., Lamarre-Vincent, N., Lippert, A., Poulin-Kerstien, K.G., Ramakrishnan, B., Qasba, P.K. and Hsieh-Wilson, L.C. (2003) A chemoenzymatic approach toward the rapid and sensitive detection of O-GlcNAc posttranslational modifications. *Journal of the American Chemical Society*, **125**, 16162–16163.

Kim, J.K., Mastronardi, F.G., Wood, D.D., Lubman, D.M., Zand, R. and Moscarello, M.A. (2003) Multiple sclerosis: an important role for post-translational modifications of myelin basic protein in pathogenesis. *Molecular & Cellular Proteomics*, **2**, 453–462.

Klushnik, T.P., Spunde, A., Yakovlev, A.G., Khuchua, Z.A., Saks, V.A. and Vartanyan, M.E. (1991) Intracellular alterations of the creatine kinase isoforms in brains of schizophrenic patients. *Molecular and Chemical Neuropathology*, **15**, 271–280.

Kobayashi, N. and Mundel, P. (1998) A role of microtubules during the formation of cell processes in neuronal and non-neuronal cells. *Cell and Tissue Research*, **291**, 163–174.

Kuster, B. and Mann, M. (1999) 18O-labeling of N-glycosylation sites to improve the identification of gel-separated glycoproteins using peptide mass mapping and database searching. *Analytical Chemistry*, **71**, 1431–1440.

Larsen, M.R., Thingholm, T.E., Jensen, O.N., Roepstorff, P. and Jorgensen, T.J. (2005) Highly selective enrichment of phosphorylated peptides from peptide mixtures using titanium dioxide microcolumns. *Molecular & Cellular Proteomics*, **4**, 873–886.

Ma, Y., Lu, Y., Zeng, H., Ron, D., Mo, W. and Neubert, T.A. (2001) Characterization of phosphopeptides from protein digests using matrix-assisted laser desorption/ionization time-of-flight mass spectrometry and nanoelectrospray quadrupole time-of-flight mass spectrometry. *Rapid Communications in Mass Spectrometry*, **15**, 1693–1700.

Maccioni, R.B., Munoz, J.P. and Barbeito, L. (2001) The molecular bases of Alzheimer's disease and other neurodegenerative disorders. *Archives of Medical Research*, **32**, 367–381.

Mandell, J.W. and Banker, G.A. (1996) Microtubule-associated proteins, phosphorylation gradients, and the establishment of neuronal polarity. *Perspectives on Developmental Neurobiology*, **4**, 125–135.

Manning, J.C., Seyrek, K., Kaltner, H., Andre, S., Sinowatz, F. and Gabius, H.J. (2004) Glycomic profiling of developmental changes in bovine testis by lectin histochemistry and further analysis of the most prominent alteration on the level of the glycoproteome by lectin blotting and lectin affinity chromatography. *Histology and Histopathology*, **19**, 1043–1060.

Marotti, L.A., Jr. Newitt, R., Wang, Y., Aebersold, R. and Dohlman, H.G. (2002) Direct identification of a G protein ubiquitination site by mass spectrometry. *Biochemistry*, **41**, 5067–5074.

Mayor, T., Lipford, J.R., Graumann, J., Smith, G.T. and Deshaies, R.J. (2005) Analysis of polyubiquitin conjugates reveals that the Rpn10 substrate receptor contributes to the turnover of multiple proteasome targets. *Molecular & Cellular Proteomics*, **4**, 741–751.

McGaugh, J.L. (2000) Memory—a century of consolidation. *Science*, **287**, 248–251.

Nawarak, J., Phutrakul, S. and Chen, S.T. (2004) Analysis of lectin-bound glycoproteins in snake venom from the Elapidae and Viperidae families. *Journal of Proteome Research*, **3**, 383–392.

Neubert, T.A. and Johnson, R.S. (1995) High-resolution structural determination of protein-linked acyl groups. *Methods in Enzymology*, **250**, 487–494.

Nishikawa, H., Ooka, S., Sato, K., Arima, K., Okamoto, J., Klevit, R.E., Fukuda, M. and Ohta, T. (2004) Mass spectrometric and mutational analyses reveal Lys-6-linked polyubiquitin chains catalyzed by BRCA1-BARD1 ubiquitin ligase. *Journal of Biological Chemistry*, **279**, 3916–3924.

Oda, Y., Nagasu, T. and Chait, B.T. (2001) Enrichment analysis of phosphorylated proteins as a tool for probing the phosphoproteome. *Nature Biotechnology*, **19**, 379–382.

Pant, H.C., Veeranna and Grant, P. (2000) Regulation of axonal neurofilament phosphorylation. *Current Topics in Cellular Regulation*, **36**, 133–150.

Pays, L. and Schwarting, G. (2000) Gal-NCAM is a differentially expressed marker for mature sensory neurons in the rat olfactory system. *Journal of Neurobiology*, **43**, 173–185.

Peng, J., Schwartz, D., Elias, J.E., Thoreen, C.C., Cheng, D., Marsischky, G., Roelofs, J., Finley, D. and Gygi, S.P. (2003) A proteomics approach to understanding protein ubiquitination. *Nature Biotechnology*, **21**, 921–926.

Pickart, C.M. (2001) Mechanisms underlying ubiquitination. *Annual Review of Biochemistry*, **70**, 503–533.

Pickart, C.M. and Fushman, D. (2004) Polyubiquitin chains: polymeric protein signals. *Current Opinion in Chemical Biology*, **8**, 610–616.

Pinkse, M.W., Uitto, P.M., Hilhorst, M.J., Ooms, B. and Heck, A.J. (2004) Selective isolation at the femtomole level of phosphopeptides from proteolytic digests using 2D-NanoLC-ESI-MS/MS and titanium oxide precolumns. *Analytical Chemistry*, **76**, 3935–3943.

Routtenberg, A. (1979) Anatomical localization of phosphoprotein and glycoprotein substrates of memory. *Progress in Neurobiology*, **12**, 85–113.

Routtenberg, A. and Rekart, J.L. (2005) Post-translational protein modification as the substrate for long-lasting memory. *Trends in Neurosciences*, **28**, 12–19.

Rush, J., Moritz, A., Lee, K.A., Guo, A., Goss, V.L., Spek, E.J., Zhang, H., Zha, X.M., Polakiewicz, R.D. and Comb, M.J. (2005) Immunoaffinity profiling of tyrosine phosphorylation in cancer cells. *Nature Biotechnology*, **23**, 94–101.

Saeki, Y., Tayama, Y., Toh-e, A. and Yokosawa, H. (2004) Definitive evidence for Ufd2-catalyzed elongation of the ubiquitin chain through Lys48 linkage. *Biochemical and Biophysical Research Communications*, **320**, 840–845.

Sanchez, C., Diaz-Nido, J. and Avila, J. (2000) Phosphorylation of microtubule-associated protein 2 (MAP2) and its relevance for the regulation of the neuronal cytoskeleton function. *Progress in Neurobiology*, **61**, 133–168.

Saragoni, L., Hernandez, P. and Maccioni, R.B. (2000) Differential association of tau with subsets of microtubules containing posttranslationally-modified tubulin variants in neuroblastoma cells. *Neurochemical Research*, **25**, 59–70.

Sarmiere, P.D. and Bamburg, J.R. (2004) Regulation of the neuronal actin cytoskeleton by ADF/cofilin. *Journal of Neurobiology*, **58**, 103–117.

Schroeder, M.J., Shabanowitz, J., Schwartz, J.C., Hunt, D.F. and Coon, J.J. (2004) A neutral loss activation method for improved phosphopeptide sequence analysis by quadrupole ion trap mass spectrometry. *Analytical Chemistry*, **76**, 3590–3598.

Shea, T.B. (2000) Microtubule motors, phosphorylation and axonal transport of neurofilaments. *Journal of Neurocytology*, **29**, 873–887.

Sprung, R., Nandi, A., Chen, Y., Kim, S.C., Barma, D., Falck, J.R. and Zhao, Y. (2005) Tagging-via-substrate strategy for probing O-GlcNAc modified proteins. *Journal of Proteome Research*, **4**, 950–957.

Starita, L.M., Machida, Y., Sankaran, S., Elias, J.E., Griffin, K., Schlegel, B.P., Gygi, S.P. and Parvin, J.D. (2004) BRCA1-dependent ubiquitination of gamma-tubulin regulates centrosome number. *Molecular and Cellular Biology*, **24**, 8457–8466.

Steen, H. and Mann, M. (2002) A new derivatization strategy for the analysis of phosphopeptides by precursor ion scanning in positive ion mode. *Journal of the American Society for Mass Spectrometry*, **13**, 996–1003.

Stensballe, A., Andersen, S. and Jensen, O.N. (2001) Characterization of phosphoproteins from electrophoretic gels by nanoscale Fe(III) affinity chromatography with off-line mass spectrometry analysis. *Proteomics*, **1**, 207–222.

Sweatt, J.D. (2001) Memory mechanisms: the yin and yang of protein phosphorylation. *Current Biology*, **11**, R391–R394.

Tai, M.H. and Zipser, B. (2002) Sequential steps of carbohydrate signaling mediate sensory afferent differentiation. *Journal of Neurocytology*, **31**, 743–754.

Vosseller, K., Trinidad, J.C., Chalkley, R.J., Specht, C.G., Thalhammer, A., Lynn, A.J., Snedecor, J.O., Guan, S., Medzihradszky, K.F., Maltby, D.A., Schoepfer, R. and Burlingame, A.L. (2006) O-linked N-acetylglucosamine proteomics of postsynaptic density preparations using lectin weak affinity chromatography and mass spectrometry. *Molecular & Cellular Proteomics*, **5**, 923–934.

Wang, D. and Cotter, R.J. (2005) Approach for determining protein ubiquitination sites by MALDI-TOF mass spectrometry. *Analytical Chemistry*, **77**, 1458–1466.

Wang, D., Kalume, D., Pickart, C., Pandey, A. and Cotter, R.J. (2006) Identification of protein ubiquitylation by electrospray ionization tandem mass spectrometric analysis of sulfonated tryptic peptides. *Analytical Chemistry*, **78**, 3681–3687.

Wu-Baer, F., Lagrazon, K., Yuan, W. and Baer, R. (2003) The BRCA1/BARD1 heterodimer assembles polyubiquitin chains through an unconventional linkage involving lysine residue K6 of ubiquitin. *Journal of Biological Chemistry*, **278**, 34743–34746.

Wuhrer, M., Catalina, M.I., Deelder, A.M. and Hokke, C.H. (2007) Glycoproteomics based on tandem mass spectrometry of glycopeptides. *Journal of Chromatography B, Analytical Technologies in the Biomedical and Life Sciences*, **849**, 115–128.

Xie, B., Zhou, G., Chan, S.Y., Shapiro, E., Kong, X.P., Wu, X.R., Sun, T.T. and Costello, C.E. (2006) Distinct glycan structures of uroplakins Ia and Ib: structural basis for the selective binding of FimH adhesin to uroplakin Ia. *Journal of Biological Chemistry*, **281**, 14644–14653.

Xu, C.F., Lu, Y., Ma, J., Mohammadi, M. and Neubert, T.A. (2005) Identification of phosphopeptides by MALDI Q-TOF MS in positive and negative ion modes after methyl esterification. *Molecular & Cellular Proteomics*, **4**, 809–818.

Zhang, G. and Neubert, T.A. (2006) Use of detergents to increase selectivity of immunoprecipitation of tyrosine phosphorylated peptides prior to identification by MALDI quadrupole-TOF MS. *Proteomics*, **6**, 571–578.

Zhang, H., Li, X.J., Martin, D.B. and Aebersold, R. (2003) Identification and quantification of N-linked glycoproteins using hydrazide chemistry, stable isotope labeling and mass spectrometry. *Nature Biotechnology*, **21**, 660–666.

Zhang, H., Yi, E.C., Li, X.J., Mallick, P., Kelly-Spratt, K.S., Masselon, C.D., Camp, D.G., II, Smith, R.D., Kemp, C.J. and Aebersold, R. (2005) High throughput quantitative analysis of serum proteins using glycopeptide capture and liquid chromatography mass spectrometry. *Molecular & Cellular Proteomics*, **4**, 144–155.

Zhou, G., Mo, W.J., Sebbel, P., Min, G., Neubert, T.A., Glockshuber, R., Wu, X.R., Sun, T.T. and Kong, X.P. (2001) Uroplakin Ia is the urothelial receptor for uropathogenic *Escherichia coli*: evidence from in vitro FimH binding. *Journal of Cell Science*, **114**, 4095–4103.

12
Proteomics of Neurodegenerative Disorders

Thorsten Müller, Florian Tribl, Michael Hamacher, André van Hall, Helmut E. Meyer and Katrin Marcus

12.1
Introduction

The brain is one of the most complex organs in mammals, consisting of numerous anatomically or functionally defined structures and cell types. To understand brain physiology as well as neuropathologies at the molecular level, the expression pattern of mRNAs and proteins in different brain structures or cell types have to be studied, for which transcriptome and proteome techniques are promising tools. Whereas transcriptomics analyses mRNA levels, proteomics tends to identify proteins, differential protein expression, and posttranslational modifications (PTMs). The human genome comprises about 30 000 genes, which encode for a dimension of several 100 000 protein species as a result of alternative splicing and PTMs (see Chapter 11). In total, there are about 300 different PTMs known (e.g. glycosylation, phosphorylation, oxidation, acetylation, ubiquitination, sulfation, and farnesylation). Therefore, the task lying ahead for neuroproteomics is very challenging: namely, the analysis of complex protein mixtures in different areas of the nervous system or even cell types (Davidsson and Sjogren, 2005; Johnson *et al.*, 2005).

As with other tissues, two strategies can be distinguished in brain proteomics: "mapping" approaches aiming at the identification of the entire set of proteins within the sample of interest and "comparative/differential" proteomics aiming at the identification of key players for development, plasticity, or disease-related changes of the nervous system. Examples include mapping studies in individual brain areas or neuronal cell types or comparative analysis of cerebral disorders such as Alzheimer's disease and Parkinson's disease, which are thought to dramatically disturb the cellular proteome.

In this article, we present a short historical review on brain proteomic methods. We then provide a flavor of the many facets of proteomics by reviewing the efforts done for the two most frequently occurring

Proteomics of the Nervous System. Edited by H.G. Nothwang and S.E. Pfeiffer
Copyright © 2008 WILEY-VCH Verlag GmbH & Co. KGaA, Weinheim
ISBN: 978-3-527-31716-5

neurodegenerative human diseases: Alzheimer's disease and Parkinson's disease. This will also illustrate the need for concerted actions and we finish by introducing two interdisciplinary mainly academic consortia: the Human Brain Proteome Project (HBPP) as part of the National Genome Research Network (NGFN) in Germany and the Brain Proteome Project under the patronage of the Human Proteome Organization (HUPO) as an international project.

12.2
History of Brain Proteomics

In general, the combination of highly specific sample fractionation and state-of-the-art proteomics is one of the most promising approaches to increase our knowledge of protein expression, function, and organization in signaling processes and regulatory networks. Over the years several studies have been performed towards a better understanding of general processes in the brain as well as the elucidation of mechanisms involved in neurodegeneration. Searching for "brain proteomics" in PubMed yields about 600 articles, of which one third were released over the last 2 years. This makes brain proteomics a major research branch with growing interest. One of the first experiments in 1999 examined the proteome of human brain samples using two-dimensional polyacrylamide-based gel electrophoresis (2D-PAGE) with subsequent identification of dysregulated proteins with mass spectrometry techniques (Lubec *et al.*, 1999). 2D-PAGE-based proteome techniques revealed the highest available resolution (up to 10 000 proteins), the possibility of detecting PTMs, good relative quantification, and high reproducibility. It thus became routine to use 2D-PAGE to identify differentially expressed proteins in tissues or in fractionated samples such as the synaptosome (Li *et al.*, 2004), clathrin-coated vesicles (Ritter *et al.*, 2003), multiprotein complexes (Grant and Husi, 2001), or cell lines (Peyrl *et al.*, 2003). In 2003, laser capture microdissection and 2D-PAGE were combined to analyze the proteome of specific cells in unstained fixed human brain samples (Mouledous *et al.*, 2003). In 2004, the fluorescence difference in-gel electrophoresis (DIGE) technique was introduced to study human postmortem brain samples for the first time and thereby increased the sensitivity to detect differentially expressed proteins between two conditions (Swatton *et al.*, 2004). To overcome the limits of 2D-PAGE (see Chapter 2) (Lohaus *et al.*, 2007), alternative methods based on chromatographic steps were developed and liquid chromatography methods have increasingly been used in brain proteomics since 2002 (Montine *et al.*, 2006). Hence, proteomics is an ongoing and developing field with the existing technologies being still further improved.

Due to this rapid progress in the field of proteomics, knowledge derived from proteomics will greatly advance our understanding of the causes of disorders in the nervous system, improve our capability of establishing a diagnosis at early onset, and finally help to pave the way toward improved treatments. In the following sections, we will review progress made with proteomics in our understanding the two most frequently neurodegenerative human diseases: Alzheimer's disease and Parkinson's disease.

12.3
Alzheimer's Disease

Alzheimer's disease is a progressive neurodegenerative disorder that currently affects 2% of the population in industrialized countries. It is neuropathologically characterized by two types of lesions: neuritic plaques and neurofibrillary tangles (Figure 12.1a,b). Plaques are mainly composed of the β-amyloid protein, which is a cleavage product of the amyloid precursor protein (APP). Neurofibrillary tangles mostly consist of the hyperphosphorylated tau protein. Beside these main players, apolipoprotein E, ubiquitin, and other factors are thought to play a role in Alzheimer's disease. Patients often show reduced sizes of brain areas involved in learning and memory processes, including the temporal and frontal lobes as a result of the degeneration of synapses and death of neurons (Mattson, 2004).

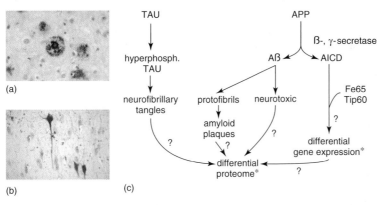

Figure 12.1 Neuropathological hallmarks and putative pathophysiological pathways in Alzheimer's disease. Reliable diagnosis of Alzheimer's disease is based upon immunohistochemical detection of extracellular amyloid plaques (a) as well as intracellular neurofibrillar tangles (b). Plaques consist of β-amyloid, which is cleaved off from the amyloid precursor protein by β- and γ-secretases (c). The intracellular domain of APP (AICD; another APP cleavage product) is believed to enter the nucleus and to alter gene expression pattern (in concert with the proteins Fe65 and Tip60). Neurofibrillary tangles mainly consist of hyperphosphorylated tau protein. (Please find a color version of this figure in the color plates.)

12.3.1
Alzheimer's Disease Proteomics with Human Samples

The identification of biomarkers and subsequent confirmed diagnosis of Alzheimer's disease is necessary for future successful drug treatment strategies (see Chapter 13). In the last 5 years, first efforts have been undertaken to study the proteomics of brain samples from Alzheimer's disease patients versus controls. Using silver-stained 2D-PAGE, the proteome of brain areas such as the hippocampus, temporal cortex, entorhinal cortex, or cerebellum as well as the proteome of the cerebrospinal fluid (CSF) was compared between Alzheimer's disease and control samples. This resulted in more or less long lists of putative differentially expressed proteins (Schonberger *et al.*, 2001; Tsuji *et al.*, 2002; Puchades *et al.*, 2003). In particular, proteins involved in synaptic transmission, stress response, and lipid transport were found to be differentially expressed. Interestingly, the relevance of disturbed lipid transport in Alzheimer's disease has been widely discussed (Poirier, 2005).

The existence of different cell types in brain tissue samples as well as interindividual basal expression differences renders those samples critical for initial proteome analysis. A combination of laser capture microdissection and 2D-PAGE might overcome those obstacles. Analysis of microdissected material from senile plaques in human Alzheimer's disease brains revealed 26 proteins enriched in the plaques of two Alzheimer's disease cases by quantitative comparison with surrounding non-plaque tissue (Liao *et al.*, 2004). Besides $A\beta$ and tau, proteins such as glial fibrillary acidic protein (GFAP), 14-3-3 kinases, and dynein heavy chain were also found to be differentially expressed.

Inbred Alzheimer's disease-related knockout or transgenic mice lines as well as cell culture models might be much better suited to the study of pathophysiological mechanisms. In the case of Alzheimer's disease, mice that differentially express APP, presenilins, or tau are of main interest.

12.3.2
Amyloid Precursor Protein and the γ-Secretase Complex

APP is a type 1 transmembrane protein composed of a large extracellular and a small intracellular domain. APP can undergo proteolytic cleavage by β- and γ-secretase activities resulting in the production of $A\beta$ (Selkoe, 1994). A summary of the APP related pathway is shown in Figure 12.1c. $A\beta$ is thought to be neurotoxic by inducing oxidative stress, inflammation, and neurodegeneration (Mattson, 2004). The intraneuronal accumulation of $A\beta$ protofibrils is thought to cause progressive neurotoxicity in cortical neurons (Hartley *et al.*, 1999). Another APP cleavage product is the APP intracellular domain (AICD), a small 6-kDa protein which arises from APP cleavage by γ-secretase activity (Octave *et al.*, 2000). More recently, AICD was shown to have transactivation potential (Cao and Sudhof, 2001). AICD levels are detectable in membrane fractions of murine total brain homogenates, and increase significantly in mice overexpressing the Swedish mutation of human APP (K595M; N596L) (Ryan and Pimplikar, 2005).

The fact that a putative transcriptionally active protein like AICD is involved in Alzheimer's disease makes differential transcriptomic and proteomic studies of APP transgenic or knockout models a promising tool to understand pathophysiological pathways in Alzheimer's disease. Indeed, transcriptome analysis of neuroblastoma cell lines identified target genes of AICD (Muller *et al.*, 2007). Proteome analysis of cortices from an Alzheimer's disease mouse model with the Swedish and London mutation (Thy1-APP751; K595M; N596L; V642I) or with the Swedish mutation alone (K595M; N596L) identified 15 and 12 different proteins, respectively, which were significantly regulated (Shin *et al.*, 2004; Sizova *et al.*, 2007). Interestingly, mice transgenic for Swedish/London APP revealed upregulation of the apolipoprotein E (ApoE), which has also been found to be differentially expressed in Alzheimer's disease vs. control brains. Moreover, increased expression of ApoE in these mice demonstrated an APP-dependent regulation of this protein.

ApoE-related physiology is of great interest in Alzheimer's disease, as the frequency of the ApoE4 isoform is higher among patients with Alzheimer's disease than in controls (Corder *et al.*, 1993). ApoE is a constituent of several different lipoprotein particles and is involved in the metabolism of lipids. Next to the liver, the largest production of apolipoproteins is found in the brain.

As in human brain samples, a combination of microdissection and 2D techniques have been used for transgenic animals. The CA1 pyramidal neuron layers of transgenic rats carrying the human APP vs. those from controls were microdissected and their proteome analyzed using DIGE (Wilson *et al.*, 2005). Over 100 proteins were found to be significantly altered.

Taken together, transgenic animals may reveal a convenient model for the study of Alzheimer's disease-related pathophysiology, minimizing interindividual variations in comparison to human samples. However, samples from animal tissue contain different cell types, which might be critical when the transgene is expressed in a cell type-specific manner. Therefore, another option would be the proteome analysis of stably transfected cell culture models. At present very few studies have used cell culture models. In one such study proteome analysis of presenilin 1 and presenilin 2-null blastocysts and wild-type controls demonstrated abnormal localization of caveolin 1, which might play a role in APP processing (Wood *et al.*, 2005).

12.3.3
Tau protein

Next to extracellular neuritic plaques, intracellular neurofibrillary tangles are the most important neuropathological hallmark of Alzheimer's disease (Hardy and Selkoe, 2002). Intracellular neurofibrillary tangles mostly consist of hyperphosphorylated tau protein (Figure 12.1b). Such modified tau protein fails to interact with microtubules and thereby destabilizes them. This might have dramatic consequences for the cells. Interestingly, in mice carrying a P301L tau mutation (resulting in accumulation of hyperphosphorylated tau protein), components of the mitochondrial respiratory chain complex, antioxidant enzymes, and synaptic proteins revealed altered expression (David *et al.*, 2005). Analysis of neurofibrillary tangles obtained by laser capture microdissection from pyramidal neurons in the hippocampal sector CA1 in patients with Alzheimer's disease using liquid chromatography coupled to mass spectrometry (LC-MS) identified proteins involved in energy and metabolism, cytoskeleton, and intracellular trafficking.

12.3.4
Alterations of Posttranslational Modifications in Alzheimer's Disease

PTMs are crucial to the molecular pathogenesis of neurodegenerative diseases. For example, as mentioned above, tau protein is hyperphosphorylated in Alzheimer's disease. Below, we emphasize proteomic approaches identifying oxidation and glycosylation in complex samples. Until now, 2D-PAGE-based phosphorylation studies have not been available for complex samples.

12.3.4.1 Oxidation

There is accumulating evidence that oxidative stress plays an important role in the pathophysiology of Alzheimer's disease. Therefore, the identification of specific targets of protein oxidation in Alzheimer's disease is of high interest. Using the oxyblot technique, proteins like the peptidyl prolyl *cis-trans* isomerase, dihydropyrimidinase related protein-2 (DRP-2), and α-enolase have been identified as significantly oxidized. This results in reduced enzyme activities in Alzheimer's disease hippocampus relative to control hippocampus samples (Sultana *et al.*, 2005) (see Chapter 14). Interestingly, DRP-2 was also oxidized in synaptosomes treated with $A\beta_{42}$ (Boyd-Kimball *et al.*, 2005) as well as in the hippocampus of 6-month-old ApoE-knockout mice (Choi *et al.*, 2004).

12.3.4.2 Glycosylation

Glycosylation influences the biological activity of proteins and affects their folding and stability. Aberrant glycosylation has been shown to be associated with Alzheimer's disease. Using affinity column chromatography specific for glycoproteins in conjunction with 2D-PAGE and matrix-assisted laser desorption ionization time-of-flight (MALDI-TOF) MS, it was demonstrated that the human glycoproteins transferrin, hemopexin, and α_1-antitrypsin were enriched in Alzheimer's disease plasma samples relative to controls (Yu *et al.*, 2003). Analyzing frontal cortex samples with ProQ Emerald staining revealed reduced glycosylation of collapsin response mediator protein 2 (CRMP-2) and increased glycosylation of glial fibrillary acidic protein (Kanninen et al., 2004).

12.4
Parkinson's Disease

Following Alzheimer's disease, Parkinson's disease is the second most frequent neurodegenerative disorder in elderly people. In Europe, about 3 million people are affected, including 1% of those in the sixth decade of life and 3% of those in the eighth decade. Parkinson's disease is a chronically progressing disorder showing characteristic motor symptoms that include akinesia, rigidity, a flexed posture, resting tremor, the "freezing" phenomenon, and a loss of postural reflexes (Hoehn and Yahr, 1967). These disabling motor symptoms result from a progressive degeneration of the pigmented dopaminergic neurons in the substantia nigra pars compacta, which entails a substantial decrease of the neurotransmitter dopamine in the striatum. The movement disorder becomes detectable at a time when approximately 80% of the substantia nigra has irreversibly been lost. The preclinical phase of Parkinson's disease is estimated to last for 10 years and is still inaccessible to therapeutic treatment. There is therefore an urgent need for biomarkers to allow a diagnosis of Parkinson's disease at the pre-motor symptomatic phase.

12.4.1
Etiology of Parkinson's Disease

The lead concepts for our understanding of Parkinson's disease have focused on the substantia nigra. Here, the most devastating pathology takes place (Figure 12.2) and leads to disabling motor symptoms. However, recent pathological data suggest an onset of this disorder outside the brain with an ascending pathology (Braak et al., 2003).

The actual causes of Parkinson's disease are currently unknown, but likely arise from complex interplays of genetic and environmental factors, which give rise to a broad range of phenomena in the Parkinson's disease brain. These include erroneous protein degradation, aggregation of proteins such as α-synuclein, the formation of Lewy bodies, an inhibition and disruption of the mitochondrial respiratory chain complexes I–III and a dramatically increased formation of free radicals, a severely disturbed iron metabolism, the disturbance of Ca^{2+} homoeostasis, an activation of microglial cells and increased nitric oxide formation, glutamate excitotoxicity, apoptosis, inflammation, and reduced neurotrophic support (Hoehn and Yahr, 1967; Gerlach et al., 1996; Jenner and Olanow, 1996; Hirsch et al., 1998; Jellinger, 2002).

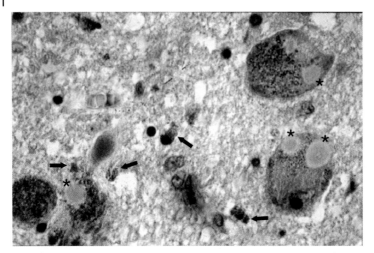

Figure 12.2 Neuromelanin and Parkinson's disease. Neurodegeneration of the substantia nigra pars compacta in Parkinson's disease is accompanied by massive loss of the pigmented neurons. During this process, the pigment neuromelanin is liberated from the neurons and phagocytosed by glial cells (arrows). Some pigmented neurons exhibit pathophysiological α-synuclein-containing protein aggregates, so-called Lewy bodies (asterisks). This figure was kindly provided by Prof. Dr. W. Paulus, Münster, Germany, and was published by the German Neuroscience Society. (Please find a color version of this figure in the color plates.)

The concept of an environmental contribution to the pathogenesis of Parkinson's disease evolved with the discovery of a parkinsonian phenotype that resulted from 1-methyl-4-phenyl-1,2,3,6-tetrahydropyridine intoxication (Davis *et al.*, 1979; Langston *et al.*, 1983). Since then an increasing number of neurotoxins have been found to induce Parkinson's disease symptoms, including paraquat, 6-hydroxydopamine, rotenone, 1,2,3,4-tetrahydroisoquinolines, β-carbolines and their respective derivatives (Collins and Neafsey, 1985; Tanner, 1989; Bringmann *et al.*, 1995; Naoi and Maruyama, 1999; Bringmann *et al.*, 2002). These neurotoxins have also been used to generate animal models of Parkinson's disease (Gerlach and Riederer, 1996).

Rare inherited forms of monogenic Parkinsonism (approximately 10–15% of all Parkinson's disease cases) have entailed the identification of an increasing number of genes and gene loci (*PARK1–PARK13*; Table 12.1) that are involved in neurodegeneration of the substantia nigra and the establishment of a parkinsonian phenotype (Gasser, 2001; Huang *et al.*, 2004; Klein and Schlossmacher, 2006).

Although the early age of onset and the symptomatology in most of these "familial" cases dramatically differ from the more common "sporadic" forms of Parkinson's disease, study of the genetics of Parkinson's disease has suggested for the first time the involvement of aberrant genes, improving

Table 12.1 Genetics of parkinsonism.

Genetic form	Mode of inheritance	Gene	Chromosomal location	Protein	Phenotype	Pathology	Comment
PARK1, 4	Autosomal dominant	*SNCA*	4q21	α-Synuclein	Parkinsonism with good response to levodopa treatment, autonomic dysfunction	Lewy body disease with neuronal degeneration	Early onset (~50 years)
PARK2	Autosomal recessive	*PARK2*	6q25.2–q27	Parkin	Juvenile parkinsonism with diurnal fluctuations, dystonia	Neuronal loss in the SN, reduced NM in the surviving neurons, no LBs	Onset before the age of 40
PARK3	Autosomal dominant	?	2p13	?	?	?	The sepiapterin reductase gene (*SPR*) may be involved
PARK5	Autosomal dominant	*UCHL1*	4p14	Ubiquitin C-terminal hydrolase L1	Late-onset parkinsonism	?	Causes the aggregation of α-synuclein in cultured cells
PARK6	Autosomal recessive	*PINK1*	1p35–p36	Serine/threonine-	Slowly progressing	?	Located in mitochondria,

(continued overleaf)

Table 12.1 (*continued*).

Genetic form	Mode of inheritance	Gene	Chromosomal location	Protein	Phenotype	Pathology	Comment
				protein kinase PINK1	parkinsonism with moderate response to levodopa	?	age of onset ranging from 20 to 60 years
PARK7	Autosomal recessive	*DJ1*	1p36	Protein DJ1	Early-onset parkinsonism, accompanied by psychiatric symptoms	?	Redox-dependent chaperone, inhibits α-synuclein aggregation
PARK8	Autosomal dominant	*LRRK2*	12q12	Leucine-rich repeat serine/threonine-protein kinase 2	Consistent with sporadic Parkinson's disease	Neuronal loss, predominantly LBs	May have GTPase activity
PARK9	Autosomal recessive	?	1p36	?	Parkinsonism with pallidopyramidal syndrome	?	
PARK10	?	?	1p32	?	Late-onset	?	
PARK11	?	?	2q36–q37	?	Sporadic Parkinson's disease?	?	
PARK12	?	?	Xq21–q25	?	?	?	
PARK13	?	*HTRA2*	2p12	Serine protease HTRA2	Bradykinesia, tremor, and muscular rigidity, good response to levodopa therapy	?	Located in mitochondria

our molecular understanding of neurodegenerative processes in Parkinson's disease (Table 12.1).

Taken together, Parkinson's disease appears to be a heterogeneous syndrome, in which multiple factors lead to various subtypes of idiopathic Parkinson's disease (Birkmayer *et al.*, 1979; Graham and Sagar, 1999; Riederer and Foley, 2002).

12.4.2
Proteomics of Animal and Cellular Models of Parkinson's Disease

In contrast to human samples, animal and cellular models are suitable for genetic or pharmacological manipulations to facilitate a proteomic and functional investigation of key players in Parkinson's disease, for example, α-synuclein, parkin, or neurotoxins.

12.4.2.1 α-Synuclein
With the discovery of a family carrying a mutation in the α-synuclein gene (Polymeropoulos *et al.*, 1997), the first protein related to parkinsonism was identified. The mutant protein aggregates in the substantia nigra and localizes to Lewy bodies (Spillantini *et al.*, 1997). Nevertheless, despite extensive efforts, the physiological function of α-synuclein remains elusive. One study attempted to tackle α-synuclein functionality using a yeast two-hybrid screen to assess its binding partners. This identified synphilin-1, which is also an aggregation-prone protein causing neurotoxicity (Eyal *et al.*, 2006). Alternatively, a proteomic approach based on affinity chromatography uncovered several α-synuclein-binding proteins that are engaged in signaling pathways or components of the ubiquitin proteasome system (UPS), for example, MAPK, PKC, BAD, ERK (Zhou *et al.*, 2004). A role of α-synuclein in protein clearance via the UPS was also suggested by the finding that heat shock protein 70 not only associated with α-synuclein, but also ameliorated rotenone-mediated cytotoxicity via decrease of α-synuclein aggregation (Zhou *et al.*, 2004).

α-Synuclein also binds to lysosomal proteins, especially to proteins of the lysosomal-associated membrane protein (LAMP) family, which recently have been identified in pigment-containing neuromelanin granules by subcellular proteomics (Tribl *et al.*, 2005). Neuromelanin granules are lysosome-related organelles in the substantia nigra (Figure 12.2) (Tribl *et al.*, 2006) that are engaged in iron storage (Jellinger *et al.*, 1992). The binding of α-synuclein to neuromelanin granules in early Parkinson's disease (Fasano *et al.*, 2003; Halliday *et al.*, 2005) might serve as an initial nucleation seed for further aggregation (Conway *et al.*, 2001; Fasano *et al.*, 2006).

12.4.2.2 Parkin

A second Parkinson's disease-linked gene (*PARK2*) was identified in individuals carrying mutations in the gene coding for parkin (Kitada *et al.*, 1998), which is a component of the multiprotein E3 ubiquitin ligase complex and thus engaged in protein turnover by the UPS (Shimura *et al.*, 2001). Intriguingly, the 22-kDa glycosylated form of α-synuclein (alpha-Sp22) is a substrate of parkin, but Lewy bodies are mostly absent in individuals carrying the *PARK2*-mutation. Although various parkin$^{-/-}$ mice exhibit an impaired nigro-striatal pathway, no neurodegeneration is observed (Goldberg *et al.*, 2003; Itier *et al.*, 2003) and the substrates of parkin are unchanged in their steady state levels. However, the proteomic analyses of the parkin$^{-/-}$ mice brains identified misregulated proteins involved in mitochondrial oxidative phosphorylation, for example, NADH-ubiquinone oxidoreductase subunits, and a decrease in peroxiredoxins, which counteract oxidative stress (Goldberg *et al.*, 2003).

12.4.2.3 Neurotoxins

Since the occurrence of parkinsonism in post-encephalitic cases of encephalitis lethargica has been reported, the exposure to viruses or bacteria at a prenatal developmental stage of the brain has been suggested to trigger Parkinson's disease (Hayase and Tobita, 1997; Dale *et al.*, 2004). Indeed, intrauterine exposure to bacterial endotoxin lipopolysaccharides dramatically reduced the number of dopaminergic neurons in the substantia nigra and ultimately may result in parkinsonian symptoms (Mattock *et al.*, 1988; Ling *et al.*, 2002).

Intoxication with neurotoxins, including 1-methyl-4-phenyl-1,2,3,6-tetrahydropyridine, 6-hydroxydopamine, rotenone, and lipopolysaccharides, entails a microglial activation (Liu and Hong, 2003), as described in Parkinson's disease (Hirsch *et al.*, 1998). Recently, a study on differential protein expression in neuroinflammation focused on a co-culture system of rat primary neurons and glial cells isolated from C57BL/6 or SWR/J mice and identified various new inflammatory mediators, for example, thioredoxin-related protein, interferon-activation protein 204, cAMP-dependent regulatory protein kinase, and the chemokine receptor type 2 (McLaughlin *et al.*, 2006). In addition, known mediators involved in the upregulation of cyclooxygenase-2 (COX-2), prostaglandin E2 (PGE$_2$), or inducible nitric oxide synthase (iNOS), for example, the nuclear factor-kappa B (NF-κB) or c-Jun N-terminal kinases (JNKs) were found to be upregulated.

Following the concept of a neuronal death-induced microglial activation (Liu and Hong, 2003), which may be mediated by cell–cell contact, Zhou and co-workers investigated proteins differentially expressed in membrane fractions of a rat mesencephalic neuronal cell line treated with 1-methyl-4-phenylpyridinium, the active metabolite of the toxin 1-methyl-4-phenyl-1,2,3,6-tetrahydropyridine, and identified potential candidates of microglial activators, for example, upregulated proteins engaged in the ubiquitin-proteasome pathway and downregulated thioredoxin-related protein 2 (Zhou *et al.*, 2005).

12.4.3
Posttranslational Modifications in Parkinson's Disease

PTMs have not so far been systematically investigated in Parkinson's disease by proteomics. The few studies available have focused on oxidatively modified proteins (see Chapter 14). Oxidative stress in Parkinson's disease entails severe lipid peroxidation giving rise to lipid fragmentation and the formation of carbonyl compounds, for example, malonedialdehyde and 4-hydroxy-2-nonenal that readily form Schiff bases with nucleophilic side-chains of proteins. As in human Parkinson's disease samples, which exhibit a reduced antioxidant capacity (Riederer *et al.*, 1989) and an increase in 4-hydroxy-2-nonenal-modified proteins (Yoritaka *et al.*, 1996), these neurochemical findings are also mirrored in parkin$^{-/-}$ mice (Palacino *et al.*, 2004), while others report no significant increase in protein oxidation in their parkin$^{-/-}$ mouse models (Periquet *et al.*, 2005). Nevertheless, a detailed investigation of PTM proteins in Parkinson's disease, for example, following 2D-PAGE, as shown for Alzheimer's disease or Parkinson's disease-related tissue or CSF are almost missing. For future experiments, it is necessary to increase the number of analyzed samples to overcome inter-individual fluctuations. However, sample acquisition from Alzheimer's disease/Parkinson's disease patients and in particular from non-affected persons is often limited.

For the future, differential proteomics is a promising tool for the analysis of pathophysiological pathways using a combination of cell culture, mouse models, as well as human brain samples. Such analysis will help us to understand the complex mechanisms leading to neurodegenerative diseases and could be instrumental in identifying drug targets with potential for treatment of the disease.

12.5
Administrative Realization of Neuroproteomics: The Brain Proteome Projects

Two interdisciplinary, mainly academic, consortia were funded in 2001 in an attempt to understand the pathophysiology of the brain: the Human Brain Proteome Project (HBPP) as part of the National Genome Research Network (NGFN), funded by the German Ministry for Education and Research (www.smp-proteomics.de), and the Brain Proteome Project (www.hbpp.org) under the patronage of the Human Proteome Organization (HUPO) as an international project. Both projects use the synergistic effects of comprehensive networks composed of complementary research approaches to engage the extensive analysis of brain proteomes.

The aim of the HBPP is to develop technology and gain knowledge that can be applied to enable the development of new strategies for the diagnosis and treatment of neurodegenerative diseases. The HBPP is a network of interdisciplinary German research groups which encompasses human genetics, cell biology, animal models, molecular biology, and biochemistry. The following goals were specifically defined for the HBPP: (i) The advancement of already established technologies to analyze the functional implications of gene mutations selected in collaborations with the clinical partners. (ii) The investigation of neurodegenerative diseases (especially Alzheimer's disease and Parkinson's disease) with a focus on the systematic analysis of protein pattern in human, primate, and mouse brain samples. (iii) The networking within the NGFN to improve collaboration between basic scientists and clinical groups as well as other theoretical technology platforms, for example, bioinformatics.

The international HUPO was established as a non-profit organization promoting proteomic research and proteome analysis of human tissues (www.hupo.org). The HBPP as part of HUPO (Meyer *et al.*, 2003) is chaired by Helmut E. Meyer at the Medizinisches Proteom-Center (MPC), Bochum, and defines its main goal as "Towards an understanding of the pathological processes of the brain proteome in neurodegenerative diseases and aging."

In order to evaluate the existing approaches in brain proteomics as well as to establish a standardized data reprocessing pipeline, pilot studies have been initiated including both mouse and human samples (Meyer and Hamacher, 2006). The combination of the generated output results in added-value, as on the one hand identified proteins can be approved, while on the other hand new proteins can be detected by the combination of the peptides identified by different groups. The separation features of the different techniques overlap and can be applied successively.

References

Birkmayer, W., Riederer, P. and Youdim, B.H. (1979) Distinction between benign and malignant type of Parkinson's disease. *Clinical Neurology and Neurosurgery*, **81**, 158–164.

Boyd-Kimball, D., Castegna, A., Sultana, R., Poon, H.F., Petroze, R., Lynn, B.C., Klein, J.B. and Butterfield, D.A. (2005) Proteomic identification of proteins oxidized by Abeta(1–42) in synaptosomes: implications for Alzheimer's disease. *Brain Research*, **1044**, 206–215.

Braak, H., Del Tredici, K., Rub, U., de Vos, R.A., Jansen Steur, E.N. and Braak, E. (2003) Staging of brain pathology related to sporadic Parkinson's disease. *Neurobiology of Aging*, **24**, 197–211.

Bringmann, G., God, R., Feineis, D., Wesemann, W., Riederer, P., Rausch, W.D., Reichmann, H. and Sontag, K.H. (1995) The TaClo concept: 1-trichloromethyl-1,2,3,4-tetrahydro-beta-carboline (TaClo), a new toxin for dopaminergic neurons. *Journal of Neural*

Transmission. *Supplementum*, **46**, 235–244.

Bringmann, G., Feineis, D., God, R., Peters, K., Peters, E.M., Scholz, J., Riederer, F. and Moser, A. (2002) 1-Trichloromethyl-1,2,3,4-tetrahydro-beta-carboline (TaClo) and related derivatives: chemistry and biochemical effects on catecholamine biosynthesis. *Bioorganic & Medicinal Chemistry*, **10**, 2207–2214.

Cao, X. and Sudhof, T.C. (2001) A transcriptionally [correction of transcriptively] active complex of APP with Fe65 and histone acetyltransferase Tip60. *Science*, **293**, 115–120.

Choi, J., Forster, M.J., McDonald, S.R., Weintraub, S.T., Carroll, C.A. and Gracy, R.W. (2004) Proteomic identification of specific oxidized proteins in ApoE-knockout mice: relevance to Alzheimer's disease. *Free Radical Biology & Medicine*, **36**, 1155–1162.

Collins, M.A. and Neafsey, E.J. (1985) Beta-carboline analogues of N-methyl-4-phenyl-1,2,5, 6-tetrahydropyridine (MPTP): endogenous factors underlying idiopathic parkinsonism? *Neuroscience Letters*, **55**, 179–184.

Conway, K.A., Rochet, J.C., Bieganski, R.M. and Lansbury, P.T. Jr. (2001) Kinetic stabilization of the alpha-synuclein protofibril by a dopamine-alpha-synuclein adduct. *Science*, **294**, 1346–1349.

Corder, E.H., Saunders, A.M., Strittmatter, W.J., Schmechel, D.E., Gaskell, P.C., Small, G.W., Roses, A.D., Haines, J.L. and Pericak-Vance, M.A. (1993) Gene dose of apolipoprotein E type 4 allele and the risk of Alzheimer's disease in late onset families. *Science*, **261**, 921–923.

Dale, R.C., Church, A.J., Surtees, R.A., Lees, A.J., Adcock, J.E., Harding, B., Neville, B.G. and Giovannoni, G. (2004) Encephalitis lethargica syndrome: 20 new cases and evidence of basal ganglia autoimmunity. *Brain*, **127**, 21–33.

David, D.C., Hauptmann, S., Scherping, I., Schuessel, K., Keil, U., Rizzu, P., Ravid, R., Drose, S., Brandt, U.,

Muller, W.E., Eckert, A. and Gotz, J. (2005) Proteomic and functional analyses reveal a mitochondrial dysfunction in P301L tau transgenic mice. *Journal of Biological Chemistry*, **280**, 23802–23814.

Davidsson, P. and Sjogren, M. (2005) The use of proteomics in biomarker discovery in neurodegenerative diseases. *Disease Markers*, **21**, 81–92.

Davis, G.C., Williams, A.C., Markey, S.P., Ebert, M.H., Caine, E.D., Reichert, C.M. and Kopin, I.J. (1979) Chronic Parkinsonism secondary to intravenous injection of meperidine analogues. *Psychiatry Research*, **1**, 249–254.

Eyal, A., Szargel, R., Avraham, E., Liani, E., Haskin, J., Rott, R. and Engelender, S. (2006) Synphilin-1A: an aggregation-prone isoform of synphilin-1 that causes neuronal death and is present in aggregates from alpha-synucleinopathy patients. *Proceedings of the National Academy of Sciences of the United States of America*, **103**, 5917–5922.

Fasano, M., Giraudo, S., Coha, S., Bergamasco, B. and Lopiano, L. (2003) Residual substantia nigra neuromelanin in Parkinson's disease is cross-linked to alpha-synuclein. *Neurochemistry International*, **42**, 603–606.

Fasano, M., Bergamasco, B. and Lopiano, L. (2006) Modifications of the iron-neuromelanin system in Parkinson's disease. *Journal of Neurochemistry*, **96**, 909–916.

Gasser, T. (2001) Genetics of Parkinson's disease. *Journal of Neurology*, **248**, 833–840.

Gerlach, M. and Riederer, P. (1996) Animal models of Parkinson's disease: an empirical comparison with the phenomenology of the disease in man. *Journal of Neural Transmission*, **103**, 987–1041.

Gerlach, M., Riederer, P. and Youdim, M.B. (1996) Molecular mechanisms for neurodegeneration. Synergism between reactive oxygen species, calcium, and excitotoxic amino acids. *Advances in Neurology*, **69**, 177–194.

Goldberg, M.S., Fleming, S.M., Palacino, J.J., Cepeda, C., Lam, H.A., Bhatnagar, A., Meloni, E.G. Wu, N.,

Ackerson, L.C., Klapstein, G.J., Gajendiran, M., Roth, B.L., Chesselet, M.F., Maidment, N.T., Levine, M.S. and Shen, J. (2003) Parkin-deficient mice exhibit nigrostriatal deficits but not loss of dopaminergic neurons. *Journal of Biological Chemistry*, **278**, 43628–43635.

Graham, J.M. and Sagar, H.J. (1999) A data-driven approach to the study of heterogeneity in idiopathic Parkinson's disease: identification of three distinct subtypes. *Movement Disorders*, **14**, 10–20.

Grant, S.G. and Husi, H. (2001) Proteomics of multiprotein complexes: answering fundamental questions in neuroscience. *Trends in Biotechnology*, **19**, S49–S54.

Halliday, G.M., Ophof, A., Broe, M., Jensen, P.H., Kettle, E., Fedorow, H., Cartwright, M.I., Griffiths, F.M., Shepherd, C.E. and Double, K.L. (2005) Alpha-synuclein redistributes to neuromelanin lipid in the substantia nigra early in Parkinson's disease. *Brain*, **128**, 2654–2664.

Hardy, J. and Selkoe, D.J. (2002) The amyloid hypothesis of Alzheimer's disease: progress and problems on the road to therapeutics. *Science*, **297**, 353–356.

Hartley, D.M., Walsh, D.M., Ye, C.P., Diehl, T., Vasquez, S., Vassilev, P.M., Teplow, D.B. and Selkoe, D.J. (1999) Protofibrillar intermediates of amyloid beta-protein induce acute electrophysiological changes and progressive neurotoxicity in cortical neurons. *Journal of Neuroscience*, **19**, 8876–8884.

Hayase, Y. and Tobita, K. (1997) Influenza virus and neurological diseases. *Psychiatry and Clinical Neurosciences*, **51**, 181–184.

Hirsch, E.C., Hunot, S., Damier, P. and Faucheux, B. (1998) Glial cells and inflammation in Parkinson's disease: a role in neurodegeneration? *Annals of Neurology*, **44**, S115–S120.

Hoehn, M.M. and Yahr, M.D. (1967) Parkinsonism: onset, progression and mortality. *Neurology*, **17**, 427–442.

Huang, Y., Cheung, L., Rowe, D. and Halliday, G. (2004) Genetic contributions to Parkinson's disease. *Brain Research. Brain Research Reviews*, **46**, 44–70.

Itier, J.M., *et al.* (2003) Parkin gene inactivation alters behaviour and dopamine neurotransmission in the mouse. *Human Molecular Genetics*, **12**, 2277–2291.

Jellinger, K.A. (2002) Recent developments in the pathology of Parkinson's disease. *Journal of Neural Transmission. Supplementum*, **62**, 347–376.

Jellinger, K., Kienzl, E., Rumpelmair, G., Riederer, P., Stachelberger, H., Ben Shachar, D. and Youdim, M.B. (1992) Iron-melanin complex in substantia nigra of parkinsonian brains: an X-ray microanalysis. *Journal of Neurochemistry*, **59**, 1168–1171.

Jenner, P. and Olanow, C.W. (1996) Oxidative stress and the pathogenesis of Parkinson's disease. *Neurology*, **47**, S161–S170.

Johnson, M.D., Yu, L.R., Conrads, T.P., Kinoshita, Y., Uo, T., McBee, J.K., Veenstra, T.D. and Morrison, R.S. (2005) The proteomics of neurodegeneration. *American Journal of Pharmacogenomics*, **5**, 259–270.

Kanninen, K., Goldsteins, G., Auriola, S., Alafuzoff, I. and Koistinaho, J. (2004) Glycosylation changes in Alzheimer's disease as revealed by a proteomic approach. *Neuroscience Letters*, **367**, 235–240.

Kitada, T., Asakawa, S., Hattori, N., Matsumine, H., Yamamura, Y., Minoshima, S., Yokochi, M., Mizuno, Y. and Shimizu, N. (1998) Mutations in the parkin gene cause autosomal recessive juvenile parkinsonism. *Nature*, **392**, 605–608.

Klein, C. and Schlossmacher, M.G. (2006) The genetics of Parkinson disease: Implications for neurological care. *Nature Clinical Practice Neurology*, **2**, 136–146.

Langston, J.W., Ballard, P., Tetrud, J.W. and Irwin, I. (1983) Chronic Parkinsonism in humans due to a product of meperidine-analog synthesis. *Science*, **219**, 979–980.

Li, K.W., Hornshaw, M.P., Van Der Schors, R.C., Watson, R., Tate, S., Casetta, B., Jimenez, C.R.,

Gouwenberg, Y., Gundelfinger, E.D., Smalla, K.H. and Smit, A.B. (2004) Proteomics analysis of rat brain postsynaptic density. Implications of the diverse protein functional groups for the integration of synaptic physiology. *Journal of Biological Chemistry*, **279**, 987–1002.

Liao, L., Cheng, D., Wang, J., Duong, D.M., Losik, T.G., Gearing, M., Rees, H.D., Lah, J.J., Levey, A.I. and Peng, J. (2004) Proteomic characterization of postmortem amyloid plaques isolated by laser capture microdissection. *Journal of Biological Chemistry*, **279**, 37061–37068.

Ling, Z., Gayle, D.A., Ma, S.Y., Lipton, J.W., Tong, C.W., Hong, J.S. and Carvey, P.M. (2002) In utero bacterial endotoxin exposure causes loss of tyrosine hydroxylase neurons in the postnatal rat midbrain. *Movement Disorders*, **17**, 116–124.

Liu, B. and Hong, J.S. (2003) Role of microglia in inflammation-mediated neurodegenerative diseases: mechanisms and strategies for therapeutic intervention. *The Journal of Pharmacology and Experimental Therapeutics*, **304**, 1–7.

Lohaus, C., Nolte, A., Bluggel, M., Scheer, C., Klose, J., Gobom, J., Schuler, A., Wiebringhaus, T., Meyer, H.E. and Marcus, K. (2007) Multidimensional chromatography: a powerful tool for the analysis of membrane proteins in mouse brain. *Journal of Proteome Research*, **6**, 105–113.

Lubec, G., Nonaka, M., Krapfenbauer, K., Gratzer, M., Cairns, N. and Fountoulakis, M. (1999) Expression of the dihydropyrimidinase related protein 2 (DRP-2) in Down syndrome and Alzheimer's disease brain is downregulated at the mRNA and dysregulated at the protein level. *Journal of Neural Transmission. Supplementum*, **57**, 161–177.

Mattock, C., Marmot, M. and Stern, G. (1988) Could Parkinson's disease follow intra-uterine influenza?: a speculative hypothesis. *Journal of Neurology, Neurosurgery, and Psychiatry*, **51**, 753–756.

Mattson, M.P. (2004) Pathways towards and away from Alzheimer's disease. *Nature*, **430**, 631–639.

McLaughlin, P., Zhou, Y., Ma, T., Liu, J., Zhang, W., Hong, J.S., Kovacs, M. and Zhang, J. (2006) Proteomic analysis of microglial contribution to mouse strain-dependent dopaminergic neurotoxicity. *Glia*, **53**, 567–582.

Meyer, H.E. and Hamacher, M. (2006) Quintessence from proteomics networks –the HUPO Brain Proteome Project Pilot Studies. *Proteomics*, **6**, 4887–4889.

Meyer, H.E., Klose, J. and Hamacher, M. (2003) HBPP and the pursuit of standardisation. *Lancet Neurology*, **2**, 657–658.

Montine, T.J., Woltjer, R.L., Pan, C., Montine, K.S. and Zhang, J. (2006) Liquid chromatography with tandem mass spectrometry-based proteomic discovery in aging and Alzheimer's disease. *NeuroRx*, **3**, 336–343.

Mouledous, L., Hunt, S., Harcourt, R., Harry, J., Williams, K.L. and Gutstein, H.B. (2003) Navigated laser capture microdissection as an alternative to direct histological staining for proteomic analysis of brain samples. *Proteomics*, **3**, 610–615.

Muller, T., Concannon, C., Ward, M., Walsh, C., Tirniceriu, A., Tribl, F., Kogel, D., Prehn, J. and Egensperger, R. (2007) Modulation of gene expression and cytoskeletal dynamics by the APP intracellular domain (AICD). *Molecular Biology of the Cell*, **18**, 201–210.

Naoi, M. and Maruyama, W. (1999) N-methyl(R)salsolinol, a dopamine neurotoxin, in Parkinson's disease. *Advances in Neurology*, **80**, 259–264.

Octave, J.N., Essalmani, R., Tasiaux, B., Menager, J., Czech, C. and Mercken, L. (2000) The role of presenilin-1 in the gamma-secretase cleavage of the amyloid precursor protein of Alzheimer's disease. *Journal of Biological Chemistry*, **275**, 1525–1528.

Palacino, J.J., Sagi, D., Goldberg, M.S., Krauss, S., Motz, C., Wacker, M., Klose, J. and Shen, J. (2004) Mitochondrial dysfunction and oxidative damage in parkin-deficient mice. *Journal*

of Biological Chemistry, **279,**
18614–18622.

Periquet, M., Corti, O., Jacquier, S. and
Brice, A. (2005) Proteomic analysis of
parkin knockout mice: alterations in
energy metabolism, protein handling
and synaptic function. *Journal of
Neurochemistry,* **95,** 1259–1276.

Peyrl, A., Krapfenbauer, K., Slavc, I.,
Strobel, T. and Lubec, G. (2003)
Proteomic characterization of the human
cortical neuronal cell line HCN-2. *Journal
of Chemical Neuroanatomy,* **26,** 171–178.

Poirier, J. (2005) Apolipoprotein E,
cholesterol transport and synthesis in
sporadic Alzheimer's disease.
Neurobiology of Aging, **26,** 355–361.

Polymeropoulos, M.H., Lavedan, C.,
Leroy, E., Ide, S.E., Dehejia, A.,
Dutra, A., Pike, B., Root, H.,
Rubenstein, J., Boyer, R., Stenroos, E.S.,
Chandrasekharappa, S.,
Athanassiadou, A., Papapetropoulos, T.,
Johnson, W.G., Lazzarini, A.M.,
Duvoisin, R.C., Di Iorio, G., Golbe, L.I.
and Nussbaum, R.L. 1997 Mutation in
the alpha-synuclein gene identified in
families with Parkinson's disease.
Science, **276,** 2045–2047.

Puchades, M., Hansson, S.F.,
Nilsson, C.L., Andreasen, N.,
Blennow, K. and Davidsson, P. (2003)
Proteomic studies of potential
cerebrospinal fluid protein markers for
Alzheimer's disease. *Brain Research.
Molecular Brain Research,* **118,** 140–146.

Riederer, P. and Foley, P. (2002)
Mini-review: multiple developmental
forms of parkinsonism. The basis for
further research as to the pathogenesis
of parkinsonism. *Journal of Neural
Transmission,* **109,** 1469–1475.

Riederer, P., Sofic, E., Rausch, W.D.,
Schmidt, B., Reynolds, G.P., Jellinger, K.
and Youdim, M.B. (1989) Transition
metals, ferritin, glutathione, and
ascorbic acid in parkinsonian brains.
Journal of Neurochemistry, **52,** 515–520.

Ritter, B., Philie, J., Girard, M., Tung, E.C.,
Blondeau, F. and McPherson, P.S. (2003)
Identification of a family of endocytic
proteins that define a new alpha-adaptin
ear-binding motif. *EMBO Reports,* **4,**
1089–1095.

Ryan, K.A. and Pimplikar, S.W. (2005)
Activation of GSK-3 and phosphorylation
of CRMP2 in transgenic mice expressing
APP intracellular domain. *The Journal of
Cell Biology,* **171,** 327–335.

Schonberger, S.J., Edgar, P.F., Kydd, R.,
Faull, R.L. and Cooper, G.J. (2001)
Proteomic analysis of the brain in
Alzheimer's disease: molecular
phenotype of a complex disease process.
Proteomics, **1,** 1519–1528.

Selkoe, D.J. (1994) Normal and abnormal
biology of the beta-amyloid precursor
protein. *Annual Review of Neuroscience,*
17, 489–517.

Shimura, H., Schlossmacher, M.G.,
Hattori, N., Frosch, M.P.,
Trockenbacher, A., Schneider, R.,
Mizuno, Y., Kosik, K.S. and Selkoe, D.J.
(2001) Ubiquitination of a new form of
alpha-synuclein by parkin from human
brain: implications for Parkinson's
disease. *Science,* **293,** 263–269.

Shin, S.J., Lee, S.E., Boo, J.H., Kim, M.,
Yoon, Y.D., Kim, S.I. and Mook-Jung, I.
(2004) Profiling proteins related to
amyloid deposited brain of Tg2576 mice.
Proteomics, **4,** 3359–3368.

Sizova, D., Charbaut, E., Delalande, F.,
Poirier, F., High, A.A., Parker, F., Van
Dorsselaer, A., Duchesne, M. and
Diu-Hercend, A. (2007) Proteomic
analysis of brain tissue from an
Alzheimer's disease mouse model by
two-dimensional difference gel
electrophoresis. *Neurobiology of Aging,*
28, 357–370.

Spillantini, M.G., Schmidt, M.L.,
Lee, V.M., Trojanowski, J.Q., Jakes, R.
and Goedert, M. (1997) Alpha-synuclein
in Lewy bodies. *Nature,* **388,** 839–840.

Sultana, R., Boyd-Kimball, D., Poon, H.F.,
Cai, J., Pierce, W.M., Klein, J.B.,
Merchant, M., Markesbery, W.R. and
Butterfield, D.A. (2005) Redox
proteomics identification of oxidized
proteins in Alzheimer's disease
hippocampus and cerebellum: An
approach to understand pathological and
biochemical alterations in AD.
Neurobiology of Aging, **27,** 1564–1576.

Swatton, J.E., Prabakaran, S., Karp, N.A.,
Lilley, K.S. and Bahn, S. (2004) Protein
profiling of human postmortem brain

using 2-dimensional fluorescence difference gel electrophoresis (2-D DIGE). *Molecular Psychiatry*, **9**, 128–143.

Tanner, C.M. (1989) The role of environmental toxins in the etiology of Parkinson's disease. *Trends in Neurosciences*, **12**, 49–54.

Tribl, F., Gerlach, M., Marcus, K., Asan, E., Tatschner, T., Arzberger, T., Meyer, H.E., Bringmann, G. and Riederer, P. (2005) "Subcellular proteomics" of neuromelanin granules isolated from the human brain. *Molecular & Cellular Proteomics*, **4**, 945–957.

Tribl, F., Marcus, K., Meyer, H.E., Bringmann, G., Gerlach, M. and Riederer, P. (2006) Subcellular proteomics reveals neuromelanin granules to be a lysosome-related organelle. *Journal of Neural Transmission*, **113**, 1041–1054.

Tsuji, T., Shiozaki, A., Kohno, R., Yoshizato, K. and Shimohama, S. (2002) Proteomic profiling and neurodegeneration in Alzheimer's disease. *Neurochemical Research*, **27**, 1245–1253.

Wilson, K.E., Marouga, R., Prime, J.E., Pashby, D.P., Orange, P.R., Crosier, S., Keith, A.B., Lathe, R., Mullins, J., Estibeiro, P., Bergling, H., Hawkins, E. and Morris, C.M. (2005) Comparative proteomic analysis using samples obtained with laser microdissection and saturation dye labelling. *Proteomics*, **5**, 3851–3858.

Wood, D.R., Nye, J.S., Lamb, N.J., Fernandez, A. and Kitzmann, M. (2005) Intracellular retention of caveolin 1 in presenilin-deficient cells. *Journal of Biological Chemistry*, **280**, 6663–6668.

Yoritaka, A., Hattori, N., Uchida, K., Tanaka, M., Stadtman, E.R. and Mizuno, Y. (1996) Immunohistochemical detection of 4-hydroxynonenal protein adducts in Parkinson disease. *Proceedings of the National Academy of Sciences of the United States of America*, **93**, 2696–2701.

Yu, H.L., Chertkow, H.M., Bergman, H. and Schipper, H.M. (2003) Aberrant profiles of native and oxidized glycoproteins in Alzheimer plasma. *Proteomics*, **3**, 2240–2248.

Zhou, Y., Gu, G., Goodlett, D.R., Zhang, T., Pan, C., Montine, T.J., Montine, K.S., Aebersold, R.H. and Zhang, J. (2004) Analysis of alpha-synuclein-associated proteins by quantitative proteomics. *Journal of Biological Chemistry*, **279**, 39155–39164.

Zhou, Y., Wang, Y., Kovacs, M., Jin, J. and Zhang, J. (2005) Microglial activation induced by neurodegeneration: a proteomic analysis. *Molecular & Cellular Proteomics*, **4**, 1471–1479.

13
The Search for Protein Biomarkers of Neurobiological Diseases

Gary M. Muschik, Haleem J. Issaq and Timothy D. Veenstra

13.1
Introduction

13.1.1
Biomarkers

Diseases such as Alzheimer's disease, Parkinson's disease, Lewy body dementia, frontotemporal dementia, amyotrophic lateral sclerosis (ALS), Creutzfeldt–Jakob disease, familial amyliodotic polyneuropathy, gliomas, schizophrenia, and stroke are diseases of the nervous system. The twentieth-century increase in life expectancy has led to an increase in neurodegenerative diseases, cancer, and stroke cases. For example, the prevalence of dementia is estimated to range from 1% for those between 65 and 69 years of age to 39% in the 90- to 95-year-old population (Jorm *et al.*, 1987). While absolute cures for many neurological disorders are lacking, the discovery of diagnostic biomarkers for the detection of early-stage disease is still critical so that available treatment to alleviate debilitating symptoms can be administered in a timely fashion.

A biomarker is a biochemical or biophysical feature that can be used to measure the presence, progress, or remission of a disease or the effect of treatment. A biomarker must have the ability to detect the presence or determine the absence of a disease, the stage of disease progression (diagnostic), and the success or failure of treatment (prognostic). A gene, RNA, protein, metabolite, image, antigen, antibody, and virus are all examples of potential disease biomarkers. The early diagnosis and prediction of a disease state depends on our ability to discover, develop, test, and validate a biomarker in large populations.

The development of a clinical biomarker is based on the laboratory search for a difference between the constituents of healthy and diseased samples, followed by years of development and subsequent Food and Drug Administration (FDA) approval in the United States, after which a validated clinical biomarker is achieved for general population screening (Sullivan *et al.*, 2001; Frank *et al.*,

Proteomics of the Nervous System. Edited by H.G. Nothwang and S.E. Pfeiffer
Copyright © 2008 WILEY-VCH Verlag GmbH & Co. KGaA, Weinheim
ISBN: 978-3-527-31716-5

2003; Rafai *et al.*, 2006). Table 13.1 summarizes the five phases involved in biomarker discovery. An ideal biomarker would be present in a readily obtainable sample, such as saliva, tears, urine, breath, sweat, hair, blood, or cerebrospinal fluid (CSF). The marker detection and quantification method should be simple and economical, and the results easily interpreted. An effective biomarker will also diagnose the targeted condition with high sensitivity and specificity. Sensitivity is defined as the percentage of positive samples identified by a model as a true positive, and it decreases with an increase in false negatives. Specificity is defined as the percentage of negative samples identified by a model as a true negative, and it decreases with an increase in false positives. An optimal biomarker should give 100% sensitivity and specificity; however, such a perfect value is not easily attainable. The sensitivity and specificity of many clinical biomarkers used today are not necessarily high. For example, the prostate-specific antigen (PSA) biomarker for prostate cancer has a sensitivity of 46% and a specificity of 91% (Gann *et al.*, 1995), the HER-2/neu biomarker for stage IV breast cancer has a sensitivity of 40% and a specificity of 98% (Cook *et al.*, 2001), and troponin I for myocardial infarction has a sensitivity of 93% and a specificity of 81% (Eggers *et al.*, 2004). Recently, it has been suggested that a panel of biomarkers may give better sensitivity and specificity than a single biomarker. For example, a leptin, prolactin, osteopontin, and IGF-II panel for the detection of ovarian cancer was reported to have a sensitivity and specificity of 95% each (Mor *et al.*, 2005). Also, a panel of CD98, fascin, sPlgR, and 14-3-3 eta for lung cancer was reported to have a sensitivity of 96% and a specificity of 77% (Xiao *et al.*, 2005).

Clinical and paraclinical evaluations, neuropsychological tests, single photon emission computer tomography (SPECT), magnetic resonance imaging (MRI), and biomarkers have been used separately and together to diagnose dementia. The onset of Alzheimer's disease pathology is thought to start 20–30 years before the clinical signs of dementia are observed (Davies *et al.*, 1988). The confirmation rate for "possible" Alzheimer's disease ranges from 63 to 88%

Table 13.1 Phases defining biomarker discovery.

Phase 1	Discovery phase: Exploratory studies to identify potentially useful biomarkers
Phase 2	Validation phase: Biomarkers are studied to determine their capacity for distinguishing between diseased and healthy people
Phase 3	Studies to assess the capacity of a biomarker to detect preclinical disease by testing the marker against tissues collected longitudinally from research cohorts
Phase 4	Prospective screening studies
Phase 5	Definitive large-scale population studies to determine the overall impact of screening on health outcomes in the target populations

From Ahn *et al.* (2004).

Table 13.2 Methods and protocols for biomarker discovery.

Method	Reference
Lectin affinity chromatography	Freeze, 1995
Liquid isoelectric focusing	Zhu *et al.*, 2003; Ahn *et al.*, 2004; Kapkova *et al.*, 2006; Kweon and Hakansson, 2006
Capillary electrophoresis	Burg and Smith, 2003; Righetti *et al.*, 2003; Issaq *et al.*, 2005
Ion-exchange HPLC	Link *et al.*, 2003; Mussalman and Speicher, 2005
Reverse-phase HPLC	Issaq *et al.*, 2005; Link *et al.*, 2003; Mussalman and Speicher, 2005; Henzel and Stults, 2001
LC/MS/MS	Mussalman and Speicher, 2005; Patterson, 1998; Lee *et al.*, 2000a, 2000b; Delahunty and Yates, 2003
Isotope-coded affinity tag (ICAT) quantification	Yi and Goodlett, 2003
Proteolytic [^{18}O] water labeling quantification	Reynolds and Fenselau, 2003
I.TRAQ	
Data bases/protein identification	Addona and Clauser, 2000; Moore *et al.*, 2000; Beavis and Fenyo, 2004; Gulcicek *et al.*, 2005; Lundgren *et al.*, 2005

and for "probable" Alzheimer's disease from 81 to 100% based on current criteria at dementia referral centers (Petrovitch *et al.* 2001). The ability to diagnose and treat patients during the early stages of pathological disease development, before clinical symptoms occur, holds great promise in that it allows for early therapeutic intervention. The discovery and validation of new neurological biomarkers could lead to the early detection and treatment of neurological diseases.

This chapter will first focus on critical aspects to be considered during sample collection, preparation, separation, quantification, and proteomic analysis using mass spectrometry for biomarker discovery. A list of currently used methods is given in Table 13.2. Finally, selected recent applications will be presented.

13.1.2
Sample Collection

13.1.2.1 Requirements for Sample Collection
Sample collection is an important aspect of biomarker discovery. Specimens collected from controls and patients should be matched as closely as possible

(age and gender) because differences in proteins, metabolites, and other biomolecules that can be identified as possible biomarkers do change with age and gender (J. Zhang *et al.*, 2005; Liu *et al.*, 2005). To date, these factors have been neither extensively studied nor adequately understood.

Also, sample collection time, method, volume, and processing methods should be closely followed in order to obtain representative samples and reproducible results. Samples should be collected in clean tubes, partitioned into appropriate aliquots, and stored as soon as possible at $-80\,^\circ$C until analyzed. Finally, written standard operating procedures for sample collection and handling are necessary, especially if more than one collection site exists.

13.1.2.2   Cerebrospinal Fluid as a Sample

CSF, which is in direct contact with the outer surface brain tissue, has been the material most studied for neurodegenerative disease biomarker discovery. The total protein concentration of CSF is 200- to 400-fold less than in blood (You *et al.*, 2005). This can be an advantage when searching for non-protein biomarkers, but a disadvantage when searching for low-concentration protein biomarkers. CSF samples should be centrifuged to remove cell debris and, if they contain more than 10 red blood cells per microliter and a serum-to-CSF apolipoprotein B ratio less than 6000, they should be excluded from the study due to blood contamination (Z. Zhang *et al.*, 2005).

13.1.2.3   Tissue as a Sample

The search for biomarkers using diseased tissue samples is problematic since these tissues are typically heterogeneous, containing both normal and diseased cells. Therefore, investigators using tissue samples are challenged with selecting only the diseased cells of interest and eliminating the normal cells that add to sample complexity and analyte dilution. Laser capture microdissection (LCM) (Liao *et al.*, 2004) is a technique that allows the researcher to select specific targeted cells for collection and study. In addition, a new procedure that uses laser capture microdissection of formalin-fixed, paraffin-embedded tissues for proteomic studies has been reported (Hood *et al.*, 2005a) making available a new source of clinical samples for biomarker discovery.

13.1.2.4   Serum as a Sample

The search for neurological disease biomarkers in serum has been difficult because of the complexity of serum. Other factors that may affect the success of biomarker discovery from serum samples include the possible biomarker dilution effect caused by the volume of serum, and the blood–brain barrier, which might prevent the transport of a biomarker into the serum. However, serum is easy to collect and is being extensively studied as a source for other disease biomarkers.

13.1.3
Techniques for Sample Preparation

Affinity chromatography is a method that can be used for depletion of the most abundant proteins or selection of specifically modified proteins. In addition, the proteins adsorbed onto the multi-affinity columns can be probed for additional biomarkers, such as proteins, peptides, and small molecules that are also present due to adsorption (Lowenthal *et al.*, 2005; Veenstra *et al.*, 2005). Several multiple-affinity spin cartridges for a one-step depletion of abundant glycoproteins are commercially available (e.g. Agilent Technologies; GenWay Biotech).

An estimated 50% of all proteins in serum and CSF are glycoproteins (Agilent Technologies). *N*-Linked and *O*-linked glycopeptides are complex structures and difficult to separate and to isolate by classical methods. Different lectins, as shown in Table 13.3, have been used to deplete, concentrate, or separate *N*- and *O*-linked glycopeptides. In addition, Yang and Hancock (2004) developed a multi-lectin affinity column that can remove additional glycoproteins.

The addition of trichloroacetic acid, acetonitrile/trifluoroacetic acid, acetonitrile, acetone, chloroform/methanol, and ammonium sulfate to plasma and serum samples has been used for selected or total protein precipitation (Chertov *et al.*, 2004; Jiang *et al.*, 2004; Want *et al.*, 2006). Some of these protein precipitation methods have also been used for CSF protein depletion.

Phosphoproteins, phosphopeptides, and organic phosphates such as sugar phosphates, nucleotides, phospholipids, and phosphorylated metabolites can be either enriched for selective analyses or depleted from a sample by using

Table 13.3 Summary of lectin chromatography affinities for glycoforms.

Lectin	Affinity	Reference
Jacalin	GalNAc *O*-glycans and high mannose *N*-glycans	Hortin, 1990; Durham and Regnier, 2006
Lotus tetragonolobus agglutinin	α-l-Fucose	Xiong *et al.*, 2003
Wheat germ agglutinin	GlcNAc *O*-glycans and sialic acid	Vosseller *et al.*, 2006; Zhao *et al.*, 2006
Concanavalin A	High mannose *N*-glycans, biantennary *N*-glycans	Durham and Regnier, 2006; Qiu and Regnier, 2005
Sambucus nigra agglutinin	terminal α-2,6-linked sialic acid	Qiu and Regnier, 2005
Elderberry	sialic acid sub-class	Zhao *et al.*, 2006
Maackia amurensis	sialic acid sub-class	Zhao *et al.*, 2006

titanium dioxide (Ikeguchi and Nakamura, 2000; Pinkse *et al.*, 2004; Larsen *et al.*, 2005; Hata *et al.*, 2006), zirconium dioxide (Kweon and Hakansson, 2006), immobilized metal ion affinity chromatography (IMAC) (Ahn *et al.*, 2004), or highly cross-linked polystyrene-divinylbenzene (Kapkova *et al.*, 2006) materials in microcolumns and beads.

Liquid-phase isoelectric focusing (IEF) has been used to fractionate proteins present in CSF samples prior to separation by two-dimensional polyacrylamide gel electrophoresis (2D-PAGE) (Davidsson *et al.*, 1999, 2001, 2002) or high-performance liquid chromatography (HPLC) (Wall *et al.*, 2000). Liquid-phase IEF separates proteins according to the differences in their isoelectric points (pI). This step reduces the complex protein mixture into simplified mixtures that improve the separation and detection of lower-abundance proteins. However, it increases by 20 times (the number of fractions collected from the Rotofor apparatus) the number of samples for analysis. Complex serum peptide mixtures (Xiao *et al.*, 2004) have also been reduced in complexity by IEF fractionation prior to 2D chromatography separation and MS identification.

13.1.4
Methods for Protein Quantification

Differences in the expression levels of biomolecules (proteins, peptides, metabolites, and so forth) in the biological fluid samples obtained from normal and diseased subjects may indicate a pathophysiological condition, and therefore might be used as a biomarker. In the event that protein expression differences exist between the normal and disease states, quantification methods are necessary. Proteins and peptides from two different disease states can be quantified together as a pooled sample by using one or more of a number of different labeling methods (see Chapter 2). A few examples of the more frequently used labeling methods are 2D-difference gel electrophoresis (DIGE) (Zhou *et al.*, 2002; Beckner *et al.*, 2005; Hu *et al.*, 2005; Wilson *et al.*, 2005), carbon isotope-coded affinity tags (cICAT) (Gygi *et al.*, 1999; D'Ascenzo *et al.*, 2005; Wu *et al.*, 2006), isobaric tags for relative and absolute quantification (iTRAQ) (Ross *et al.*, 2004; D'Ascenzo *et al.*, 2005; Wu *et al.*, 2006), and $^{18}O/^{16}O$ proteolytic labeling (Yao *et al.*, 2001; Hood *et al.*, 2005b; Blonder *et al.*, 2006). Comparative studies have suggested that these methods identify different proteins and should therefore be considered to be complementary (Blonder *et al.*, 2006; Wu *et al.*, 2006).

13.1.5
Separation Techniques

Due to the large differences in biomolecule sample concentration dynamic range and the sample complexity, there is not a single simple comprehensive platform for biomolecule separation and biomarker discovery. A majority of investigators have used 2D-PAGE, DIGE, or 2D-HPLC to achieve comprehensive separations. In certain cases, such as searching for low-abundance proteins, it is necessary to remove the high-abundance proteins and fractionate the samples before attempting additional separations.

The method of choice for biologists is 2D-PAGE, which has been widely employed as a separation platform for protein biomarker discovery in CSF (Puchades *et al.*, 2003; Terry and Desiderio, 2003; Hakansson *et al.*, 2003; Maccarrone *et al.*, 2004; Hu *et al.*, 2005; Castano *et al.*, 2006), serum (Li *et al.*, 2005), and tissue samples (Freeman and Hemby, 2004; Fountoulakis, 2004) obtained from patients with neurodegenerative diseases. However, 2D-PAGE has certain limitations with respect to co-migrating proteins and proteins with extreme pH, size or hydrophobicity (see Chapter 2).

Capillary electrophoresis is an analytical separation technique that can resolve charged and neutral biomolecules (Hempel, 2003). This technique can separate a wide range of different endogenous molecules such as metabolites (Rada *et al.*, 1999; Rajda *et al.*, 2005), nucleic acids (Dorschner *et al.*, 2002), amino acids, and peptides (Viglio *et al.*, 2001; Varesio *et al.*, 2002; Wittke *et al.*, 2005). It is also used as a solution-based proteomic analysis method for the separation of complex peptide mixtures generated by enzymatic digestion of protein samples for biomarker and proteome studies (D'Ascenzo *et al.*, 2005; Issaq *et al.*, 2005; Amon *et al.*, 2006).

One of the most frequently used proteome and metabolome sample separation techniques is HPLC. A wide range of potential biomarker molecules such as metabolites (Cavus *et al.*, 2005; Comai *et al.*, 2006; Mackay *et al.*, 2006), peptides (Du *et al.*, 2005; Bateman *et al.*, 2006), nucleic acids (Schmidt *et al.*, 2005) and others (Bicikova *et al.*, 2004; Misra *et al.*, 2005) have been separated by this technique. Currently, it is the separation method of choice for solution-based proteome analysis. Due to protein posttranslational modification complexities and the large number of peptides present after digestion, multi-dimensional separation strategies employing 2D-HPLC have been developed to achieve separation prior to analysis by mass spectrometry (Washburn *et al.*, 2001; Issaq *et al.*, 2002; Xiao *et al.*, 2004; Yu *et al.*, 2004; Alvarez-Manilla *et al.*, 2006). Recently, multi-dimensional HPLC separation, prior to tandem mass spectrometry (MS/MS) detection and identification has been used for brain disease biomarker discovery (Baraniuk *et al.*, 2005; Cheng *et al.*, 2006; Jin *et al.*, 2006; Lukas *et al.*, 2006).

13.1.6
Selected Applications of Biomarker Discovery

The literature has numerous applications of the techniques discussed for proteomic analysis and biomarker discovery using CSF, tissue, and serum samples. Here we present selected neurological biomarker discovery applications using CSF or serum to demonstrate the utility of the different techniques.

13.1.6.1 Cerebrospinal Fluid

Global quantitative proteomics analysis of CSF from Alzheimer's disease and control patients to determine detectable differences in protein concentrations was reported by Z. Zhang *et al.* (2005). The patients were clinically characterized as having probable Alzheimer's disease; and the age-appropriate controls were free of any symptoms of neurological disease prior to CSF collection. The collected CSF samples were screened for red blood cells (<10 RBC per mL) and a serum-to-CSF apolipoprotein B ratio >6000. Equal volumes of screened CSF samples were pooled to make a single disease and control samples for proteomics analysis. Acetonitrile was used to precipitate albumin and immunoglobulin, while leaving the lower abundance proteins in solution. The cICAT method was used for protein quantification and consisted of labeling the disease protein samples with heavy (^{13}C) and the controls with light (^{12}C) reagents, followed by enzymatic digestion, affinity isolation, sample pooling, 2D-microcapillary HPLC separation, and MS/MS detection and quantification of the labeled pairs. The relative levels of 163 proteins were quantified between the Alzheimer's disease and control pooled CSF samples. The results indicated that 78 proteins were at comparative levels. Of the remaining 85 proteins, 39 had a relative concentration of $\geq 120\%$ and 46 had a relative concentration of $\leq 80\%$ than the Alzheimer's disease CSF proteins. The authors confirmed the relative concentration accuracy of the cICAT method by Western blot analysis and optical quantification of four of the identified proteins using commercially available antibodies. These results demonstrate that quantitative proteomic analyses of CSF could yield a panel of biomarkers that, after extensive validation, could hold promise for distinguishing Alzheimer's disease patients from normal aging patients.

13.1.6.2 Serum

2D-PAGE and gel imaging analysis was used by Goldknopf *et al.* (2006) to analyze serum proteins in 422 samples from neurodegenerative disease and control patients in a search for biomarkers. Thirty-four 2-DGE protein spot differences were identified after digital image analysis of samples from ALS, Parkinson's disease, and control samples. The 34 protein spots were removed from the gels with a robotic gel cutter and subjected to tryptic digestion. Matrix assisted laser desorption ionization-time of flight (MALDI-TOF)/MS peptide fingerprint analysis and nanoLC-MS/MS peptide fragmentation analysis were used to identify nine of the spots. This work determined that complement C3 components C3c and C3dg and a complement factor H component were overexpressed in ALS and Parkinson's disease patients' serum. The authors concluded that inflammatory processes involving complement activation were associated with ALS and Parkinson's disease, and may lead to future useful biomarker discoveries.

13.2
Methodology

Detailed methods for performing many of the procedures discussed in this chapter can be found in the references cited in Table 13.2 and in the text references. The reader is encouraged to read these sources for additional experimental details. Selected protocols for sample preparation, detection, and identification are provided in the following sections.

13.2.1
Sample Preparation

Depending on the type of sample, sample preparation may involve fractionation, extraction, dissolution, or homogenization. Also, the selected sample preparation procedure will vary with the type of molecules of interest, depending on whether the biomolecules are proteins, peptides, posttranslational modified proteins, or metabolites, and so forth. Large molecular weight proteins that are abundant in CSF, plasma, and tissue homogenates can be either depleted or concentrated using antibody-based affinity immunodepletion materials. The following two techniques will be described in more detail: the removal of high-abundance proteins from CSF using the multiaffinity removal system (MARS) from Agilent Technologies, Palo Alto, CA, USA as reported by Hu *et al.* (2005), and sample fractionation using liquid-phase IEF as developed by Davidsson *et al.* (1999).

13.2.1.1 CSF Immunoaffinity Column Depletion
The purpose of this depletion step is to reduce the complexity and concentration dynamic range of proteins in the CSF, enabling the detection of low-abundance proteins.

Requirements

Reagents: Multiaffinity removal system (MARS, Agilent Technologies); 22 µm spin filters (Millipore).

Instrumentation: Centrifuge; an HPLC/UV system.
  1. Concentrate and buffer exchange 1–2 mL of CSF three times using buffer A (supplied by the manufacturer) to approximately 50 µL using a 5- or 10-kDa molecular weight membrane filter; then bring the sample to a final volume of 200 µL using additional buffer A.
  2. Pass the sample through a 22-µm spin filter at $16\,000 \times g$ for 1 min to remove particulates.

3. Inject the 200 µL sample onto a 4.6 × 50-mm MARS column equilibrated with buffer A at a flow rate of 0.25 mL min^{-1} at room temperature using an HPLC system. Monitor column effluents at 280 nm with an appropriate cell size in-line HPLC/UV detector.
4. Collect the CSF lower abundance proteins that pass through the column for further analysis.
5. Elute the higher abundance proteins captured by the MARS column using buffer B. The higher abundance protein fraction can be probed for additional biomarkers, such as proteins, peptides, and other small molecules that might be adsorbed onto these abundant proteins.
6. An aliquot of each protein flow-through can be used directly for one-dimensional gel electrophoresis (1D-PAGE) analysis. All samples should be stored at −80 °C until future use.

13.2.1.2 Liquid Isoelectric Focusing
Liquid isoelectric focusing can be used with unprocessed CSF or CSF after depletion of abundant proteins.

Requirements

Chemicals: Urea; dithiothreitol (DTT); diethyl ether; ethanol; ampholyte (pH range 3–10).

Solutions: 10% Trichloroacetic acid.

Instrumentation: Rotofor apparatus (Bio-Rad Laboratories, Hercules, CA, USA); refrigerated water bath.
1. Precipitate CSF proteins using 10% trichloroacetic acid (or any other protein precipitation method) while cooling the sample in an ice/water bath, then centrifuge at 2000 × g for 10 min to pellet the proteins.
2. Wash the pellet twice with ether/ethanol (1 : 1 v/v) followed by centrifugation and drying.
3. Dissolve the protein pellet in 12 mL of a 6–8 M urea, 20 mM DTT, and 2% ampholyte, pH range 3–10, solution.
4. Place the prepared CSF protein sample into an assembled Rotofor cell. A constant power of 10 W is applied for 2–4 h, or until the voltage stabilizes, with apparatus cooling provided by a circulating refrigerated water bath. Each protein-containing fraction is aspirated simultaneously with vacuum into appropriately labeled, individual test tubes.
5. Confirm the formation of a pH gradient by measuring the pH of each collected fraction.
6. Determine the protein concentration of each fraction using Lowry or equivalent method.

7. Additional analysis using either 1D-PAGE or HPLC-MS is recommended to characterize the protein composition of each fraction.

13.2.2
Quantitative Comparison by Carbon Isotope-Coded Affinity Tags

Sample labeling is another aspect of sample preparation prior to final analysis. When using biomarkers in a diagnostic setting, an important measurement is their abundance in the disease-affected patient compared to a healthy patient. Relative protein abundance difference ratios between normal and disease samples can be obtained using a protein quantification method such as the cICAT method. The cICAT procedure involves labeling proteins from two different disease states with heavy (^{13}C) and light (^{12}C) reagents, followed by enzymatic digestion, affinity isolation, sample pooling, HPLC separation, and MS/MS detection and quantification of the labeled pairs. The following cICAT method uses protein pellets obtained from non-treated and treated primary cortical neuron cultures established from newborn mice as reported by Yu *et al.* (2004).

Requirements

Reagents: cICAT-^{12}C$_9$ and cICAT-^{13}C$_9$ reagents (ABI, Framingham, MA, USA); acetonitrile; D-salt Excellulose plastic desalting column (Pierce, Rockford, IL, USA); trypsin (Promega, Madison, WI, USA); phenylmethanesulfonyl fluoride; avidin columns (Applied Biosystems, Foster City, CA, USA); methanol.

Solutions: Denaturing reagent (6 M guanidine hydrochloride in 50 mM ammonium bicarbonate, pH 8.3); reducing reagent (100 mM Tris (2-carboxyethyl)phosphine hydrochloride); 50 mM ammonium bicarbonate, pH 8.3; PBS (0.2 M sodium phosphate, 0.3 M NaCl, pH 7.2); 50 mM ammonium bicarbonate/20% acetonitrile, pH 8.3; 30% (v/v) acetonitrile/0.4% (v/v) formic acid.

Instrumentaiton: Water bath; lyophilizer.
1. Label 800 µg of non-treated and treated cortical neuron sample protein pellets with the light (cICAT-^{12}C$_9$) and heavy (cICAT-^{13}C$_9$) cICAT reagent according to the manufacturer's instructions.
2. Place each sample in separate tubes and dissolve it in 80 µL of denaturing reagent.
3. Add 1 µL of reducing reagent, and reduce each sample by boiling for 10 min in a water bath.
4. Transfer each reduced sample to a separate vial containing a 10-fold excess of either cICAT-^{12}C$_9$ or cICAT-^{13}C$_9$ reagent to protein-free

sulfhydryl groups (with a minimum final cICAT reagent concentration of 1.2 mM) dissolved in 20 μL of acetonitrile and heat for 2 h at 37 °C.

5. Add a 10-fold excess of reducing agent to each sample to react with the unreacted cICAT reagent.

6. Combine the two samples into one and buffer exchange it into a 50 mM ammonium bicarbonate buffer (pH 8.3) using a D-Salt Excellulose plastic desalting column followed by trypsin digestion overnight at 37 °C using a 1 : 50 (w/w) enzyme-to-protein ratio.

7. Quench the digestion by boiling the sample for 10 min in a water bath and add phenylmethanesulfonyl fluoride to a 1 mM final concentration.

8. Load the cICAT-labeled combined peptides sample onto an avidin column and allow to equilibrate at room temperature for 15 min before eluting.

9. Wash the column with 2× PBS, 1× PBS, and 50 mM ammonium bicarbonate/20%/acetonitrile, pH 8.3.

10. Elute the cICAT-labeled biotin-tagged peptides using 30% (v/v) acetonitrile/0.4% (v/v) formic acid.

11. Cleave the biotin tags from the modified peptides according to the manufacturer's instructions using the provided cleaving reagents A and B.

12. Lyophilize the resulting peptide mixture to dryness.

13. Equilibrate a second avidin column with 20% methanol and load the peptide mixture dissolved in 20% methanol on the column. The cICAT-labeled peptides begin to elute from the column during the loading step. An additional two column volumes of 20% methanol are required to insure the complete elution of the peptides. Note: the impurities remain bound to the column under these conditions and do not elute with the cICAT-labeled peptides.

14. Dry the purified cICAT-labeled peptide solution by vacuum lyophilization. The peptide samples are stored at −80 °C until analysis by HPLC-MS/MS.

13.2.3
Sample Detection and Identification

This procedure is patterned after the method of Yu *et al.* (2004), in which micro-reversed-phase liquid chromatography (μRP-HPLC)/ESI-MS/MS was used for the detection and identification of peptides from untreated and treated primary cortical neuron cultures.

Requirements

Reagents: Formic acid; acetonitrile; isopropanol; HPLC grade water.

Material and Instrumentation: An empty 75-μm ID fused-silica capillary column (Polymicro Technologies, Phoenix, AZ, USA); Jupiter C18, 5 μm

Protein	Disease		Reference
Transthyretin (Val → Met)	FAP	u	Bergquist et al., 2000
S-cysteinylated	FTD	u	Ruetschi et al., 2005
Transthyretin ubiquitin	AD	–	Davidsson et al., 2002; Davidsson and Sjogren, 2006
Kininogen	AD	d	Puchades et al., 2003; Davidsson and Sjogren, 2006
β Glycoprotein (1)	AD	d	Puchades et al., 2003; Davidsson and Sjogren, 2006
apoJ (2)	AD	d	Puchades et al., 2003; Davidsson and Sjogren, 2006
apoE (3)	AD, FTD	d	Davidsson et al., 2002; Davidsson and Sjogren, 2006
apoA1 (2)	AD	d	Puchades et al., 2003; Davidsson and Sjogren, 2006
β-trace	AD	d	Puchades et al., 2003; Davidsson and Sjogren, 2006
Cell cycle progression eight protein	AD	d	Puchades et al., 2003; Davidsson and Sjogren, 2006
Retinol binding protein	AD, FTD	v	Davidsson et al., 2002; Puchades et al., 2003; Davidsson and Sjogren, 2006
α-1-antitrypsin (1)	AD	u	Davidsson and Sjogren, 2006; Davidsson et al., 2002
α-2-HS Glycoprotein	AD	d	Puchades et al., 2003
Transferrin precursor	AD	d	Puchades et al., 2003
Albumin precursor	AD	d	Puchades et al., 2003
albumin	FTD	–	Puchades et al., 2003; Castano et al., 2006
Granin-like neuroendocrine precursor	FTD	d	Davidsson et al., 2002

(continued overleaf)

Table 13.4 *(continued)*.

Marker	Disease	Regulation	Reference
Pigment-epithelium derived factor	FTD	d	Davidsson *et al.*, 2002
Haptoglobin	FTD	d	Davidsson *et al.*, 2002
14-3-3	MS	v	Teunissen *et al.*, 2005
Actin	MS	u	Teunissen *et al.*, 2005
Truncated cystatin C	FTD, MS	v	Ruetschi *et al.*, 2005; Irani *et al.*, 2006
Fragment of neurosecretory protein	FTD	d	Ruetschi *et al.*, 2005
Chromogranin	FTD	d	Ruetschi *et al.*, 2005
Epstein–Barr virus	MS	positive	Lunemann *et al.*, 2006
Blood/serum:			
24S-Hydroxycholesterol	MS	d	Teunissen *et al.*, 2005
apoE	AD	d	Siest *et al.*, 2000
Brain tissue:			
Ubiquitin C-terminal hydrolase L1 (UCH-L1)	AD, PD	d	Gong *et al.*, 2006
ε4 allele frequency	AD	U	Berg *et al.*, 1998

v, varies between diseases; u, increased from normal; d, decreased from normal; nc, no observed change; AD, Alzheimer's disease; AIS, acute ischemic stroke; PD, Parkinson's disease; LBD, Lewy body dementia; ALS, amyotrophic lateral sclerosis; MS, multiple sclerosis; FTD, frontotemporal dementia; MCI, mild cognitive impairment; DS, Down's syndrome; FAP, familial amyloidotic polyneuropathy.

biomarker discovery is a long and costly endeavor, but one that is necessary for detecting and treating disease in the early stages, where the patient will benefit the most.

Acknowledgments

This project has been funded in whole or in part with federal funds from the National Cancer Institute, National Institutes of Health, under Contract N01-CO-12400. The content of this publication does not necessarily reflect the views or policies of the Department of Health and Human Services, nor does mention of trade names, commercial products, or organizations imply endorsement by the United States Government.

References

Addona, T. and Clauser, K. (2000) De Novo peptide sequencing via manual interpretation of MS/MS spectra, in *Current Protocols in Protein Science* (eds J.E. Coligan, B.M. Dunn, D.W. Speicher and P.T. Wingfield), John Wiley & Sons, Inc., New York, pp. 16.11.1–16.11.19.

Ahn, Y.H., Park, E.J., Chu, K., Kim, J.Y., Ha, S.H., Ryu, S.H. and Yoo, J.S. (2004) Dynamic identification of phosphopeptides using immobilized metal ion affinity chromatography enrichment, subsequent partial β-elimination/chemical tagging and matrix-assisted laser desorption/ionization mass spectrometric analysis. *Rapid Communications in Mass Spectrometry*, **18**, 2495–2501.

Alvarez-Manilla, G., Atwood, J., III, Guo, Y., Warren, N.L., Orlando, R. and Pierce, M. (2006) Tools for glycoproteomic analysis: size exclusion chromatography facilitates identification of tryptic glycopeptides with N-linked glycosylation sites. *Journal of Proteomic Research*, **5**, 701–708.

Amon, S., Plemati, A. and Rizzi, A. (2006) Capillary zone electrophoresis of glycopeptides under controlled electroosmotic flow conditions coupled to electrospray and matrix-assisted laser desorption/ionization mass

spectrometry. *Electrophoresis*, **27**, 1209–1219.

Baraniuk, J.N., Casado, B., Maiback, H., Clauw, D.J., Pannell, L.K. and Hess, S. (2005) A chronic fatigue syndrome-related proteome in human cerebrospinal fluid. *BMC Neurology*, **5**, 22–41.

Bateman, R.J., Munsell, L.Y., Morris, J.C., Swarm, R., Yarasheski, K.E. and Holtzman, D.M. (2006) Human amyloid-β synthesis and clearance rates as measured in cerebrospinal fluid *in vivo*. *Nature Medicine*, **12**, 856–861.

Beavis, R. and Fenyo, D. (2004) Finding protein sequences using PROWL, in *Current Protocols in Bioinformatics* (eds A.D. Baxevanis, D.B. Davison, R.D.M. Page, G.A. Petsko, L.D. Stein and G.D. Stormo), John Wiley & Sons, Inc., New York, pp. 13. 2.1–13.2.20.

Beckner, M.E., Chen, X., An, J., Day, B.W. and Pollack, I.F. (2005) Proteomic characterization of harvested pseudopodia with differential gel electrophoresis and specific antibodies. *Laboratory Investigation*, **85**, 316–327.

Berg, L., McKeel, D.W., Miller, J.P., Storandt, M., Rubin, E.H., Morris, J.C., Baty, J., Coats, M., Norton, J., Goate, A.M., Price, J.L., Gearing, M., Mirra, S.S. and Saunders, A.M. (1998) Clinicopathologic studies in cognitively healthy aging and Alzheimer's disease. *Archives of Neurology*, **55**, 326–335.

Bergquist, J., Andersen, O. and Westman, A. (2000) Rapid method to characterize mutations in transthyretin in cerebrospinal fluid from familial amyloidotic polyneuropathy patients by use of matrix-assisted laser desorption/ionization time-of-flight mass spectrometry. *Clinical Chemistry*, **46**, 1293–1300.

Bicikova, M., Ripova, D., Hill, M., Jirak, R., Havlikova, H., Tallova, J. and Hampl, R. (2004) Plasma levels of 7-hydroxylated dehydroepiandrosterone (DHEA) metabolites and selected amino-thiols as discriminatory tools of Alzheimer's disease vascular dementia. *Clinical Chemistry and Laboratory Medicine*, **42**, 518–524.

Blonder, J., Yu, L.-R., Radeva, G., Chan, K.C., Lucas, D.A., Waybright, T.J., Issaq, H.J., Sharom, F.J. and Veenstra, T.D. (2006) Combined chemical and enzymatic stable isotope labeling for quantitative profiling of detergent-insoluble membrane proteins isolated using Triton X-100 and Brij-96. *Journal of Proteome Research*, **5**, 349–360.

Brettschneider, J., Petzold, A., Sussmuth, S.D., Ludolph, A.C. and Tumani, H. (2006) Axonal damage markers in cerebrospinal fluid are increased in ALS. *Neurology*, **66**, 852–856.

Burg, D. and Smith, A.J. (2003) Capillary electrophoresis of proteins and peptides, in *Current Protocols in Protein Science* (eds J.E. Coligan, B.M. Dunn, D.W. Speicher and P.T. Wingfield), John Wiley & Sons, Inc., New York, pp. 10.9.1–10.9.13.

Castano, E.M., Roher, A.E., Esh, C.L., Kokjohn, T.A. and Beach, T. (2006) Comparative proteomics of cerebrospinal fluid in neuropathologically-confirmed Alzheimer's disease and non-demented elderly sublects. *Neurological Research*, **28**, 155–163.

Cavus, I., Kasoff, W.S., Cassaday, M.P., Jacob, R., Gueorguieva, R., Sherwin, R.S., Krystal, J.H., Spencer, D.D. and Abi-Saab, W.M. (2005) Extracellular metabolites in the cortex and hippocampus of epileptic patients. *Annals of Neurology*, **57**, 226–235.

Cheng, D., Hoogenraad, C.C., Rush, J., Ramm, E., Schlager, M.A., Duong, D.M., Xu, P., Wijayawardana, S.R., Hanfelt, J., Nakagawa, T., Sheng, M. and Peng, J. (2006) Relative and absolute quantification of postsynaptic density proteome isolated from rat forebrain and cerebellum. *Molecular and Cellular Proteomics: MCP*, **5**, 1158–1170.

Chertov, O., Biragyn, A., Kwak, L.W., Simpson, J.T., Boronina, T., Hoang, V.M., Prieto, D.A., Conrads, T.P., Veenstra, T.D. and Fisher, R.J. (2004) Organic solvent extraction of proteins and peptides from serum as an effective sample preparation for detection and identification of biomarkers by mass spectrometry. *Proteomics*, **4**, 1195–2003.

Comai, S., Longatti, P., Perin, A., Bertazzo, A., Ragazzi, E., Costa, C.V.L. and Allegri, G. (2006) Study of tryptophan metabolism via serotonin in cerebrospinal fluid of patients with noncommunicating hydrocephalus using a new endoscopic technique. *Journal of Neuroscience Research*, **84**, 683–692.

Cook, G.B., Neaman, I.E., Goldblatt, J.L., Cambetas, D.R., Hussain, M., Luftner, D., Yeung, K.K., Chan, D.W., Schwartz, M.K. and Allard, W.J. (2001) Clinical utility of serum HER-2/neu testing on the Bayer Immuno 1® automated system in breast cancer. *Anticancer Research*, **21**, 1465–1470.

Davidsson, P., Folkesson, S., Christiansson, M., Lindbjer, M., Dellheben, B., Blennow, K. and Westman-Brinkmalm, A. (2002) Identification of proteins in human cerebrospinal fluid using liquid-phase isoelectric focusing as a prefractionation step followed by two-dimensional gel electrophoresis and matrix assisted laser desorption/ionization mass spectrometry. *Rapid Communications in Mass Spectrometry*, **16**, 2083–2088.

D'Ascenzo, M., Relkin, N.R. and Lee, K.H. (2005) Alzheimer's disease cerebrospinal fluid biomarker discovery: a proteomics approach. *Current Opinion in Molecular Therapeutics*, **7**, 557–564.

Davidsson, P. and Sjogren, M. (2006) Proteome studies of CSF in AD patients. *Mechanisms of Ageing and Development*, **127**, 133–137.

Davidsson, P., Westman, A., Puchades, M., Nilsson, C.L. and Blennow, K. (1999) Characterization of proteins from human cerebrospinal fluid by a combination of preparative two-dimensional liquid-phase electrophoresis and matrix- assisted laser desorption/ionization time-of-flight mass spectrometry. *Analytical Chemistry*, **71**, 642–647.

Davidsson, P., Paulson, L., Hesse, C., Blennow, K. and Nilsson, C.L. (2001) Proteome studies of human cerebrospinal fluid and brain tissue using a preparative two- dimensional electrophoresis approach prior to mass spectrometry. *Proteomics*, **1**, 444–452.

Davidsson, P., Sjogren, M., Andreasen, N., Lindbjer, M., Nilsson, C.L., Westman-Brinkmalm, A. and Blennow, K. (2002) Studies of the pathophysiological mechanisms in frontotemporal dementia by proteome analysis of CSF proteins. *Molecular Brain Research*, **109**, 128–133.

Davies, L., Wolska, B., Hilbich, C., Multhaup, G., Martins, R., Simms, G., Beyreuther, K. and Masters, C.L. (1988) A4 amyloid protein deposition and the diagnosis of Alzheimer's disease. *Neurology*, **38**, 1688–1693.

Delahunty, C. and Yates, J.R. III (2003) Identification of proteins in complex mixtures using liquid chromatography and mass spectrometry, in *Current Protocols in Cell Biology* (J.S. Bonifacino, M. Dasso, J.B. Harford, J. Lippincott-Schwartz and M. Yamada), John Wiley & Sons, Inc., New York, pp. 5.6.1–5.6.17.

Dorschner, M.O., Barden, D. and Stephens, K. (2002) Diagnosis of five spinocerebellar ataxia disorders by multiplex amplification and capillary electrophoresis. *The Journal of Molecular Diagnostics*, **4**, 108–113.

Du, C., Ramaley, C., McLean, H., Leonard, S.C. and Miller, J. (2005) High-performance liquid chromatography coupled with tandem mass spectrometry for the detection of amyloid beta peptide related with Alzheimer's. *Journal of Biomolecular Techniques*, **16**, 354–363.

Durham, M. and Regnier, F.E. (2006) Targeted glycoproteomics: serial affinity chromatography in the selection of O-glycosylation sites on proteins from the human blood proteome. *Journal of Chromatography A*, **1132**, 165–173.

Eggers, K.M., Oldgren, J., Nordenskjold, A. and Lindahl, B. (2004) Diagnostic value of serial measurement of cardiac markers in patients with chest pain: limited value of adding myoglobin to troponin I for exclusion of myocardial infarction. *American Heart Journal*, **148**, 574–581.

Frank, R.A., Galasko, D., Hampel, H., Hardy, J., deLeon, M.J., Mehta, P.D., Rogers, J., Siemers, E. and Trojanowski, J.Q. (2003) Biological markers for therapeutic trails in Alzheimer's disease. Proceedings of the biological markers working group; NIA initiative on neuroimaging in Alzheimer's disease. *Neurobiology of Aging*, **24**, 521–536.

Freeman, W.M. and Hemby, S.E. (2004) Proteomics for protein expression profiling in neuroscience. *Neurochemical Research*, **29**, 1065–1081.

Freeze, H.H. (1995) Lectin affinity chromatography, in *Current Protocols in Protein Science* (eds J.E. Coligan, B.M. Dunn, D.W. Speicher and P.T. Wingfield), John Wiley & Sons, Inc., New York, pp. 9.1.1–9.1.9.

Fountoulakis, M. (2004) Application of proteomics technologies in the investigation of the brain. *Mass Spectrometry Reviews*, **23**, 231–258.

Gann, P.H., Hennekens, C.H. and Stampfer, M.J. (1995) A prospective evaluation of plasma prostate-specific antigen for the detection of prostate cancer. *Journal of the American Medical Association*, **273**, 289–294.

Goldknopf, I.L., Sheta, E.A., Bryson, J., Folsom, B., Wilson, C., Duty, J., Yen, A.A. and Appel, S.H. (2006) Complement C3a and related protein biomarkers in amyotrophic lateral sclerosis and Parkinson's disease. *Biochemical and Biophysical Research Communications*, **342**, 1034–1039.

Gong, B., Cao, Z., Zheng, P., Vitolo, O.V., Liu, S., Staniszewski, A., Moolman, D., Zhang, H., Shelanski, M. and Arancio, O. (2006) Ubiquitin hydrolase UchL1 rescues β-amyloid-induced decrease in synaptic function and contextual memory. *Cell*, **126**, 775–788.

Gulcicek, E.E., Colangelo, C.M., McMurray, W., Stone, K., Williams, K., Wu, T., Zhao, H., Spratt, H., Kurosky, A. and Wu, B. (2005) Proteomics and the analysis of proteomic data: an overview of current protein-protein technologies, in *Current Protocols in Bioinformatics* (eds A.D. Baxevanis, D.B. Davison, R.D.M Page, G.A. Petsko, L.D. Stein and G.D. Stormo), John Wiley & Sons, Inc., New York, pp. 13.1.1–13.1.31.

Gygi, S.P., Rist, R., Gerber, S.A., Turecek, F., Gelb, M. and Aebersold, R. (1999) Quantitative analysis of complex protein mixtures using isotope-coded tags. *Nature Biotechnology*, **17**, 994–999.

Hata, K., Morisaka, H., Hara, K., Mima, J., Yumoto, N., Tatsu, Y., Furuno, M., Ishizuka, N. and Ueda, M. (2006) Two-dimensional HPLC on-line analysis of phosphopeptides using titania and monolithic columns. *Analytical Biochemistry*, **350**, 292–297.

Hempel, G. (2003) Biomedical application of capillary electrophoresis. *Clinical Chemistry and Laboratory Medicine*, **41**, 720–723.

Henzel, W.J. and Stults, J.T. (2001) Reversed-phase isolation of peptides, in *Current Protocols in Protein Science* (eds J.E. Coligan, B.M. Dunn, D.W. Speicher and P.T. Wingfield), John Wiley & Sons, Inc., New York, pp. 11.6.1–11.6.16.

Hood, B.L., Darfler, M.M., Guiel, T.G., Furusato, B., Lucas, D.A., Ringeisen, B.R., Sesterhenn, I.A., Conrads, T.P., Veenstra, T.D. and Krizman, D.B. (2005a) Proteomic analysis of formalin-fixed prostate cancer tissue. *Molecular and Cellular Proteomics*, **4**, 1741–1753.

Hood, B.L., Lucas, D.A., Kim, G., Chan, K.C., Blonder, J., Issaw, H.J.,

Veenstra, T.D., Conrads, T.P., Pollet, I. and Karsan, A. (2005b) Quantitative analysis of the low molecular weight serum proteome using ^{18}O stable isotope labeling in a lung tumar xenograph mouse model. *Journal of the American Society for Mass Spectrometry*, **16**, 1221–1230.

Hakansson, K., Emmette, M.R., Marshall, A.G., Davidsson, P. and Nilsson, C.L. (2003) Structural analysis of 2D-gel-separated glycoproteins from human cerebrospinal fluid by tandem high-resolution mass spectrometry. *Journal of Proteome Research*, **2**, 581–588.

Hesse, C., Rosengren, L., Andreasen, N., Davidsson, P., Vanderstichele, H., Vanmechelen, E. and Blennow, K. (2001) Transient increase in total tau but not phospho-tau in human cerebrospinal fluid after acute stroke. *Neuroscience Letters*, **297**, 187–190.

Hortin, G.L. (1990) Isolation of glycopeptides containing O-linked oligosaccharides by lectin affinity chromatography on jacalin-agarose. *Analytical Biochemistry*, **191**, 262–267.

Hu, Y., Malone, J.P., Fagan, A.M., Townsend, R.R. and Holtzman, D.M. (2005) Comparative proteomic analysis of intra- and interindividual variation in human cerebrospinal fluid. *Molecular and Cellular Proteomics*, **4**, 2000–2009.

Ikeguchi, Y. and Nakamura, H. (2000) Selective enrichment of phospholipids by titania. *Analytical Sciences*, **16**, 541–543.

Irani, D.N., Anderson, C., Gundry, R., Cotter, R., Moore, S., Kerr, D.A., McArthur, J.C., Sacktor, N., Pardo, C.A., Jones, M., Calabresi, P.A. and Nath, A. (2006) Cleavage of Cystatin C in the cerebrospinal fluid of patients with multiple sclerosis. *Annals of Neurology*, **59**, 237–247.

Issaq, H.J., Conrads, T.P., Janini, G.M. and Veenstra, T.D. (2002) Methods for fractionation, separation and profiling of proteins and peptides. *Electrophoresis*, **23**, 3048–3061.

Issaq, H.J., Chan, K.C., Janini, G.M., Conrads, T.P. and Veenstra, T.D. (2005) Multidimensional separation of peptides for effective proteomic analysis. *Journal of Chromatography B*, **817**, 35–47.

Jiang, L., He, L. and Fountoulakis, M. (2004) Comparison of protein precipitation methods for sample preparation prior to proteomic analysis. *Journal of Chromatography A*, **1023**, 317–320.

Jin, J., Hulette Wang, C.Y., Zhang, T., Pan, C., Wadhwa, R. and Zhang, J. (2006) Proteomic identification of a stress protein. Mortalin/mthsp70/ GRP75. *Molecular and Cellular Proteomics*, **5**, 1193–1204.

Johnson, G., Brane, D., Block, W., van Kammen, D.P., Gurklis, J., peters, J.L., Wyatt, R.J., Kirch, D.G., Ghanbari, H.A. and Merril, C.R. (1992) Cerebrospinal fluid protein variations in common to Alzheimer's disease and schizophrenia. *Applied and Theoretical Electrophoresis*, **3**, 47–53.

Jorm, A.F., Korten, A.E. and Henderson, A.S. (1987) The prevalence of dementia: a quantitative intergration of the literature. *Acta Psychiatrica Scand*, **76**, 465–479.

Kanemaru, K., Kameda, N. and Yamanouchi, H. (2000) Decreased CSF amyloid [beta]42 and normal tau levels in dementia with Lewy bodies. *Neurology*, **54**, 1875–1876.

Kapaki, E., Paraskevas, G.P., Zalonis, I. and Zournas, C. (2003) CSF tau protein and β-amyloid (1–42) in Alzheimer's disease diagnosis: discrimination from normal ageing and other dementias in the Greek population. *European Journal of Neurology*, **10**, 119–128.

Kapkova, P., Lattova, E. and Perreault, H. (2006) Nonretentive solid-phase extraction of phosphorylated peptides from complex peptide mixtures for detection by matrix-assisted laser desorption/ionization mass spectrometry. *Analytical Chemistry*, **78**, 7027–7033.

Kweon, H.K. and Hakansson, K. (2006) Selective zirconium dioxide-based enrichment of phosphorylated peptides for mass spectrometric analysis. *Analytical Chemistry*, **78**, 1743–1749.

Larsen, M.R., Thingholm, T.E., Jensen, O.N., Roepstorff, P. and Jorgensen, T.J.D. (2005) Highly selective enrichment of phosphorylated peptides from peptide mixtures using titanium

dioxide microcolumns. *Molecular and Cellular Proteomics*, **4**, 873–886.

Lee, T.D., Moore, R.E. and Young, M.K. (2000a) Introducing samples directly into electrospray ionization mass spectrometers using a nanospray interface, in *Current Protocols in Protein Science* (eds J.E. Coligan, B.M. Dunn, D.W. Speicher and P.T. Wingfield), John Wiley & Sons, Inc., New York, pp. 16.8.1–16.8.5.

Lee, T.D., Moore, R.E. and Young, M.K. (2000b) Introducing samples directly into electrospray ionization mass spectrometers using microscale capillary liquid chromatography, in *Current Protocols in Protein Science* (eds J.E. Coligan, B.M. Dunn, D.W. Speicher and P.T. Wingfield), John Wiley & Sons, Inc., New York, pp. 16.9.1–19.9.7.

Li, X., Gong, Y., Wang, Y., Wu, S., Cai, Y., He, P., Lu, Z., Ying, W., Zhang, Y., Jiao, L., He, H., Zhang, Z., He, F., Zhao, X. and Qian, X. (2005) Comparison of alternative analytical techniques for the characterization of the human serum proteome in HUPO Plasma Proteome Project. *Proteomics*, **5**, 3423–3441.

Liao, L., Cheng, D., Wang, J., Duong, D.M., Losik, G., Gearing, M., Rees, H.D., Lah, J.J., Levey, A.I. and Peng, J. (2004) Proteomic characterization of postmortem amyloid plaques isolated by laser capture microdissection. *The Journal of Biological Chemistry*, **279**, 37061–37068.

Link, A.J., Jennings, J.L. and Washburn, M.P. (2003) Analysis of protein composition using multidimensional chromatography and mass spectrometry, in *Current Protocols in Protein Science* (eds J.E. Coligan, B.M. Dunn, D.W. Speicher and P.T. Wingfield), John Wiley & Sons, Inc., New York, pp. 23.1.1–23.1.25.

Moore, R.E., Young, M.K. and Lee, T.D. (2000) Protein identification using a quadrupole ion trap mass spectrometer and SEQUEST database matching, in *Current Protocols in Protein Science* (eds J.E. Coligan, B.M. Dunn, D.W. Speicher and P.T. Wingfield), John Wiley & Sons, Inc., New York, pp. 16.10.1–16.10.9.

Liu, H., Harrell, L.E., Shenvi, S., Hagen, T. and Liu, R.-M. (2005) Gender differences in glutathione metabolism in Alzheimer's disease. *Journal of Neuroscience Research*, **79**, 861–867.

Lowenthal, M.S., Metha, A.I., Frogfale, K., Bandle, R.W., Araujo, R.P., Hood, B.L., Veenstra, T.D., Conrads, T.P., Goldsmith, P., Fishman, D., Petricoin, E.F., III and Liotta, L.A. (2005) Analysis of albumin-associated peptides and proteins from ovarian cancer patients. *Clinical Chemistry*, **51**, 1933–1945.

Lundgren, D.H., Eng, J.K. and Han, D.K. (2005) Protein identification using TurboSEQUEST, in *Current Protocols in Bioinformatics* (eds A.D. Baxevanis, D.B. Davison, R.D.M. Page, G.A. Petsko, L.D. Stein and G.D. Stormo), John Wiley & Sons, Inc., New York, pp. 13.3.1–13.3.13.

Lukas, T.J., Luo, W.W., Mao, H., Cole, N. and Siddique, T. (2006) Informatics-assisted protein profiling in a transgenic mouse model of amyotrophic lateral sclerosis. *Molecular and Cellular Proteomics*, **5**, 1233–1244.

Lunemann, J.D., Edwards, N., Muraro, P.A., Hayashi, S., Cohen, J.I., Munz, C. and Martin, R. (2006) Increased frequency and broadened specificity of latent EBV nuclear antigen-l-specific T cells in multiple sclerosis. *Brain*, **129**, 1493–1506.

Maccarone, G., Milfay, D., Birg, I., Rosenhagen, M., Holsboer, F., Grimm, R., Bailley, R., Zolotarjova, N. and Turck, C.W. (2004) Mining the human cerebrospinal fluid proteome by immunodepletion and shotgun mass spectrometry. *Electrophoresis*, **25**, 2402–2412.

Mackay, G.M., Forrest, C.M., Stoy, N., Christofides, J., Egerton, M., Stone, T.W. and Darlinton, L.G. (2006) Tryptophan metabolism and oxidative stress in patients with chronic brain injury. *European Journal of Neurology*, **13**, 30–42.

Misra, U.K., Kalita, J., Pandey, S., Khanna, V.K. and Babu, G.N. (2005) Cerebrospinal fluid catecholamine levels in Japanese encephalitis patients with movement disorders. *Neurochemical Research*, **30**, 1075–1078.

Mor, G., Visintin, I., Lai, Y., Zhao, H., Schwartz, P., Rutherford, T., Yue, L., Bray-Ward, P. and Ward, D.C. (2005) Serum protein markers for early detection of ovarian cancer. *Proceedings of the National Academy of Sciences of the United States of America*, **102**, 7677–7682.

Mussalman, I. and Speicher, D.W. (2005) Human serum and plasma proteomics, in *Current Protocols in Protein Science* (eds J.E. Coligan, B.M. Dunn, D.W. Speicher and P.T. Wingfield), John Wiley & Sons, Inc., New York, pp. 24.1.1–24.1.18.

Parnetti, L., Lanari, A., Silvestrelli, G., Saggese, E. and Reboldi, P. (2006) Diagnosing prodromal Alzheimer's disease: role of CSF biochemical markers. *Mechanisms of Ageing and Development*, **127**, 129–132.

Patterson, S.D. (1998) Protein identification and characterization by mass spectrometry, In: *Current Protocols in Molecular Biology* (eds F.M. Ausubel, R. Brent, R.E. Kingston, D.D. Moore, J.G. Seidman, J.A. Smith and K. Struhl), John Wiley & Sons, Inc., New York, pp. 10.22.1–10.22.24.

Petrovitch, H., White, L.R., Ross, G.W., Steinhorn, S.C., Li, C.Y., Masaki, K.H., Davis, D.G., Nelson, J., Hardman, J., Curb, J.D., Blanchette, P.L., Launer, L.J., Yano, K. and Markesbery, W.R. (2001) Accuracy of clinical criteria for AD in the Honolulu-Asia Aging Study, a population-based study. *Neurology*, **57**, 226–234.

Pinkse, M.W.H., Uitto, P.M., Hilhorst, M.J., Ooms, B. and Heck, A.J.R. (2004) Selective isolation at the femtomole level of phosphopeptides from proteolytic digests using 2D-nanoLC-ESI-MS/MS and titanium dioxide precolumns. *Analytical Chemistry*, **76**, 3935–3943.

Puchades, M., Folkesson, S.F., Nilsson, C.L., Andreasen, N., Blennow, K. and Davidsson, P. (2003) Proteomic studies of potential cerebrospinal fluid protein markers for Alzheimer's disease. *Molecular Brain Research*, **118**, 140–146.

Qiu, R. and Regnier, F.E. (2005) Comparative glycoproteomics of N-linked complex- type glycoforms containing sialic acid in human serum. *Analytical Chemistry*, **77**, 7225–7231.

Rada, R., Tucci, S., Teneud, L., Paez, X., Perez, J., Alba, G., Garcia, Y., Sacchettoni, S., del Corral, J. and Hernandez, L. (1999) Monitoring γ-aminobutyric acid in human brain and plasma microdialysates using micellar electrokinetic chromatography and laser-induced fluorescence detection. *Journal of Chromatography B*, **735**, 1–10.

Rafai, N., Gillette, M.A. and Carr, S.A. (2006) Protein biomarker discovery and validation: the long and uncertain path to clinical utility. *Nature Biotechnology*, **24**, 971–983.

Rajda, C., Dibo, G., Vecsei, L. and Bergguist, J. (2005) Increased dopamine content in lymphocytes from high-dose L-Dopa-treated Parkinson's disease patients. *Neuroimmunomodulation*, **12**, 81–84.

Reynolds, K.J. and Fenselau, K. (2003) Quantitative protein analysis using proteolytic [^{18}O] water labeling, in *Current Protocols in Protein Science* (eds J.E. Coligan, B.M. Dunn, D.W. Speicher and P.T. Wingfield), John Wiley & Sons, Inc., New York, pp. 23.4.1–23.4.8.

Righetti, G.P., Bossi, A. and Gelfi, C. (2003) Capillary electrophoresis of peptides and proteins using isoelectric buffers, in *Current Protocols in Protein Science* (eds J.E. Coligan, B.M. Dunn, D.W. Speicher and P.T. Wingfield), John Wiley & Sons, Inc., New York, pp. 10.13.1–10.13.16.

Rosengren, L.E., Karlsson, J.-E., Karlsson, J.-O., Persson, L.I. and Wikkelso, C. (1996) Patients with amyotrophic lateral sclerosis and other neurodegenerative diseases have increased levels of neurofilament protein in CSF. *Journal of Neurochemistry*, **67**, 2013–2018.

Ross, L., Huang, Y.N., Marchese, J.N., Williamson, B., Parker, K., Hattan, S., Khainovski, N., Pillai, S., Dey, S., Daniels, S., Purkayastha, S., Juhasz, P., Martin, S., Bartlet-Jones, M., He, F., Jacobson, A. and Pappin, D.J. (2004) Multiplexed protein quantitation in Saccharomyces cerevisiae using amine-reactive isobaric tagging reagents. *Molecular and Cellular Proteomics*, **3**, 1154–1169.

Ruetschi, U., Zetterberg, H., Podust, V.N., Gottfries, J., Li, S., Simonsen, A.H., McGuire, J., Karlsson, M., Rymo, L., Davies, H., Minthon, L. and Blennow, K. (2005) Identification of CSF biomarkers for frontotemporal dementia using SELDI-TOF. *Experimental Neurology*, **196**, 273–281.

Schmidt, C., Hofmann, U., Kohlmuller, D., Murdter, T., Zanger, U.M., Schwab, M. and Hoffmann, G.F. (2005) Comprehensive analysis of pyrimidine metabolism in 450 children with unspecific neurological symptoms using high-pressure liquid chromatography-electrospray ionization tandem mass spectrometry. *Journal of Inherited Metabolic Disease*, **28**, 1109–1122.

Siest, G. *et al.* (2000) Apolipoprotein E polymorphism and serum concentration in Alzheimer's disease in nine European centres: the ApoEurope Study. *Clinical Chemistry and Laboratory Medicine*, **38**, 721–730.

Sullivan Pepe, M., Etzioni, R., Feng, Z., Potter, J.D., Thompson, M.L., Thornquist, M., Winget, M. and Yasui, Y. (2001) Phases of biomarker development for early detection of cancer. *Journal of the National Cancer Institute*, **93**, 1054–1061.

Terry, D.E. and Desiderio, D.M. (2003) Between-gel reproducibility of the human cerebrospinal fluid proteome. *Proteomics*, **3**, 1962–1979.

Teunissen, C.E., Dijkstra, C. and Polman, C. (2005) Biological markers in CSF and blood for axonal degeration in multiple sclerosis. *Lancet Neurology*, **4**, 32–41.

Varesio, E., Rudaz, S., Krause, K.H. and Veuthey, J.-L. (2002) Nanoscale liquid chromatography and capillary electrophoresis coupled to electrospray mass spectrometry for the detection of amyloid-β peptide related to Alzheimer's disease. *Journal of Chromatography A*, **974**, 135–142.

Veenstra, T.D., Conrads, T.P., Hood, B.L., Avellino, A.M., Ellenbogen, R.G. and Morrison, R.S. (2005) Biomarkers: mining the biofluid proteome. *Molecular and Cellular Proteomics*, **4**, 409–418.

Vosseller, K., Trinidad, J.C., Chalkley, R.J., Specht, C.G., Thalhammer, A., Lynn, A.J., Snedecort, J.O., Gaun, S. and Burlingame, A.L. (2006) O-Linked N-acetylglucosamine proteomics of postsynaptic density preparations using lectin weak affinity chromatography. *Molecular and Cellular Proteomics*, **5**, 923–934.

Viglio, S., Marchi, E., Wisniewski, K., Casado, B., Cetta, G. and Ladarola, P. (2001) Diagnosis of late-infantile neuronal ceroid lipofuscinosis: a new sensitive method to assay lysosomal pepstatin-insensitive proteinase activity in human and animal specimens by capillary electrophoresis. *Electrophoresis*, **22**, 2343–2350.

Wall, D.B., Kachman, M.T., Gong, S., Hinderer, R., Parus, S., Misek, D.E., Hanash, S.M. and Lubman, D.M. (2000) Isoelectric focusing nonporous RP HPLC: a two- dimensional liquid-phase separation method for mapping of cellular proteins with identification using MALDI-FOF mass spectrometry. *Analytical Chemistry*, **72**, 1099–1111.

Want, E., O'Maille, G., Smith, C., Brandon, T.R., Uritboonthai, W., Qin, C., Trauger, S.A. and Siuzdak, G. (2006) Solvent-dependent metabolite distribution, clustering, and protein extraction for serum profiling with mass spectrometry. *Analytical Chemistry*, **78**, 743–752.

Washburn, M.P., Wolters, D., and Yates, J.R., III (2001) Large-scale analysis of the yeast proteome by multidimensional protein identification technology. *Nature Biotechnology*, **19**, 242–247.

Wilson, K.E., Marouga, R., Prime, J.E., Pashby, D.P., Orange, P.R., Crosier, S., Keith, A.B., Lathe, R., Mullins, J., Estibeiro, P., Bergling, H., Hawkins, E. and Morrid, C.M. (2005) Comparative proteomic analysis using samples obtained with laser microdissection and saturation dye labelling. *Proteomics*, **5**, 3851–3858.

Wittke, S., Mischak, H., Walden, M., Kolch, W., Radler, T. and Wiedemann, K. (2005) Discovery of biomarkers in human urine and cerebrospinal fluid by capillary electrophoresis coupled to mass spectromerty: toward new diagnostic and therapeutic approaches. *Electrophoresis*, **26**, 1476–1487.

Wu, W.W., Wang, G., Baek, S.J. and Shen, R.-F. (2006) Comparative study of three quantitative methods, DIGE, cICAT, and iTRAQ, using 2D gel- or LC-MALDI TOF/TOF. *Journal of Proteome Research*, **5**, 651–658.

Xiao, T., Ying, W., Li, L., Hu, Z., Ma, Y., Jiao, L., Ma, J., Cai, Y., Lin, D., Guo, S., Han, N., Di, X., Li, M., Zhang, D., Su, K., Yaun, J., Zheng, H., Gao, M., He, J., Shi, S., Li, W., Xu, N., Zhang, H., Lui, Y., Zhang, K., Gao, Y., Qian, X. and Cheng, S. (2005) An approach to studying lung cancer-related proteins in human blood. *Molecular and Cellular Proteomics*, **10**, 1480–1486.

Xiao, Z., Conrads, T.P., Lucas, D.A., Janini, G.M., Schaefer, C.F., Buetow, K.H., Issaq, H.J. and Veenstra, T.D. (2004) Direct ampholyte-free liquid-phase isoelectric peptide focusing: application to the human serum proteome. *Electrophoresis*, **25**, 128–133.

Xiong, L., Andrews, D. and Regnier, F. (2003) Comparative proteomics of glycoproteins based on lectin selection and isotope coding. *Journal of Proteome Research*, **2**, 618–625.

Yang, Z. and Hancock, W.S. (2004) Approch to the comprehensive analysis of glycoproteins isoalted from human serum using a multi-lectin affinity column. *Journal of Chromatography. A*, **1053**, 79–88.

Yao, X., Freas, A., Ramirez, J., Demirev, P.A. and Fenselau, C. (2001) Proteolytic ^{18}O labeling for comparative proteomics: model studies with two serotypes of Adenovirus. *Analytical Chemistry*, **73**, 2836–2842.

Yi, E.C. and Goodlett, D.R. (2003) Quantitative protein profile comparisons using the isotope-coded affinity tag method, in *Current Protocols in Protein Science* (eds Coligan, J.E., Dunn, B.M., Speicher, D.W. and Wingfield, P.T.), John Wiley & Sons, Inc., New York, pp. 23.2.1–23.2.11.

You, J.-S., Gelfanova, V. and Knierman, M.D. (2005) The impact of blood contamination on the proteome of cerebrospinal fluid. *Proteomics*, **5**, 290–296.

Yu, L.R., Conrads, T.P., Uo, T., Kinoshita, Y., Morrison, R.S., Lucas, D.A., Chan, K.C., Blonder, J., Issaq, H.J. and Veenstra, T.D. (2004) Global analysis of the cortical neuron proteome. *Molecular and Cellular Proteomics*, **3**, 896–907.

Yu, L.R., Conrads, T.P., Uo, T., Issaq, H.J., Morrison, R.S. and Veenstra, T.D. (2004) Evaluation of the acid-cleavable isotope-codes affinity tag reagent: application to camptothecin-treated cortical neurons. *Journal of Proteomic Research*, **3**, 469–477.

Zhang, J., Goodlett, D.R., Peskind, E.R., Quinn, J.F., Zhou, Y., Wang, J., Pan, C., Yi, E., Eng, J., Aebersold, R.H. and Montine, T.J. (2005) Quantitative proteomics of age-related changes in human cerebrospinal fluid. *Neurobiology of Aging*, **26**, 207–227.

Zhang, J., Goodlett, D.R., Quinn, J.F., Peskind, E., Kaye, J.A., Zhou, Y., Pan, C.,

Yi, E., Eng, J., Wang, Q., Aebersold, R.H. and Montine, T.J. (2005) Quantitative proteomics of cerebrospinal fluid from patients with Alzheimer's disease. *Journal of Alzheimer's Disease*, **7**, 125–133.

Zhao, H., Simeone, D.M., Heidt, D., Anderson, M.A. and Lubman, D.M. (2006) Comparative serum glycoproteomics using lectin selected sialic acid glycoproteins with mass spectrometric analysis: applications to pancreatic cancer serum. *Journal of Proteome Research*, **5**, 1792–1802.

Zhou, G., Li, H., DeCamp, D., Chen, S., Shu, H., Gong, Y., Flaig, M., Gillespie, J.W., Hu, N., Taylor, P.R., Emmert-buck, M.R., Liotta, L.A., Petricoin, E.F. and Zhao, Y. (2002) 2D Differential in-gel electrophoresis for the identification of esophageal scans cell cancer-specific protein markers. *Molecular and Cellular Proteomics*, **1**, 117–124.

Zhu, K., Yan, F., O'Neil, K.A., Hamler, R., Lubman, D.M., Lin, L. and Barder, T.J. (2003) Protein analysis using 2-D liquid separations of intact proteins from whole-cell lysates, in *Current Protocols in Protein Science Science* (eds J.E. Coligan, B.M. Dunn, D.W. Speicher and P.T. Wingfield), John Wiley & Sons, Inc., New York, pp. 23.3.1–23.3.28.

14

Redox Proteomics: Applications to Age-Related Neurodegenerative Disorders

Rukhsana Sultana, Shelley F. Newman and D. Allan Butterfield

14.1
Introduction

14.1.1
Protein Oxidation

Oxidative stress occurs due to an imbalance in pro- and antioxidants either by a decrease in antioxidants or an increase in pro-oxidants. Also, loss of degradation potential of oxidized proteins, for example, loss of proteasomal activity, can lead to elevated markers of oxidative stress. Pro-oxidants include reactive oxygen species (ROS) and reactive nitrogen species (RNS), which are highly reactive with biomolecules, including proteins and lipids (Butterfield, 1997). A specific example of an ROS is superoxide ($O_2^{-\cdot}$) that leaks from complex I and complex III in mitochondria (Chen *et al.*, 2003). Superoxide can react with other biomolecules to cause direct damage or indirect damage by producing other pro-oxidant molecules such as a hydroxide radical (HO$^{\cdot}$). Oxidative damage leads to cellular dysfunctions (Mark *et al.*, 1997; Markesbery, 1997; Smith *et al.*, 1997; Lovell and Markesbery, 2001; Butterfield, 2002; Butterfield and Lauderback, 2002; Butterfield *et al.*, 2002; Castegna *et al.*, 2004a). Markers of oxidative stress commonly observed in biological samples include protein carbonyls, protein-bound 3-nitrotyrosine (3-NT), and 4-hydroxy-2-*trans*-nonenal (HNE)-modified proteins.

Protein carbonyls are a relatively stable modification and are widely used as markers to determine the extent of protein oxidation (Berlett and Stadtman, 1997; Butterfield and Stadtman, 1997; Stadtman and Levine, 2003; Dalle-Donne *et al.*, 2006). Protein carbonyl groups are generated by direct oxidation of specific amino acid side-chains (i.e. Lys, Arg, Pro, Thr, and His, etc.), peptide backbone scission, Michael addition reactions of His, Lys, and Cys residues with α,β-unsaturated aldehydes, or glycol-oxidation of Lys amino groups (Berlett and Stadtman, 1997; Butterfield and Stadtman, 1997; Stadtman and Levine, 2003; Dalle-Donne *et al.*, 2005, 2006). Protein carbonyl levels can be

Proteomics of the Nervous System. Edited by H.G. Nothwang and S.E. Pfeiffer
Copyright © 2008 WILEY-VCH Verlag GmbH & Co. KGaA, Weinheim
ISBN: 978-3-527-31716-5

determined experimentally by derivatization of the carbonyl groups with 2,4-dinitrophenylhydrazine (DNPH), followed by immunochemical detection of the resulting hydrazone product (Levine *et al.*, 1994; Butterfield and Stadtman, 1997; Dalle-Donne *et al.*, 2006).

One consequence of protein oxidation are conformational changes, which may expose hydrophobic residues to an aqueous environment. This can result in loss of structural or functional activity, and aggregation, thereby disrupting cellular function. Another consequence is the overexpression of inducible nitric oxide synthase (iNOS) and neuronal NOS (nNOS) that increase the production of nitric oxide via the catalytic conversion of arginine to citrulline. Nitric oxide reacts with superoxide anion (O_2^-) to produce peroxynitrite ($ONOO^-$), which rapidly reacts with a variety of substrates depending upon its cellular environment. If a free tyrosine residue is available, peroxynitrite in the presence of CO_2 produces 3-NT (Koppenol *et al.*, 1992), which is a marker of nitrosative stress in a variety of disease conditions (Beckman and Koppenol, 1996; Ischiropoulos, 2003).

14.1.2
Neurological Disorders and Oxidative Stress

Alzheimer's disease, Parkinson's disease, amyotrophic lateral sclerosis (ALS), and Huntington's disease are all major neurodegenerative disorders where oxidative stress is implicated. Alzheimer's disease is an age-related disorder that is characterized clinically by a progressive loss of memory and cognitive functions (Mirra *et al.*, 1991) (see Chapter 12). Neuropathologically, Alzheimer's disease hallmarks include the accumulation of two types of insoluble fibrous material: extracellular amyloid-β peptide deposited in senile plaques and intracellular neurofibrillary tangles primarily compiled of abnormal and hyperphosphorylated tau protein (Selkoe, 2001). Mild cognitive impairment (MCI) is considered as a transition stage between normal and Alzheimer's disease pathogenesis. Parkinson's disease is a progressive disorder with dopaminergic neuronal loss in the substantia nigra as well as Lewy body formation (Pearce *et al.*, 1997). Clinically, Parkinson's disease affects motor control causing rigidity, uncontrolled tremors, and potentially loss of movement. ALS is one of the most common neuromuscular diseases worldwide and is marked by gradual degeneration of the upper and lower motor neurons that control voluntary muscle movement (Carri *et al.*, 2003). Finally, Huntington's disease is a hereditary neurodegenerative disorder distinguished by motor, psychiatric, and cognitive symptoms (Beal *et al.*, 1993a, 1993b; Browne *et al.*, 1999). All of these diseases are connected by an increase in oxidative stress that damages neurons.

The identification of oxidatively modified proteins, especially in neurodegenerative diseases, is the ongoing pursuit of redox proteomics (Butterfield and Boyd-Kimball, 2004; Butterfield *et al.*, 2006a). Many proteomics studies have provided confirmation of the oxidative damage of particular proteins in neurodegenerative diseases (Smith *et al.*, 1994, 1997; Wang *et al.*, 2005). Using redox proteomics we have evaluated the changes in brain protein carbonyls, HNE adducts, and the nitration of tyrosine residues in Alzheimer's disease, MCI, and models of Alzheimer's disease, Huntington's disease, ALS and Parkinson's disease (Castegna *et al.*, 2002a, 2002b, 2003; Perluigi *et al.*, 2005b; Poon *et al.*, 2005a, 2005b; Butterfield *et al.*, 2006b; Sultana *et al.*, 2006b, 2006c).

14.1.3
Principles of Redox Proteomics

Redox proteomics has been employed in our laboratory to identify significant oxidation of brain proteins from a subject with a neurodegenerative disease (Alzheimer's disease) compared to those from an age-matched neurologically normal control. As practised in our laboratory, redox proteomics couples two-dimensional polyacrylamide gel electrophoresis (2D-PAGE) with immunoblotting to detect proteins that are oxidized more in disease than in control samples (Figure 14.1). Interesting proteins are then identified by mass spectrometry.

To maximize results in our laboratory, chaotropic agents such as urea and thiourea are coupled with non-ionic or zwitterionic detergents to solubilize proteins and to avoid protein precipitation during 2D-PAGE. Experience has shown that the use of immobilized pH isoelectric focusing (IEF) strips instead of tube gels avoids catalytic drift, thereby improving reproducibility between samples. Narrow-range IEF strips have been incorporated to give higher resolution separation in a particular area of interest of a 2D-PAGE map. However, one should bear in mind that 2D-PAGE hardly displays membrane and highly basic proteins (see Chapter 2). Oxidatively modified proteins are subsequently detected by immunoblot analysis using specific antibodies against protein carbonyls derivatized by DNPH, HNE-modified proteins, or nitrated proteins indexed by 3-NT. These blots are then matched to 2D-PAGE of the same sample stained with Sypro Ruby using computer-assisted image analysis (Figure 14.2).

14.1.4
Redox Proteomics in Alzheimer's Disease and Mild Cognitive Impairment

Our redox proteomics studies accomplished the identification of oxidatively modified proteins, indexed either by increased carbonyl levels or by increased 3-NT levels, in the inferior parietal lobule and in the hippocampus of patients with Alzheimer's disease (Table 14.1). Both brain regions are rich in β-amyloid. In contrast, we did not observe protein oxidation in the cerebellum, which shows low levels of β-amyloid and is little affected in Alzheimer's disease. In this section, we discuss the putative role of selected oxidized proteins in the pathogenesis of Alzheimer's disease.

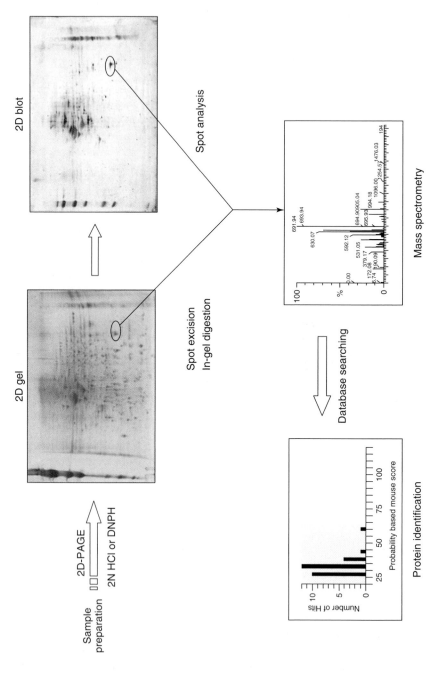

Figure 14.1 Schematic workflow of the basic protocol for the identification of oxidized proteins by redox proteomics.

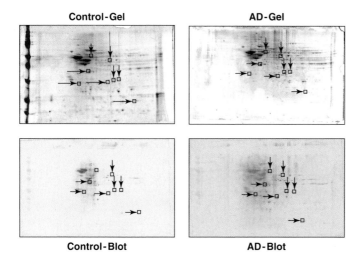

Control-Gel **AD-Gel**

Control-Blot **AD-Blot**

Figure 14.2 Images of Sypro Ruby-stained 2D gels (a and c) and blots probed for protein carbonyls (b and d) from control and Alzheimer's disease subjects, respectively. The arrows within the boxed areas indicate a number of oxidized proteins, both in a qualitative and quantitative manner. (Please find a color version of this figure in the color plates.)

Table 14.1 Oxidatively modified proteins identified in brain from Alzheimer's disease and/or mild cognitive impairment patients using redox proteomics.

Protein functions	Oxidized proteins
Energy-related enzymes	CK, Enolase, TPI, PGM1, LDH, GAPDH, PK
Neurotransmitter-related proteins	EAAT2, GS
Proteasome-related proteins	UCH-L1, HSC 71
Cholinergic system	Neuropolypeptide h3
pH regulation-protein	CA2 II
Structural proteins	DRP2, β-actin
Cell cycle; Tau phosphorylation	Pin1
Synaptic abnormalities and LTP	Gamma-SNAP
Mitochondrial abnormalities	ATP synthase alpha chain, VDAC-1

CK, creatine kinase BB; TPI, triose phosphate isomerase; PK, pyruvate kinase; PGM1, phosphoglycerate mutase 1; LDH, lactate dehydrogenase; EATT2, excitatory amino acid transporter 2; GS, glutamine synthase; UCH-L1, ubiquitin C-terminal hydrolase L-1; HSC 71, heat shock cognate 71; DRP2, dihydropyrimidinase-related protein 2; Pin1, peptidyl-prolyl *cis-trans* isomerase; gamma-SNAP, gamma-soluble NSF-attachment proteins; VDAC, voltage-dependent anion channel protein.

Numerous studies using positron emission tomography (PET) and other methods have demonstrated reduced glucose utilization and decreased activity of glucose metabolism enzymes in Alzheimer's disease (Iwangoff *et al.*, 1980; Meier-Ruge *et al.*, 1984; Messier and Gagnon, 1996; Vanhanen and Soininen, 1998; Rapoport, 1999; Watson and Craft, 2004; Sultana *et al.*, 2006b). Using redox proteomics, we have identified in brain tissue from Alzheimer's disease patients a number of oxidatively modified proteins that are involved in energy metabolism, such as creatine kinase, alpha-enolase (ENO1), triosephosphate isomerase (TPI), glyceraldehyde 3-phosphate dehydrogenase (GAPDH), phosphoglycerate mutase 1 (PGM1), voltage-dependent anion channel protein 1 (VDAC-1), and α-ATPase (Table 14.1) (Castegna *et al.*, 2002a, 2002b, 2003; Sultana *et al.*, 2006b, 2006c).

Interestingly, in the brains of MCI patients we also identified oxidation of two proteins important for energy metabolism: enolase and pyruvate kinase (Butterfield *et al.*, 2006b) (Table 14.1). Since MCI is considered to be a transition stage between normal and Alzheimer's disease pathogenesis, the identification of enolase as a common target for oxidation in the hippocampus from Alzheimer's disease and MCI patients suggests that this protein is highly sensitive to oxidative modification and that the energy pathway is among the first to be compromised during the progression of this disease.

One of the hallmarks of the pathogenesis of Alzheimer's disease is the presence of protein aggregates such as amyloid in the form of plaques or tau in the form of tangles. Using redox proteomics we identified carbonic anhydrase II (CA2), peptidyl prolyl *cis-trans* isomerase (Pin1), and ubiquitin C-terminal hydrolase L1 (UCH-L1) as oxidized proteins in Alzheimer's disease (Table 14.1) (Castegna *et al.*, 2002a; Sultana *et al.*, 2006b, 2006c). CA2 plays a crucial role in regulating intracellular pH and has been shown to display decreased activity in Alzheimer's disease (Meier-Ruge *et al.*, 1984). Since intracellular pH is important for the structure and function of proteins, decreased CA2 activity favors the formation of protein aggregation. The oxidation of Pin1 may increase phosphorylation of tau via its action on phosphatases, thereby potentially contributing to tangle formation. In addition, Pin1 has been reported to show decreased expression and activity in brain from both MCI and Alzheimer's disease patients (Lu *et al.*, 1999; Butterfield *et al.*, 2006b; Sultana *et al.*, 2006a). Finally, UCH-L1 belongs to the ubiquitin-proteasome system (UPS) and plays an important role in protein degradation (Castegna *et al.*, 2004b). Oxidized UCH-L1 suggests that the UPS might be functionally constrained, leading to protein aggregation and finally synaptic degeneration as reported in brain from Alzheimer's disease patients (Castegna *et al.*, 2002a; Sultana *et al.*, 2006b). The presence of oxidized UCH-L1 in brain from Alzheimer's disease patients has been confirmed by others (Choi *et al.*, 2004).

Another set of oxidized proteins that might be involved in impaired neurotransmission and learning and memory formation in Alzheimer's disease patients includes oxidized dihydropyrimidinase-related protein 2 (DRP2), β-actin, gamma-SNAP, glutamine synthase, and the glutamate transporter EAAT2 (Glt-1) (Table 14.1) (Lauderback *et al.*, 2001; Castegna *et al.*, 2002a; Castegna *et al.*, 2002b, 2003; Sultana *et al.*, 2006b). Decreased activities of the EAAT2 and glutamine synthase may in addition lead to increased excitotoxicity, which might be involved in the pathogenesis of synaptic damage and neurodegeneration in Alzheimer's disease.

Finally, we identified the neuropolypeptide h3 as being oxidized (Table 14.1). This protein plays an important role in regulating choline acetyl transferase (ChAT) and may be involved in maintaining phospholipid asymmetry. Both processes are important for normal mitochondrial and plasma membrane function. Our results correlate well with a previous study that reported decreased activity of ChAT in Alzheimer's disease brain (Davies *et al.*, 1999).

14.1.5
Redox Proteomics in Models of Parkinson's Disease, Huntington's Disease, Amyotrophic Lateral Sclerosis: Similarities and Difference to Alzheimer's Disease

Similar redox proteomics analyses of brains from rodent models of the age-related neurodegenerative disorders Parkinson's disease, Huntington's disease, and ALS have been conducted. A list of oxidized proteins is provided in Table 14.2. In each case, the proteins identified as being oxidatively modified are consistent with the known biochemical and/or pathological alterations in these disorders.

One oxidized protein common to Alzheimer's disease, Huntington's disease, Parkinson's disease, and the G93A-SOD1 transgenic mice model of heritable or familial ALS (fALS) is alpha-enolase (Tables 14.1 and 14.2) (Castegna *et al.*, 2002a, 2002b, 2003; Perluigi *et al.*, 2005a, 2005b; Poon *et al.*, 2005a, 2005b; Sultana *et al.*, 2006b, 2006c). The identification of oxidized alpha-enolase in all four conditions analyzed suggests a high susceptibility of this protein to oxidative modification. Consequently, energy pathways are among the most vulnerable to oxidative impairment in all these pathologies.

Further oxidized proteins shared between Alzheimer's disease and Huntington's disease include the previously discussed proteins VDAC-1, gamma-enolase, and CK (Castegna *et al.*, 2002a, 2003; Perluigi *et al.*, 2005b; Sultana *et al.*, 2006c). Consistent with the oxidative modification of CK is the reported decrease in CK activity both in Alzheimer's disease and Huntington's disease (Aksenov *et al.*, 2000; Castegna *et al.*, 2002a). Furthermore, creatine therapy provides neuroprotection and delays motor symptoms in a transgenic animal model of Huntington's disease (Dedeoglu *et al.*, 2003). These findings suggest that enhancement of cerebral energy metabolism is a protective mechanism against neurodegeneration. The identification of oxidized VDAC-1 both in Alzheimer's disease and in Huntington's disease might shed some light on the mechanistic cause underlying altered mitochondrial Ca^{2+} homeostasis in these two conditions, as the channel provides a route for calcium to cross the outer mitochondrial membrane. In contrast to the above mentioned proteins, aconitase

Table 14.2 Oxidatively modified brain proteins identified in Parkinson's disease, amyotrophic lateral sclerosis, and Huntington's disease mouse models using redox proteomics.

Oxidatively modified proteins	PD model	HD model	ALS model
Carbonic anhydrase 2	X		
Alpha-enolase	X	X	X
Gamma-enolase		X	
Lactate dehydrogenase	X		
Creatine kinase		X	
Aconitase		X	
HSP90		X	
Voltage-dependent anion channel protein 1		X	
αB crystalline			X
Transcriptionally controlled tumor protein 1			X
Cu,Zn-superoxide dismutase			X
Ubiquitin C-terminal hydrolase isozyme L1			X
Dihydropyrimidinase-related protein			X
Hsp70			X

ALS, amyotrophic lateral sclerosis; PD, Parkinson's disease; HD, Huntington's disease.

and HSP90 are proteins that were found to be oxidatively modified in Huntington's disease but not in Alzheimer's disease (Table 14.2) (Perluigi *et al.*, 2005b).

When comparing Alzheimer's disease and Parkinson's disease, lactate dehydrogenase was found to be oxidized in both disorders (Castegna *et al.*, 2003; Poon *et al.*, 2005a). LDH is a glycolytic protein that catalyzes the reversible NAD-dependent interconversion of pyruvate to lactate. Under post-ischemic/hypoxia conditions, lactate competes with glucose as an oxidizible energy substrate to support neuronal recovery (Schurr *et al.*, 1997; Murata *et al.*, 2000; Cater *et al.*, 2003).

UCH-L1 and DRP-2 are oxidized proteins in common between Alzheimer's disease and ALS (Table 14.2) (Castegna *et al.*, 2002a; Perluigi *et al.*, 2005a; Poon *et al.*, 2005b). UCH-L1 plays an important role in the UPS. Its oxidation may lead to impaired protein degradation and accumulation of aggregated and damaged proteins, which are observed in both disorders (Castegna *et al.*, 2002a; Perluigi *et al.*, 2005a; Poon *et al.*, 2005b).

In summary, redox proteomics results suggest that in Alzheimer's disease and related disease models, oxidative modifications are more pronounced in proteins that are related directly or indirectly to mitochondria, making mitochondria the prime target of oxidative stress.

14.2
Methods

14.2.1
Sample Preparation

It is often necessary to isolate particular brain areas of interest for proteomic studies as disease-based alterations are often very local. Microdissection is one method of obtaining the desired substructures (Sitek *et al.*, 2005). Careful sample handling including complete freezing from the moment the sample is obtained is crucial to the integrity of the results. Protein degradation can profoundly affect the visualized protein pattern (Fountoulakis and Takacs, 2001). The fundamental goal of sample preparation is to have efficient, quantitative solubilization of cellular proteins. The simplest procedure reduces the occurrence of unspecific protein loss and alterations in protein structure. Coupled to this prerequisite for proper proteomic analysis is the necessity to have a rapid autopsy in the case of human samples and to obtain fresh brain tissue in the case of animals.

14.2.2
Preparation of Samples

Requirements

Solutions: Medium I (10 mM HEPES buffer (pH 7.4) containing 137 mM NaCl, 4.6 mM KCl, 1.1 mM KH_2PO_4, 0.6 mM $MgSO_4$, and proteinase inhibitors: leupeptin (0.5 mg mL^{-1}), pepstatin (0.7 µg mL^{-1}), type IIS soybean trypsin inhibitor (0.5 µg mL^{-1}), and PMSF (40 µg mL^{-1}); 10 mM DNPH prepared in 2 N HCl; 2 N HCl; 30% ice-cold trichloroacetic acid (TCA); ethanol:ethyl acetate (1 : 1).
1. Homogenize the samples (10% w/v) in ice-cold medium I.
2. Centrifuge the homogenates 14 000 × g for 10 min. This will remove unbroken cells and debris.
3. The supernatant is used for proteomics analysis, whereas the pellet is discarded.
4. Protein concentration in the supernatant is determined by the Pierce BCA method.

14.2.3
Sample Derivatization

1. Split the sample into two aliquots (referred to as A and B) each containing 100–150 µg protein.
2. For detection of carbonylated proteins, incubate aliquot A with 4 times the sample volume of 10 mM 2,4-dinitrophenylhydrazone, vortex the

sample and incubate at room temperature for 30 min. This aliquot will later be used for immunoblot analysis.

3. Add 4 times the volume of 2 N HCl to aliquot B, followed by incubation at room temperature for 30 min. This aliquot will be used for Sypro Ruby staining.
4. Add 30% ice-cold TCA to both aliquots and incubate for 10 min on ice. Samples for HNE and 3-NT are also TCA precipitated.
5. Centrifuge for 5 min at $14\,000 \times g$ at $4\,°C$ and discard the supernatant.
6. Wash the pellet 4 times with ice-cold ethanol:ethyl acetate $(1:1)$. This will remove lipids, excess TCA and salts from the samples.

14.2.4
Two-Dimensional Protein Gel Electrophoresis

14.2.4.1 First Dimension (Isoelectric Focusing)

Requirements

Material: IPG readystrip (pH 3–10; Bio-Rad Laboratories, Hercules, CA, USA); mineral oil.

Solutions: Rehydration buffer (8 M urea, 2 M thiourea, 2% CHAPS, 0.2% (v/v) biolytes, 50 mM dithiothreitol (DTT), and traces of bromophenol blue).

Instrumentation: Isoelectric focusing unit (e.g. protean IEF cell (Bio-Rad)).
1. Add 200 μL of rehydration buffer to the pellet and incubate for 1 h at room temperature with continuous vortexing.
2. Sonicate the samples for 10 s and then apply 180 μL of sample to an IPG tray and place the IPG readystrip, positive side of the strip facing the positive side of the IEF tray and gel-side facing down.
3. Start active rehydration for 1 h at $20\,°C$. At the end of 1 h add 2 mL of mineral oil on to the IPG strip and then continue active rehydration for 16 h at 50 V and $20\,°C$ with the protean IEF cell.
4. After 16 h, carry out IEF at $20\,°C$ as follows: 800 V for 2 h using a linear gradient, 1200 V for 4 h using a slow gradient, 8000 V for 8 h using again a linear gradient, 8000 V for 10 h using a rapid gradient.

14.2.4.2 Second Dimension (SDS-PAGE)

Requirements

Material: Gradient precast Criterion Tris-HCl gel (8–16%; Bio-Rad); agarose overlay buffer (Bio-Rad); protein standard; Sypro Ruby (Bio-Rad).

Solutions: Equilibration solution A (50 mM Tris-HCl (pH 6.8), 6 M urea, 1% (M/V) SDS, 30% (v/v) glycerol, and 0.5% DTT); equilibration solution B (50 mM Tris-HCl (pH 6.8), 6 M urea, 1% (M/V) SDS, 30% (v/v) glycerol, and 4.5% iodoacetamide), sodium dodecyl sulfate polyacrylamide-based gel electrophoresis (SDS-PAGE) running buffer.

1. Following IEF, equilibrate the IPG strips in equilibration solution A for 10 min in dark at room temperature.
2. Re-equilibrate the IPG strips in equilibration solution B, again for 10 min in the dark.
3. Quick wash the IPG strips in running buffer (1×) and place the strips on a linear gradient precast Criterion Tris-HCl gel (8–16%).
4. Pour agarose overlay buffer to cover the strips. Make sure there are no bubbles in the agarose solution and a proper contact is established between IPG strip and gel. Load 2.5 μL of precision protein standards (Bio-Rad) in the well. This will provide a visual marker of the approximate molecular weight on the blot.
5. Carry out the second dimension electrophoresis at 200 V for 65 min. Ideally, the gel and the gel that is transferred to a blot for each sample are run together so that there is minimal difference between their protein separations.
6. One gel is blotted for immunochemical detection (see Section 14.2.3), the other gel is stained with Sypro Ruby (Bio-Rad) according to the manufacturer's instruction. Stained gels are visualized using a UV transilluminator (Molecular Dynamics, Sunnyvale, CA, USA) with wavelengths of λ_{ex} 470 nm, λ_{em} 618 nm. The images are then saved in tiff format.

14.2.5
Immunochemical Detection of Protein Carbonyls, HNE and 3-NT

Requirements

Materials and reagents: Whatman filter paper, nitrocellulose membrane; anti-DNPH (Chemicon International, Temecula, CA, USA), anti-HNE (Alpha Diagnostic International, San Antonio, TX, USA), and anti-3-NT (Sigma, St. Louis, MO, USA); SigmaFast tablets (BCIP/NBT) (Sigma).

Solutions: Blotting transfer buffer; PBS-T (PBS with 3% bovine serum albumin, 0.01% (w/v) sodium azide and 0.2% (v/v) Tween 20).

Equipment: Blotting apparatus (e.g. Transblot BlotSD Semi-dry Transfer cell (Bio-Rad)).

1. Soak the gels for blotting in the transfer buffer.

2. For transfer, arrange in the following order: filter paper–gel–nitrocellulose membrane–filter paper, and transfer the gels at 15 mA for 2 h using Transblot-BlotSD Semi-Dry Transfer Cell.
3. Block the membrane in PBS-T for 1 h at room temperature.
4. Incubate the membrane with the primary antibody specific for the investigated modification in PBS-T (1 : 100 for anti-DNPH or 1 : 1000 for anti-HNE or anti-3-NT) for 2 h at room temperature.
5. Wash the membrane 3 × 5 min in PBS-T.
6. Incubate with a secondary antibody (alkaline phosphatase) (1 : 10 000) in PBS-T for ~1 h at room temperature.
7. Rinse 3 × 5 min with PBS-T.
8. Develop the membrane with SigmaFast tablets. The intensity of the color correlates to the amount of protein oxidation.
9. Dry the blots and scan them using Adobe Photoshop. Save the images as tiff files.

14.2.6
Image Analysis

The 2D gel images and the 2D Western blots are analyzed by Parkinson's disease Quest image software (BioRad) under conditions of background subtraction. This sophisticated software offers a comparative analysis of many gels and blots obtained under identical experimental conditions. After completing spot matching, the spot intensity values obtained on the blots are divided by the spot intensity value on the gels to obtain the level of specific protein oxidation. This procedure allows for protein concentration changes between subject and control samples. The specific protein oxidation of each spot from individual samples is compared between groups using statistical analysis to determine significance.

14.3
Future Directions

Proteomics provides opportunities for identification of oxidized or altered proteins directly or indirectly involved in Alzheimer's disease. Oxidation alters the structure and functions of proteins and may eventually lead to Alzheimer's disease pathology. Some of the identified proteins like enolase, glutamine synthetase, and Pin1, oxidatively modified both in Alzheimer's disease and in MCI, will help in further delineating the progression of Alzheimer's disease. The limitations of proteomics technology will hopefully be overcome and will provide researchers with biomarkers for early detection. Furthermore, redox proteomics will aid in the development of therapeutic approaches to prevent or delay the progression from MCI to Alzheimer's disease. A future objective of our research is to link the role of oxidation to disease pathogenesis using animal models. Similar considerations apply to other age-related neurodegenerative disorders studied.

Acknowledgments

This work was supported in part by NIH grants to D.A.B. [AG-05119; 10836].

References

Aksenov, M., Aksenova, M., Butterfield, D.A. and Markesbery, W.R. (2000) Oxidative modification of creatine kinase BB in Alzheimer's disease brain. *Journal of Neurochemistry*, **74**, 2520–2527.

Beal, M.F., Brouillet, E., Jenkins, B., Henshaw, R., Rosen, B. and Hyman, B.T. (1993a) Age-dependent striatal excitotoxic lesions produced by the endogenous mitochondrial inhibitor malonate. *Journal of Neurochemistry*, **61**, 1147–1150.

Beal, M.F., Brouillet, E., Jenkins, B.G., Ferrante, R.J., Kowall, N.W., Miller, J.M., Storey, E., Srivastava, R., Rosen, B.R. and Hyman, B.T. (1993b) Neurochemical and histologic characterization of striatal excitotoxic lesions produced by the mitochondrial toxin 3-nitropropionic acid. *The Journal of Neuroscience*, **13**, 4181–4192.

Beckman, J.S. and Koppenol, W.H. (1996) Nitric oxide, superoxide, and peroxynitrite: the good, the bad, and ugly. *The American Journal of Physiology*, **271**, C1424–C1437.

Berlett, B.S. and Stadtman, E.R. (1997) Protein oxidation in aging, disease, and oxidative stress. *The Journal of Biological Chemistry*, **272**, 20313–20316.

Browne, S.E., Ferrante, R.J. and Beal, M.F. (1999) Oxidative stress in Huntington's disease. *Brain Pathology*, **9**, 147–163.

Butterfield, D.A. (1997) beta-Amyloid-associated free radical oxidative stress and neurotoxicity: implications for Alzheimer's disease. *Chemical Research in Toxicology*, **10**, 495–506.

Butterfield, D.A. (2002) Amyloid beta-peptide (1–42)-induced oxidative stress and neurotoxicity: implications for neurodegeneration in Alzheimer's disease brain. A review. *Free Radical Research*, **36**, 1307–1313.

Butterfield, D.A. and Boyd-Kimball, D. (2004) Proteomics analysis in Alzheimer's disease: new insights into mechanisms of neurodegeneration. *International Review of Neurobiology*, **61**, 159–188.

Butterfield, D.A. and Lauderback, C.M. (2002) Lipid peroxidation and protein oxidation in Alzheimer's disease brain: potential causes and consequences involving amyloid beta-peptide-associated free radical oxidative stress. *Free Radical Biology & Medicine*, **32**, 1050–1060.

Butterfield, D.A. and Stadtman, E.R. (1997) Protein oxidation processes in aging brain. *Advances in Cell Aging and Gerontology*, **2**, 161–191.

Butterfield, D.A., Castegna, A., Lauderback, C.M. and Drake, J. (2002) Evidence that amyloid beta-peptide-induced lipid peroxidation and its sequelae in Alzheimer's disease brain contribute to neuronal death. *Neurobiology of Aging*, **23**, 655–664.

Butterfield, D.A., Perluigi, M. and Sultana, R. (2006a) Oxidative stress in Alzheimer's disease brain: new insights from redox proteomics. *European Journal of Pharmacology*, **545**, 39–50.

Butterfield, D.A., Poon, H.F., St Clair, D., Keller, J.N., Pierce, W.M., Klein, J.B. and

Markesbery, W.R. (2006b) Redox proteomics identification of oxidatively modified hippocampal proteins in mild cognitive impairment: insights into the development of Alzheimer's disease. *Neurobiology of Disease*, **22**, 223–232.

Carri, M.T., Ferri, A., Cozzolino, M., Calabrese, L. and Rotilio, G. (2003) Neurodegeneration in amyotrophic lateral sclerosis: the role of oxidative stress and altered homeostasis of metals. *Brain Research Bulletin*, **61**, 365–374.

Castegna, A., Aksenov, M., Aksenova, M., Thongboonkerd, V., Klein, J.B., Pierce, W.M., Booze, R., Markesbery, W.R. and Butterfield, D.A. (2002a) Proteomic identification of oxidatively modified proteins in Alzheimer's disease brain. Part I: creatine kinase BB, glutamine synthase, and ubiquitin carboxy-terminal hydrolase L-1. *Free Radical Biology & Medicine*, **33**, 562–571.

Castegna, A., Aksenov, M., Thongboonkerd, V., Klein, J.B., Pierce, W.M., Booze, R., Markesbery, W.R. and Butterfield, D.A. (2002b) Proteomic identification of oxidatively modified proteins in Alzheimer's disease brain. Part II: dihydropyrimidinase-related protein 2, alpha-enolase and heat shock cognate 71. *Journal of Neurochemistry*, **82**, 1524–1532.

Castegna, A., Thongboonkerd, V., Klein, J.B., Lynn, B., Markesbery, W.R. and Butterfield, D.A. (2003) Proteomic identification of nitrated proteins in Alzheimer's disease brain. *Journal of Neurochemistry*, **85**, 1394–1401.

Castegna, A., Lauderback, C.M., Mohmmad-Abdul, H. and Butterfield, D.A. (2004a) Modulation of phospholipid asymmetry in synaptosomal membranes by the lipid peroxidation products, 4-hydroxynonenal and acrolein: implications for Alzheimer's disease. *Brain Research*, **1004**, 193–197.

Castegna, A., Thongboonkerd, V., Klein, J., Lynn, B.C., Wang, Y.L., Osaka, H., Wada, K. and Butterfield, D.A. (2004b) Proteomic analysis of brain proteins in the gracile axonal dystrophy (gad) mouse, a syndrome that emanates from dysfunctional ubiquitin carboxyl-terminal hydrolase L-1, reveals oxidation of key proteins. *Journal of Neurochemistry*, **88**, 1540–1546.

Cater, H.L., Chandratheva, A., Benham, C.D., Morrison, B. and Sundstrom, L.E. (2003) Lactate and glucose as energy substrates during, and after, oxygen deprivation in rat hippocampal acute and cultured slices. *Journal of Neurochemistry*, **87**, 1381–1390.

Chen, Q., Behar, K.L., Xu, T., Fan, C. and Haddad, G.G. (2003) Expression of Drosophila trehalose-phosphate synthase in HEK-293 cells increases hypoxia tolerance. *The Journal of Biological Chemistry*, **278**, 49113–49118.

Choi, J., Levey, A.I., Weintraub, S.T., Rees, H.D., Gearing, M., Chin, L.S. and Li, L. (2004) Oxidative modifications and down-regulation of ubiquitin carboxyl-terminal hydrolase L1 associated with idiopathic Parkinson's and Alzheimer's diseases. *The Journal of Biological Chemistry*, **279**, 13256–13264.

Dalle-Donne, I., Scaloni, A., Giustarini, D., Cavarra, E., Tell, G., Lungarella, G., Colombo, R., Rossi, R. and Milzani, A. (2005) Proteins as biomarkers of oxidative/nitrosative stress in diseases: the contribution of redox proteomics. *Mass Spectrometry Reviews*, **24**, 55–99.

Dalle-Donne, I., Scaloni, A. and Butterfield, D.A. (2006) *Redox Proteomics: From Protein Modifications to Cellular Dysfunction and Diseases*, John Wiley & Sons, Inc., Hoboken, NJ.

Davies, M.J., Fu, S., Wang, H. and Dean, R.T. (1999) Stable markers of oxidant damage to proteins and their application in the study of human disease. *Free Radical Biology & Medicine*, **27**, 1151–1163.

Dedeoglu, A., Kubilus, J.K., Yang, L., Ferrante, K.L., Hersch, S.M., Beal, M.F. and Ferrante, R.J. (2003) Creatine therapy provides neuroprotection after onset of clinical symptoms in Huntington's disease transgenic mice. *Journal of Neurochemistry*, **85**, 1359–1367.

Fountoulakis, M. and Takacs, B. (2001) Effect of strong detergents and chaotropes on the detection of proteins in two-dimensional gels. *Electrophoresis*, **22**, 1593–1602.

Ischiropoulos, H. (2003) Biological selectivity and functional aspects of protein tyrosine nitration. *Biochemical and Biophysical Research, Communications*, **305**, 776–783.

Iwangoff, P., Armbruster, R., Enz, A. and Meier-Ruge, W. (1980) Glycolytic enzymes from human autoptic brain cortex: normal aged and demented cases. *Mechanisms of Ageing and Development*, **14**, 203–209.

Koppenol, W.H., Moreno, J.J., Pryor, W.A., Ischiropoulos, H. and Beckman, J.S. (1992) Peroxynitrite, a cloaked oxidant formed by nitric oxide and superoxide. *Chemical Research in Toxicology*, **5**, 834–842.

Lauderback, C.M., Hackett, J.M., Huang, F.F., Keller, J.N., Szweda, L.I., Markesbery, W.R. and Butterfield, D.A. (2001) The glial glutamate transporter, GLT-1, is oxidatively modified by 4-hydroxy-2-nonenal in the Alzheimer's disease brain: the role of Abeta1-42. *Journal of Neurochemistry*, **78**, 413–416.

Levine, R.L., Williams, J.A., Stadtman, E.R. and Shacter, E. (1994) Carbonyl assays for determination of oxidatively modified proteins. *Methods in Enzymology*, **233**, 346–357.

Lovell, M.A. and Markesbery, W.R. (2001) Ratio of 8-hydroxyguanine in intact DNA to free 8-hydroxyguanine is increased in Alzheimer disease ventricular cerebrospinal fluid. *Archives of Neurology*, **58**, 392–396.

Lu, P.J., Wulf, G., Zhou, X.Z., Davies, P. and Lu, K.P. (1999) The prolyl isomerase Pin1 restores the function of Alzheimer-associated phosphorylated tau protein. *Nature*, **399**, 784–788.

Mark, R.J., Lovell, M.A., Markesbery, W.R., Uchida, K. and Mattson, M.P. (1997) A role for 4-hydroxynonenal, an aldehydic product of lipid peroxidation, in disruption of ion homeostasis and neuronal death induced by amyloid beta-peptide. *Journal of Neurochemistry*, **68**, 255–264.

Markesbery, W.R. (1997) Oxidative stress hypothesis in Alzheimer's disease. *Free Radical Biology & Medicine*, **23**, 134–147.

Meier-Ruge, W., Iwangoff, P. and Reichlmeier, K. (1984) Neurochemical enzyme changes in Alzheimer's and Pick's disease. *Archives of Gerontology Geriatrics*, **3**, 161–165.

Messier, C. and Gagnon, M. (1996) Glucose regulation and cognitive functions: relation to Alzheimer's disease and diabetes. *Behavioural Brain Research*, **75**, 1–11.

Mirra, S.S., Heyman, A., McKeel, D., Sumi, S.M., Crain, B.J., Brownlee, L.M., Vogel, F.S., Hughes, J.P., van Belle, G. and Berg, L. (1991) The Consortium to Establish a Registry for Alzheimer's Disease (CERAD). Part II. Standardization of the neuropathologic assessment of Alzheimer's disease. *Neurology*, **41**, 479–486.

Murata, T., Omata, N., Fujibayashi, Y., Waki, A., Sadato, N., Yoshimoto, M., Wada, Y. and Yonekura, Y. (2000) Posthypoxic reoxygenation-induced neurotoxicity prevented by free radical scavenger and NMDA/non-NMDA antagonist in tandem as revealed by dynamic changes in glucose metabolism with positron autoradiography. *Experimental Neurology*, **164**, 269–279.

Pearce, R.K., Owen, A., Daniel, S., Jenner, P. and Marsden, C.D. (1997) Alterations in the distribution of glutathione in the substantia nigra in Parkinson's disease. *Journal of Neural Transmission*, **104**, 661–677.

Perluigi, M., Fai Poon, H., Hensley, K., Pierce, W.M., Klein, J.B., Calabrese, V., De Marco, C. and Butterfield, D.A. (2005a) Proteomic analysis of 4-hydroxy-2-nonenal-modified proteins in G93A-SOD1 transgenic mice-a model of familial amyotrophic lateral sclerosis. *Free Radical Biology & Medicine*, **38**, 960–968.

Perluigi, M., Poon, H.F., Maragos, W., Pierce, W.M., Klein, J.B., Calabrese, V., Cini, C., De Marco, C. and Butterfield, D.A. (2005b) Proteomic analysis of protein expression and oxidative modification in r6/2 transgenic mice: a model of Huntington disease. *Molecular & Cellular Proteomics*, **4**, 1849–1861.

Poon, H.F., Frasier, M., Shreve, N., Calabrese, V., Wolozin, B. and Butterfield, D.A. (2005a) Mitochondrial associated metabolic proteins are selectively oxidized in A30P alpha-synuclein transgenic mice—a model of familial Parkinson's disease. *Neurobiology of Disease*, **18**, 492–498.

Poon, H.F., Hensley, K., Thongboonkerd, V., Merchant, M.L., Lynn, B.C., Pierce, W.M., Klein, J.B., Calabrese, V. and Butterfield, D.A. (2005b) Redox proteomics analysis of oxidatively modified proteins in G93A-SOD1 transgenic mice—a model of familial amyotrophic lateral sclerosis. *Free Radical Biology & Medicine*, **39**, 453–462.

Rapoport, S.I. (1999) In vivo PET imaging and postmortem studies suggest potentially reversible and irreversible stages of brain metabolic failure in Alzheimer's disease. *European Archives of Psychiatry and, Clinical Neuroscience*, **249**(Suppl 3), 46–55.

Schurr, A., Payne, R.S., Miller, J.J. and Rigor, B.M. (1997) Glia are the main source of lactate utilized by neurons for recovery of function posthypoxia. *Brain Research*, **774**, 221–224.

Selkoe, D.J. (2001) Alzheimer's disease: genes, proteins, and therapy. *Physiological Reviews*, **81**, 741–766.

Sitek, B., Luttges, J., Marcus, K., Kloppel, G., Schmiegel, W., Meyer, H.E., Hahn, S.A. and Stuhler, K. (2005) Application of fluorescence difference gel electrophoresis saturation labelling for the analysis of microdissected precursor lesions of pancreatic ductal adenocarcinoma. *Proteomics*, **5**, 2665–2679.

Smith, M.A., Taneda, S., Richey, P.L., Miyata, S., Yan, S.D., Stern, D., Sayre, L.M., Monnier, V.M. and Perry, G. (1994) Advanced Maillard reaction end products are associated with Alzheimer disease pathology. *Proceedings of the National Academy of Sciences of the United States of America*, **91**, 5710–5714.

Smith, M.A., Richey Harris, P.L., Sayre, L.M., Beckman, J.S. and Perry, G. (1997) Widespread peroxynitrite-mediated damage in Alzheimer's disease. *The Journal of Neuroscience*, **17**, 2653–2657.

Stadtman, E.R. and Levine, R.L. (2003) Free radical-mediated oxidation of free amino acids and amino acid residues in proteins. *Amino Acids*, **25**, 207–218.

Sultana, R., Boyd-Kimball, D., Poon, H.F., Cai, J., Pierce, W.M., Klein, J.B., Markesbery, W.R., Zhou, X.Z., Lu, K.P. and Butterfield, D.A. (2006a) Oxidative modification and down-regulation of Pin1 in Alzheimer's disease hippocampus: A redox proteomics analysis. *Neurobiology of Aging*, **27**, 918–925.

Sultana, R., Boyd-Kimball, D., Poon, H.F., Cai, J., Pierce, W.M., Klein, J.B., Merchant, M., Markesbery, W.R. and Butterfield, D.A. (2006b) Redox proteomics identification of oxidized proteins in Alzheimer's disease hippocampus and cerebellum: An approach to understand pathological and biochemical alterations in AD. *Neurobiology of Aging*, **27**, 1564–1576.

Sultana, R., Poon, H.F., Cai, J., Pierce, W.M., Merchant, M., Klein, J.B., Markesbery, W.R. and Butterfield, D.A. (2006c) Identification of nitrated proteins in Alzheimer's disease brain using a redox proteomics approach. *Neurobiology of Disease*, **22**, 76–87.

Vanhanen, M. and Soininen, H. (1998) Glucose intolerance, cognitive impairment and Alzheimer's disease. *Current Opinion in Neurology*, **11**, 673–677.

Wang, Q., Woltjer, R.L., Cimino, P.J., Pan, C., Montine, K.S., Zhang, J. and Montine, T.J. (2005) Proteomic analysis of neurofibrillary tangles in Alzheimer disease identifies GAPDH as a detergent-insoluble paired helical filament tau binding protein. *The FASEB Journal*, **19**, 869–871.

Watson, G.S. and Craft, S. (2004) Modulation of memory by insulin and glucose: neuropsychological observations in Alzheimer's disease. *European Journal of Pharmacology*, **490**, 97–113.

15
Paranode Structure and Function

Yasuhiro Ogawa and Matthew N. Rasband

15.1
Introduction

The rapid and efficient conduction of electrical signals in the mammalian nervous system depends on axons that are ensheathed by myelin membranes. Myelin performs both active and passive functions. First, myelin passively regulates the electrical properties of the axon by decreasing the membrane capacitance and by increasing the membrane resistance. Myelin actively regulates the electrical properties of the axon by clustering ion channels at regularly spaced gaps in the myelin membrane which are called nodes of Ranvier. Further, myelin directly regulates the expression of distinct types of ion channels in axons. Nodes of Ranvier are of central importance to action potential conduction because nodes are the sites of all transmembrane currents in the myelinated axon. Since many demyelinating diseases and/or injuries result in disruption of nodes of Ranvier and conduction block (Rasband *et al.*, 1998; Craner *et al.*, 2004; Devaux and Scherer, 2005), it is important to understand the molecular mechanisms underlying node formation and axon–glia interaction.

Myelin is made by oligodendrocytes in the central nervous system and by Schwann cells in the peripheral nervous system. Myelination and node of Ranvier formation both depend on a complex set of interactions between neurons and glia that result in profound molecular, morphological, and functional changes in both cell types. Myelinated axons can be subdivided into several distinct domains including the node, paranode, juxtaparanode, and internode (Figure 15.1). The node of Ranvier is characterized by high densities of voltage-gated Na^+ and K^+ channels (Nav channels and Kv channels, respectively) and is responsible for the transmembrane currents that mediate saltatory AP conduction. Flanking nodes are the paranodal or axoglial junctions. These domains are the principal sites of contact between the axon and the myelinating glia and are the site where the myelin is firmly anchored to the axon. The juxtaparanode is located adjacent to the paranode beneath the myelin membrane. It is approximately 5–15 μm in length and is characterized by a high density of Kv channels whose functions remain enigmatic (Rasband,

Proteomics of the Nervous System. Edited by H.G. Nothwang and S.E. Pfeiffer
Copyright © 2008 WILEY-VCH Verlag GmbH & Co. KGaA, Weinheim
ISBN: 978-3-527-31716-5

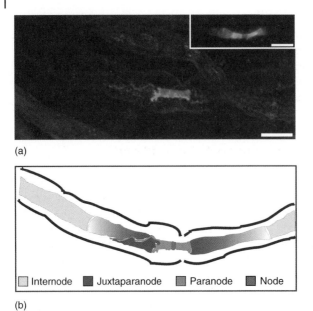

(a)

(b)

| ☐ Internode | ■ Juxtaparanode | ■ Paranode | ■ Node |

Figure 15.1 Myelinated axons are divided into polarized membrane domains including nodes, paranodes, juxtaparanodes, and internodes. (a) Nodes of Ranvier in the peripheral nervous system are characterized by a high density of Nav channels (red) flanked by paranodal junctions consisting of the cell adhesion molecules Caspr (green), contactin, and NF-155. Inset: CNS node of Ranvier immunostained using antibodies against juxtaparanodal Kv1 channels (red), paranodal Caspr (green), and nodal Nav channels (blue). (b) Cartoon illustrating the different domains of a myelinated axon. The black outline delineates the outer aspect of the myelin sheath. Scale bars = 10 μm. (Please find a color version of this figure in the color plates.)

2004). The remainder of the axonal membrane beneath the myelin is called the internode and has only a very low density of ion channels.

Nodes, paranodes, and juxtaparanodes each have a unique set of proteins that are important for neuron–glia interactions, stabilizing and anchoring the transmembrane protein complexes, and in the case of nodes and juxtaparanodes, for clustering of ion channels (Poliak and Peles, 2003; Salzer, 2003). Experimental results from many laboratories suggest a general mechanism used to establish and maintain these polarized domains in myelinated axons. In general, glial cell adhesion molecules (CAMs) interact with and position axonal CAMs at precise locations along the axon. The axonal CAMs function as attachment sites for scaffolding proteins. These scaffolds in turn bind to ion channels and the cytoskeleton, causing the accumulation of ion channels and stabilizing the entire protein complex by linking it to the underlying cytoskeleton (Schafer and Rasband, 2006).

Among the domains described above, the paranodal junction has several unique functional and molecular properties. Therefore, we have recently utilized biochemical and proteomic methods to gain important insights into the composition and function of the paranodes. This chapter will first describe what we know about these junctions, provide examples of how mutant animals and new proteomic methods have extended our understanding of these domains, and finally give a protocol for isolation of membrane fractions highly enriched in proteins associated with paranodal junctions.

15.1.1
Structure and Molecular Composition of the Paranodal Junction

The paranodal junctions formed between the axon and the myelinating glial cell are the largest known vertebrate junctional adhesion complex (Peters *et al.*, 1976; Rosenbluth, 1995). On the glial side, the myelin membranes split to form a pocket of cytoplasm that wraps helically around the axon. The paranodal junction is formed by the close apposition between axonal and glial membranes. Images of paranodal junctions using electron microscopy revealed a set of electron-dense transverse bands that connect the glial and axonal membranes.

The paranodal junction is structurally, molecularly, and functionally homologous to the invertebrate septate junctions (Einheber *et al.*, 1997). For example, the septate junctions in *Drosophila*, which form between epithelia, have electron-dense bands and function as a paracellular ion diffusion barrier. Further, *Drosophila* septate junctions consist of several CAMs including neurexin, Dcontactin, and neuroglian, and a cytoskeletal scaffold called coracle. Flies with mutations in these proteins fail to form proper epithelial septate junctions (Genova and Fehon, 2003; Faivre-Sarrailh *et al.*, 2004; Banerjee *et al.*, 2006). Each of the protein components of *Drosophila* septate junctions has a homolog at the vertebrate paranodal junction. The mammalian homolog of neurexin is the contactin-associated protein (Caspr, also known as paranodin or NCP1) (Menegoz *et al.*, 1997; Peles *et al.*, 1997), Dcontactin's mammalian counterpart is contactin (Faivre-Sarrailh *et al.*, 2004), neuroglian's homolog is neurofascin (Banerjee *et al.*, 2006), and coracle is called protein 4.1B in vertebrates (Genova and Fehon, 2003).

The CAMs Caspr and contactin are both axonal and located at paranodal junctions. Genetic ablation of either component results in failure to form paranodal junctions and transverse bands (Bhat *et al.*, 2001; Boyle *et al.*, 2001). A 155-kDa splice variant of neurofascin (NF-155) is also located at the paranode, but on the glial side of the junction. This CAM is required for recruitment of both Caspr and contactin and junction formation (Sherman *et al.*, 2005). Some data indicate that the basis of the neuron–glia interactions at the paranode is a heterotrimeric protein complex consisting of Caspr, contactin, and NF-155 (Charles *et al.*, 2002). However, more work is required since other data suggest that glial NF-155 binds only to axonal contactin and that Caspr actually inhibits NF-155 binding to Caspr (Gollan *et al.*, 2003). It is clear, however, that all three CAMs are required since loss of any one results in disruption of the paranodal junction.

The precise location of integral membrane proteins often occurs through binding to scaffolding or cytoskeletal proteins. It is therefore not surprising that scaffolding proteins have been identified on both the glial and axonal sides of the paranodal junction. On the axonal side, Caspr has been shown to colocalize and interact with protein 4.1B, while on the glial side, protein 4.1 G was recently shown to be enriched at paranodes, although its binding partner has not been identified (Ohara *et al.*, 2000; Denisenko-Nehrbass *et al.*, 2003; Ohno *et al.*, 2006). The 4.1 family of proteins links membrane proteins to the actin/spectrin-based cytoskeleton. We will have more to say about cytoskeletal interactions at paranodal junctions below.

15.1.2
Paranodal Mutants Reveal the Functions of the Paranodal Junction

Some of the functions of the paranodal junction have been determined through the use of paranodal mutant mice. Genetic disruption of Caspr, contactin, and neurofascin results in loss of paranodal septate junctions, although myelination is unaffected. Functionally, this results in compromised AP conduction, widened Nav channel clusters, and disruption of axonal membrane polarization. One of the most striking observations in paranodal mutants is that the Kv channels and their associated proteins (e.g. Caspr2 and TAG-1), normally restricted to juxtaparanodal domains, invade into paranodal zones (Bhat *et al.*, 2001; Boyle *et al.*, 2001; Poliak *et al.*, 2001). This result indicates that paranodal junctions restrict the lateral diffusion of axonal membrane proteins.

The paranodal junctions also play important roles in directly regulating the types of Nav channels located at nodes of Ranvier. During early development, Nav1.2 is the main Nav channel found at newly forming nodes of Ranvier. However, subsequent to myelination, these Nav1.2 channels are removed from nodes and replaced with Nav1.6 (Boiko *et al.*, 2001; Schafer *et al.*, 2006). In paranodal mutants, this developmental switch is compromised such that many nodes in the adult nervous system have Nav1.2 (Rios *et al.*, 2003). Thus, axoglial interactions at the paranodal junction regulate the localization of distinct Nav channel subtypes at nodes of Ranvier.

Myelin membranes are highly enriched in galactolipids. Therefore, it was a surprise to discover that mice lacking the enzymes that catalyze production of these galactolipids have normal myelin (Coetzee *et al.*, 1996). However, there was no formation of paranodal junctions (Dupree *et al.*, 1998; Ishibashi *et al.*, 2002). As with the Caspr-, contactin-, and neurofascin-null mice, galactolipid-deficient mice have reduced AP conduction velocities and altered ion channel localization. One potential explanation for these results is that galactolipids contribute to the proper organization of the paranodal junction either by directly binding to other proteins, or by regulating the lipid environment found at paranodal junctions.

To test these possibilities, Schafer *et al.* (2004) examined the biochemical properties of NF-155, since it is the most affected paranodal CAM in galactolipid-deficient mice (Poliak *et al.*, 2001). Specifically, they used several biochemical tests to investigate the association of NF-155 with lipids. First, they showed that NF-155 is insoluble in 1% Triton X-100 at 4 °C, but soluble at 37 °C. Second, they showed that NF-155 is soluble in 1% Triton X-100 at 4 °C if cholesterol is chelated from the membranes. And finally, they showed that the NF-155 in the Triton X-100 detergent-resistant membranes floats at low sucrose densities on sucrose gradients. Together, these criteria are typically used to empirically define lipid raft membrane fractions (Taylor *et al.*, 2002). Importantly, NF-155 acquired these biochemical properties only after formation of paranodal junctions and only after interacting with its axonal ligand. Consistent with the idea that axon–glia interactions are required for NF-155 to partition into lipid rafts, it does not have any of the biochemical properties of a lipid raft-associated protein in the Caspr-null mutant mice (M.N.R., unpublished results). Taken together, these results indicate that interactions between glial NF-155 and axonal ligands results in the formation of a paranodal lipid raft assembly that includes galactolipids. Furthermore, axoglial interactions likely depend not only on protein–protein interactions, but also on protein–lipid interactions.

15.1.3
Molecular Dissection of the Paranodal Junction

Since paranodal NF-155 could be isolated based on its properties as a lipid raft-associated protein, we determined that both Caspr and contactin co-fractionated with NF-155 upon formation of paranodes (Schafer *et al.*, 2004). These results suggested that the paranodal junction protein complex remained intact during the subcellular fractionation procedures and isolation of the paranodal lipid raft assemblies. If true, this presents a novel opportunity to identify additional components of paranodal junctions. Ogawa *et al.* (2006) tested this possibility by making lipid rafts from optic nerve membrane homogenates. The selection of optic nerves as source material for the membranes was important since optic nerves are highly enriched in nodes of Ranvier but lack synapses, avoiding the complication of lipid rafts derived from synapses. Liquid chromatography coupled to tandem mass spectrometry (LC-MS/MS) analysis resulted in the identification of Caspr, contactin, NF-155, and protein 4.1B (Ogawa *et al.*, 2006), confirming the enrichment of known paranodal proteins in the membrane fractions. In addition, three other cytoskeletal and scaffolding proteins were identified with very high amino acid coverage: αII spectrin, βII spectrin, and ankyrinB (ankB). The identification of these proteins was interesting since all three have been shown to comprise a protein complex in other cell types, and protein 4.1B is a binding partner of βII spectrin (Bennett and Baines, 2001).

Additional experiments confirmed the interaction of αII spectrin, βII spectrin, ankB, and protein 4.1B in axons, and that these protein complexes are highly enriched at paranodal junctions in both the CNS and PNS. The organization of this cytoskeletal protein complex is disrupted in Caspr-null mice, indicating that neuron–glia interactions regulate not only the localization of membrane proteins, but also the organization of the cytoskeleton at paranodes. The importance of neuron–glia interactions in regulating cytoskeletal properties and function is further underscored by the observation that there is dramatic cytoskeletal disruption and axon degeneration in Purkinje neurons of Caspr-null and galactolipid-deficient mice (Garcia-Fresco *et al.*, 2006). It is tempting to speculate that demyelination and loss of paranodal junctions may contribute to the axon loss seen in demyelinating diseases such as multiple sclerosis.

In summary, the paranodal junction is the principal site of interaction between axons and myelinating glia. As described above it consists of CAMs and cytoskeletal and scaffolding proteins. It is interesting to note that this molecular organization is very similar to that of other axonal membrane domains. For example, nodes of Ranvier have not only ion channels, but also high densities of the CAM NF-186 (NF-186 participates in neuron–glia interactions necessary for node formation) and a specialized nodal cytoskeleton that includes ankyrinG and βIV spectrin. Thus, nodes and paranodes both have high densities of CAMs and specialized cytoskeletons that consist of different isoforms of ankyrins and spectrins. Finally, in addition to a common protein organization, lipids may also play important structural roles in both domains. For example, βIV spectrin may function as a scaffold not only to link nodal membrane proteins to the cytoskeleton, but also to regulate the appropriate lipid composition and quantity. This hypothesis is consistent with the observation that deletion of the pleckstrin homology domain of βIV spectrin (PH domains interact with phosphoinositides and permit binding of cytosolic proteins to the plasma membrane (Lemmon *et al.*, 2002)) results in nodal membrane protrusions and broader nodes of Ranvier.

15.2
Protocols

The isolation of membranes highly enriched in paranodal proteins is based on the fact that lipid rafts are resistant to extraction in 1% Triton X-100 at 4 °C. Therefore, this protocol is separated into three parts: (i) crude optic nerve membrane preparation, (ii) Triton X-100-insoluble fraction preparation, and (iii) fractionation of the detergent-resistant membranes (DRMs) using a sucrose gradient.

15.2.1
Crude Membrane Preparation

Requirements

Material: ~100 optic nerves from adult rats.

Solutions: Homogenization buffer (320 mM sucrose, 5 mM sodium phosphate pH 7.4); protease inhibitors (leupeptin (1 µg mL^{-1} final); antipain (2 µg mL^{-1} final); benzamidine (10 µg mL^{-1} final), and 0.5 mM phenylmethyl sulfonylfluoride (PMSF).

Instrumentation: Dounce type homogenizer.

1. Add 3 mL homogenization buffer to optic nerves from 50 adult rats and homogenize by 20–30 strokes on ice. Do not use a polytron tissue homogenizer.
2. Centrifuge at 600 × g for 10 min at 4 °C to sediment nuclei.
3. After centrifugation, three layers can be seen from top to bottom: a liquid-rich (transparent), membrane-rich (white color), and nuclei layer. Transfer the liquid- and membrane-rich layers into a new tube on ice.
4. Mix the liquid- and membrane-rich layer using the dounce homogenizer.
5. Centrifuge at 21 000 × g for 90 min at 4 °C.
6. Remove the clear supernatant. Resuspend the pellet in 500 µL of homogenization buffer by pipetting and vortexing.
7. Determine the protein concentration and store the optic nerve membranes at −80 °C.

15.2.2
Triton X-100 Insoluble Fraction Preparation

Requirements

Solution: Lysis buffer (1% Triton X-100; 20 mM Tris-HCl, pH 8.0; 10 mM EDTA; 0.15 M NaCl; 10 mM iodoacetamide; protease inhibitors; 0.5 mM PMSF).

1. Add 3 mL lysis buffer to 3 mg optic nerve membrane.
2. Rotate for 1 h at 4 °C by end-over-end rotation.
3. Centrifuge at 13 000 × g for 30 min at 4 °C.
4. Remove the supernatant and resuspend the pellet in 1 mL lysis buffer without Triton X-100.
5. Keep the suspension (Triton X-100 insoluble) on ice.

15.2.3
Separation of Membrane Fraction from Triton X-100-Insoluble Fraction by Sucrose Gradient Centrifugation

Requirements

Chemicals: Peroxidase-conjugated cholera toxin B subunit.

Solution: 2 M sucrose, 1 M sucrose, 0.2 M sucrose in water.

Instrumentation: Ultracentrifuge tubes (Ultra-Clear 1/2 × 2 in (13 × 51 mm)), ultracentrifuge (e.g. Optima LE-80 K with SW51 Ti rotor).

1. Mix 1 mL Triton X-100 insoluble fraction and 1 mL 2 M sucrose in ultracentrifuge tube.
2. Carefully overlay 2 mL 1 M sucrose.
3. Carefully overlay 1.5 mL 0.2 M sucrose.
4. Centrifuge at 192 000 × g for 16–19 h at 4 °C.
5. Collect 0.4-mL fractions from the top of the tube. A white band will be present at the fourth–fifth fraction.
6. Mix each fraction by vortexing, then determine the lipid raft fraction by dot blot analysis using peroxidase-conjugated cholera toxin B subunit. Cholera toxin will bind to GM1 gangliosides, a prominent component of lipid rafts.
7. If desired, the percent sucrose in each fraction can be determined by refractometry.

15.3
Outlook

The paranodal junction is a fascinating structure that epitomizes the reciprocal interactions between neurons and glia necessary for proper nervous system function. We have described proteomics methods used to perform a molecular dissection of these domains. Nevertheless, many additional questions regarding the structure and function of paranodal junctions remain. For example, very few glial components of the paranodes have been identified. What cytoskeletal proteins are found in paranodes? What signaling complexes exist that inform myelinating glia that paranodal structures are intact? The answers to these important questions will require additional proteomics efforts to define the complex community of proteins that mediate neuron–glia interactions at paranodal junctions.

References

Banerjee, S., Pillai, A.M., Paik, R., Li, J. and Bhat, M.A. (2006) Axonal ensheathment and septate junction formation in the peripheral nervous system of Drosophila. *The Journal of Neuroscience*, **26**, 3319–3329.

Bennett, V. and Baines, A.J. (2001) Spectrin and ankyrin-based pathways: metazoan inventions for integrating cells into tissues. *Physiological Reviews*, **81**, 1353–1392.

Bhat, M.A., Rios, J.C., Lu, Y., Garcia-Fresco, G.P., Ching, W., St Martin, M., Li, J., Einheber, S., Chesler, M., Rosenbluth, J., Salzer, J.L. and Bellen, H.J. (2001) Axon-glia interactions and the domain organization of myelinated axons requires neurexin IV/Caspr/Paranodin. *Neuron*, **30**, 369–383.

Boiko, T., Rasband, M.N., Levinson, S.R., Caldwell, J.H., Mandel, G., Trimmer, J.S. and Matthews, G. (2001) Compact myelin dictates the differential targeting of two sodium channel isoforms in the same axon. *Neuron*, **30**, 91–104.

Boyle, M.E., Berglund, E.O., Murai, K.K., Weber, L., Peles, E. and Ranscht, B. (2001) Contactin orchestrates assembly of the septate-like junctions at the paranode in myelinated peripheral nerve. *Neuron*, **30**, 385–397.

Charles, P., Tait, S., Faivre-Sarrailh, C., Barbin, G., Gunn-Moore, F., Denisenko-Nehrbass, N., Guennoc, A.M., Girault, J.A., Brophy, P.J. and Lubetzki, C. (2002) Neurofascin is a glial receptor for the paranodin/Caspr-contactin axonal complex at the axoglial junction. *Current Biology*, **12**, 217–220.

Coetzee, T., Fujita, N., Dupree, J., Shi, R., Blight, A., Suzuki, K. and Popko, B. (1996) Myelination in the absence of galactocerebroside and sulfatide: normal structure with abnormal function and regional instability. *Cell*, **86**, 209–219.

Craner, M.J., Newcombe, J., Black, J.A., Hartle, C., Cuzner, M.L. and Waxman, S.G. (2004) Molecular changes in neurons in multiple sclerosis: altered axonal expression of Nav1.2 and Nav1.6 sodium channels and Na+/Ca2+ exchanger. *Proceedings of the National Academy of Sciences of the United States of America*, **101**, 8168–8173.

Denisenko-Nehrbass, N., Oguievetskaia, K., Goutebroze, L., Galvez, T., Yamakawa, H., Ohara, O., Carnaud, M. and Girault, J.A. (2003) Protein 4.1B associates with both Caspr/paranodin and Caspr2 at paranodes and juxtaparanodes of myelinated fibres. *The European Journal of Neuroscience*, **17**, 411–416.

Devaux, J.J. and Scherer, S.S. (2005) Altered ion channels in an animal model of Charcot-Marie-Tooth disease type IA. *The Journal of Neuroscience*, **25**, 1470–1480.

Dupree, J.L., Coetzee, T., Blight, A., Suzuki, K. and Popko, B. (1998) Myelin galactolipids are essential for proper node of Ranvier formation in the CNS. *The Journal of Neuroscience*, **18**, 1642–1649.

Einheber, S., Zanazzi, G., Ching, W., Scherer, S., Milner, T.A., Peles, E. and Salzer, J.L. (1997) The axonal membrane protein Caspr, a homologue of neurexin IV, is a component of the septate-like paranodal junctions that assemble during myelination. *The Journal of Cell Biology*, **139**, 1495–1506.

Faivre-Sarrailh, C., Banerjee, S., Li, J., Hortsch, M., Laval, M. and Bhat, M.A. (2004) Drosophila contactin, a homolog of vertebrate contactin, is required for septate junction organization and paracellular barrier function. *Development*, **131**, 4931–4942.

Garcia-Fresco, G.P., Sousa, A.D., Pillai, A.M., Moy, S.S., Crawley, J.N., Tessarollo, L., Dupree, J.L. and Bhat, M.A. (2006) Disruption of axo-glial junctions causes cytoskeletal disorganization and degeneration of Purkinje neuron axons. *Proceedings of the National Academy of Sciences of the United States of America*, **103**, 5137–5142.

Genova, J.L. and Fehon, R.G. (2003) Neuroglian, Gliotactin, and the Na+/K+ ATPase are essential for septate junction function in Drosophila. *The Journal of Cell Biology*, **161**, 979–989.

Gollan, L., Salomon, D., Salzer, J.L. and Peles, E. (2003) Caspr regulates the processing of contactin and inhibits its binding to neurofascin. *The Journal of Cell Biology*, **163**, 1213–1218.

Ishibashi, T., Dupree, J.L., Ikenaka, K., Hirahara, Y., Honke, K., Peles, E., Popko, B., Suzuki, K., Nishino, H. and Baba, H. (2002) A myelin galactolipid, sulfatide, is essential for maintenance of ion channels on myelinated axon but not essential for initial cluster formation. *The Journal of Neuroscience*, **22**, 6507–6514.

Lemmon, M.A., Ferguson, K.M. and Abrams, C.S. (2002) Pleckstrin homology domains and the cytoskeleton. *FEBS Letters*, **513**, 71–76.

Menegoz, M., Gaspar, P., Le Bert, M., Galvez, T., Burgaya, F., Palfrey, C., Ezan, P., Arnos, F. and Girault, J.A. (1997) Paranodin, a glycoprotein of neuronal paranodal membranes. *Neuron,* **19**, 319–331.

Ogawa, Y., Schafer, D.P., Horresh, I., Bar, V., Hales, K., Yang, Y., Susuki, K., Peles, E., Stankewich, M.C. and Rasband, M.N. (2006) Spectrins and ankyrinB constitute a specialized paranodal cytoskeleton. *The Journal of Neuroscience,* **26**, 5230–5239.

Ohara, R., Yamakawa, H., Nakayama, M. and Ohara, O. (2000) Type II brain 4.1 (4.1B/KIAA0987), a member of the protein 4.1 family, is localized to neuronal paranodes. *Brain Research Molecular Brain Research,* **85**, 41–52.

Ohno, N., Terada, N., Yamakawa, H., Komada, M., Ohara, O., Trapp, B.D. and Ohno, S. (2006) Expression of protein 4.1 G in Schwann cells of the peripheral nervous system. *Journal of Neuroscience Research,* **84**, 568–577.

Peles, E., Nativ, M., Lustig, M., Grumet, M., Schilling, J., Martinez, R., Plowman, G.D. and Schlessinger, J. (1997) Identification of a novel contactin-associated transmembrane receptor with multiple domains implicated in protein–protein interactions. *The EMBO Journal,* **16**, 978–988.

Peters, A., Palay, S.L. and Webster, H.d. (1976) *The Fine Structure of the Nervous System: The Neurons and Supporting Cells,* W.B. Saunders Company, Philadelphia, PA.

Poliak, S. and Peles, E. (2003) The local differentiation of myelinated axons at nodes of Ranvier. *Nature Reviews Neuroscience,* **4**, 968–980.

Poliak, S., Gollan, L., Salomon, D., Berglund, E.O., Ohara, R., Ranscht, B. and Peles, E. (2001) Localization of Caspr2 in myelinated nerves depends on axon-glia interactions and the generation of barriers along the axon. *The Journal of Neuroscience,* **21**, 7568–7575.

Rasband, M.N. (2004) It's 'juxta' potassium channel. *Journal of Neuroscience Research,* **76**, 749–757.

Rasband, M.N., Trimmer, J.S., Schwarz, T.L., Levinson, S.R., Ellisman, M.H., Schachner, M. and Shrager, P. (1998) Potassium channel distribution, clustering, and function in remyelinating rat axons. *The Journal of Neuroscience,* **18**, 36–47.

Rios, J.C., Rubin, M., St Martin, M., Downey, R.T., Einheber, S., Rosenbluth, J., Levinson, S.R., Bhat, M. and Salzer, J.L. (2003) Paranodal interactions regulate expression of sodium channel subtypes and provide a diffusion barrier for the node of Ranvier. *The Journal of Neuroscience,* **23**, 7001–7011.

Rosenbluth, J. (1995) Glial membranes and axoglial junctions, in *Neuroglia,* Oxford University Press, New York.

Salzer, J.L. (2003) Polarized domains of myelinated axons. *Neuron,* **40**, 297–318.

Schafer, D.P. and Rasband, M.N. (2006) Glial regulation of the axonal membrane at nodes of Ranvier. *Current Opinion in Neurobiology,* **16**, 508–514.

Schafer, D.P., Bansal, R., Hedstrom, K.L., Pfeiffer, S.E. and Rasband, M.N. (2004) Does paranode formation and maintenance require partitioning of neurofascin 155 into lipid rafts? *The Journal of Neuroscience,* **24**, 3176–3185.

Schafer, D.P., Custer, A.W., Shrager, P. and Rasband, M.N. (2006) Early events in node of Ranvier formation during myelination and remyelination in the PNS. *Neuron Glia Biology,* **2**, 69–79.

Sherman, D.L., Tait, S., Melrose, S., Johnson, R., Zonta, B., Court, F.A., Macklin, W.B., Meek, S., Smith, A.J., Cottrell, D.F. and Brophy, P.J. (2005) Neurofascins are required to establish axonal domains for saltatory conduction. *Neuron,* **48**, 737–742.

Taylor, C.M., Coetzee, T. and Pfeiffer, S.E. (2002) Detergent-insoluble glycosphingolipid/cholesterol microdomains of the myelin membrane. *Journal of Neurochemistry,* **81**, 993–1004.

Index